RENEGOTIATING HEALTH CARE

RENEGOTIATING HEALTH CARE

Resolving Conflict to Build Collaboration

LEONARD J. MARCUS
BARRY C. DORN
ERIC J. McNULTY

SECOND EDITION

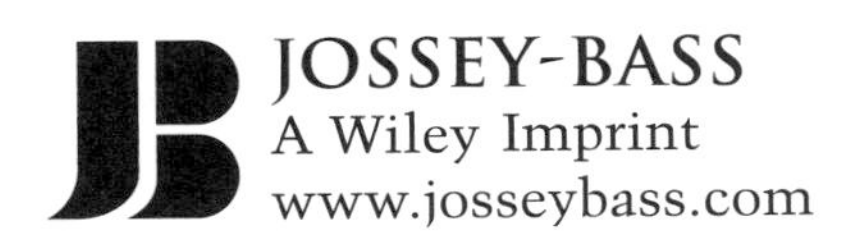

Published by Jossey-Bass
A Wiley Imprint
989 Market Street, San Francisco, CA 94103-1741—www.josseybass.com

Jossey-Bass books and products are available through most bookstores. To contact Jossey-Bass directly call our Customer Care Department within the U.S. at 800-956-7739, outside the U.S. at 317-572-3986, or fax 317-572-4002.

Jossey-Bass also publishes its books in a variety of electronic formats. Some content that appears in print may not be available in electronic books.

Library of Congress Cataloging-in-Publication Data

Marcus, Leonard J.

Renegotiating health care : resolving conflict to build collaboration / Leonard J. Marcus, Barry C. Dorn, Eric J. McNulty.—2nd ed.

p. ; cm.

Includes bibliographical references and index.

ISBN 978-0-470-56220-8 (pbk.); 978-1-118-02155-2 (ebk.); 978-1-118-02156-9 (ebk.); 978-1-118-02157-6 (ebk.)

1. Health planning—Decision making. 2. Conflict management. 3. Negotiation. 4. Medical policy—Decision making. 5. Medical care—Decision making. 6. Conflict management—Decision making—Case studies. 7. Negotiation—Case studies. 8. Medical policy—Decision making—Case studies. 9. Medical care—Decision making—Case studies. 10. Health planning—Decision making—Case studies. I. Dorn, Barry C. II. McNulty, Eric J. III. Title.

[DNLM: 1. Health Facility Administration. 2. Conflict (Psychology) 3. Interprofessional Relations. 4. Negotiating. 5. Professional-Patient Relations. WX 155]

RA394.9.M365 2011

362.1—dc22

2011011130

Printed in the United States of America

SECOND EDITION

PB Printing 10 9 8 7 6 5 4 3 2 1

CONTENTS

Part Four Evolving Health Care Practice

Part Five Shaping Purpose

PREFACE

In the fifteen years since the first edition of this book appeared, its basic premises have not changed. First, conflicts and differences are an inevitable part of your work and relationships in health care. Second, how you handle those differences affects what you can and cannot accomplish as a person and as a professional. Third, to benefit from those differences, you must not only be prepared to change what you do, you must also be ready to examine and perhaps shift the very assumptions that impel you to do it.

Much, however, has changed. New treatments, technologies, business models, and regulations have tangibly transformed the substance of health care negotiation. The United States is coming to grips with the massive health care overhaul legislation that became law in 2010. The human elements of health care—the training and work of nurses, doctors, administrators, researchers, technicians, and others as well as the expectations of patients—have also evolved as new discoveries have become available and as demographics shift. And even though the substantive questions about which people negotiate and find themselves in conflict have fluctuated, the presence and importance of these very human sides of the enterprise have not.

Health care work is a constant negotiation. You are continuously engaged in making decisions, taking actions, and selecting options—sometimes on your own and many times under the direction of others. You exchange intangibles such as information, expertise, opinion, knowledge, and skill as well as tangibles such as money, equipment, space, supplies, and personnel. Because your responsibilities are so closely intertwined with those of others, orchestrating mutual involvement is largely a matter of negotiation. That differences and sometimes conflict emerge along the way is to be expected. The effectiveness of your work is dependent on the proficiency of those exchanges and interactions.

In your hands is a set of tools in the shape of a book. Its purpose is to provide you, as a health professional, with a range of choices for what you negotiate and how you go about negotiating it. These tools are designed to fit the specific circumstances of your work: what it is you strive to accomplish set in parallel with that of others. As health and health care are increasingly team endeavors, the necessary balance of expectations among people working together is achieved using models and methods intended to construct pragmatic collaboration. And for those circumstances when differences ignite into disruptive conflict, there are strategies presented that will guide you toward resolution or, when necessary, toward a dignified exit affording you minimum pain.

This book is entitled *Renegotiating Health Care*. Why *re*negotiating? Because the changes emerging in health care today require us to do much more than improve our day-to-day negotiations. These changes are affecting the very premises, expectations, relationships, and motivations that have influenced the way health care has been conducted for many years. The ground rules that guided associations between clinicians and managers, managers and insurers, and also patients and clinicians, to name but a few, are all changing. Demands for higher quality and lower costs are bringing a closer examination of every element in the system. Orthodoxies are being challenged and assumptions being questioned at every turn. New behaviors and incentives are being negotiated to satisfy the mutual expectations of all those who have a stake in the process. These new ground rules then become the basis for continued negotiation. The intention here is to speak to the change, the *renegotiation*, mindful of the ways in which this transformation affects ongoing *negotiation*.

The subtitle, *Resolving Conflict to Build Collaboration*, points to our fundamental purpose as health professionals. That is, *conflict resolution*, as a process, is considered here not only as a method for cooling a boiling dispute but also as a regular function of your work. You negotiate your differences every day. Some of these differences are resolved routinely, without much notice. In other cases these very same issues can explode into major confrontations. Such confrontations usually have their beginnings in simple negotiations that might have been better handled. Conflict resolution therefore is viewed as an integrated aspect of what you are continually doing to balance the array of expertise, values, and aspirations attending even the simplest of decisions.

The word *collaboration* in our subtitle refers to the combined activity of the host of individuals and organizations necessary for the work of health care. In the emerging health care reality, those groups and enterprises most likely to succeed are those best able to achieve efficient and effective collaboration. Whether it be two organizations forming a partnership, three physicians devising a primary specialty care alliance or a floor of nurses creating a better-coordinated work environment, those people who do collaborate—and do it well—are those who are most likely to survive and thrive. These successful collaborations foster quality, enhance productivity, improve patient safety, reduce health disparities, and cultivate satisfaction both for those who provide health care services and for those who receive them. Technology is already beginning to enable collaboration between professionals in different cities, states, and even regions of the world. Outcome data are being aggregated to help better inform decisions. The capacity to work together will distinguish those able to leverage wider advantages and benefits from those who will not.

You need to *build* collaboration because negotiation is an ongoing process that you formulate and reformulate every day. The set of negotiation tools this book offers will serve your building process.

Who Should Read This Book

Because the purpose here is to highlight aspects of negotiation and conflict resolution particularly germane to health care and to present a model that fits its unique demands and dimensions, this book is written primarily for those who work in the field. Nonetheless, those who are consumers of health services will likely also find the insights useful, just as those who are interested in general aspects of negotiation and conflict resolution may find the dynamics of health care to inform general theoretical and methodological understanding.

How This Book Is Organized

This work is really three books in one. First, it is a guide to the concepts, methods, and techniques of negotiation and conflict resolution. This discussion ranges from the theoretical to the practical, with an emphasis on how you can build interest-based negotiation into your everyday professional repertoire.

Second, the text examines major, long-term trends that will shape the context in which you practice, from advances in technology to changes in the workforce, in patients, and in the system. This material is found mainly in Part Four, which is completely new to the second edition, and it incorporates the perspectives of a range of health care stakeholders, from frontline nurses and doctors to hospital CEOs and policymakers. The four chapters in this part are not designed to inform you about the scope and advances for each topic that they cover: changes are continual and occurring too rapidly for a comprehensive cataloguing of them here. Rather, these chapters are designed to expand your understanding of particular tectonic shifts and their potential to reframe negotiation, generate conflict, and offer fresh opportunities for collaboration and growth.

Third, this book contains a "novel"—a set of parables that play out in the context of the typical dilemmas, conflicts, and negotiations that face people working in health care settings. These stories are interwoven throughout the text and are the greatest departure from the standard format of a textbook.

People often seem compelled to create neat lists, categories, cases, and concepts to describe and understand matters of negotiation, mediation, and organization. In this organizing process it is easy to forget that each of these activities is essentially about people—what they say and do, how they feel and react, and what complex and sometimes fluky interactions they have with each other in the course of elaborate and highly consequential decision making. An approach that turns people into precisely defined objects risks creating further confusion and misunderstanding. Our novel is here to remind you of the inherently human aspects of negotiation, to illustrate those human aspects, and to inspire you by example.

A word of caution about reading the novel—it is not intended to illustrate or represent the *typical* nurse, doctor, manager, patient, or policymaker. It is also not intended to idolize, impugn, or trivialize any particular profession or type of person. Rather, it is intended to place into a plausible human dimension the considerations, problems, and consequences that arise as people work together in health care environments. Earlier, we called these sections *parables*, that is, brief and fictitious stories meant to illustrate ideas and principles. Read them as such. Do not take them too literally. Instead, ponder, contemplate, and perhaps discuss with others the insights you find in these stories and how you can generalize from them to your own situations. Because you will be reading the novel serially rather than straight through, to help you recall who's who in the various episodes, each character's first and last names alliterate (for example, *Artie Ashwood*). Remember, look for the meaning and allow yourself to engage with these characters both for who they are and for what they represent. The Appendix is a list of characters in the novel.

There is much more that is new in this second edition. For example, we have added a chapter on meta-leadership, as we find that people at all levels of organizations are increasingly being called upon to demonstrate leadership. Leadership certainly is a critical component of both negotiation and conflict resolution, and the meta-leadership framework can assist you in building the collaboration and the leverage necessary to accomplish a wider connectivity of effort. At the same time, we have, of course, kept the first-edition material that is still relevant and useful.

Why We Wrote This Book

We view the human condition as a continuous process of evolution, shaped by individuals' many intersecting journeys. We each can contribute or detract from that evolution in the paths we pursue and in the manner we conduct ourselves in our travel. This passage through life is one of exploration, discovery, learning, convergences, and departures. We make our contributions; we impose our costs. We cast our goals, set our destinations, and fulfill our aspirations. The trip sees its accomplishments and its disappointments.

Our life's journey will be marked by its many meetings: intersections with others defined by our negotiations. All our origins are varied, just as our destinations are different. The question is whether we can constructively conduct those meetings so they enhance and do not detract from the virtues we each hope to attain.

As a health care professional, you have chosen a special path for your work. You will deal with life and the quality of life. The society and the people who come for service will depend upon you to do well, to extend and enhance the value of their own journeys.

Our own work has brought us into contact with everyone from world-renowned specialists pushing the frontiers of medicine to paramedics who hit the lonely streets each night ready to serve whenever and wherever called. This has given us an appreciation for the immense breadth and depth of this endeavor called health care as well as for the character, dedication, intelligence, and caring ability of those who embrace it as their life's calling.

We hope this book nourishes you for your journey and helps you to progress through intersecting pathways in ways that enhance the ongoing process of health care change and evolution.

Happy travels.

October 2010
Cambridge, Massachusetts

Leonard J. Marcus
Barry C. Dorn
Eric J. McNulty

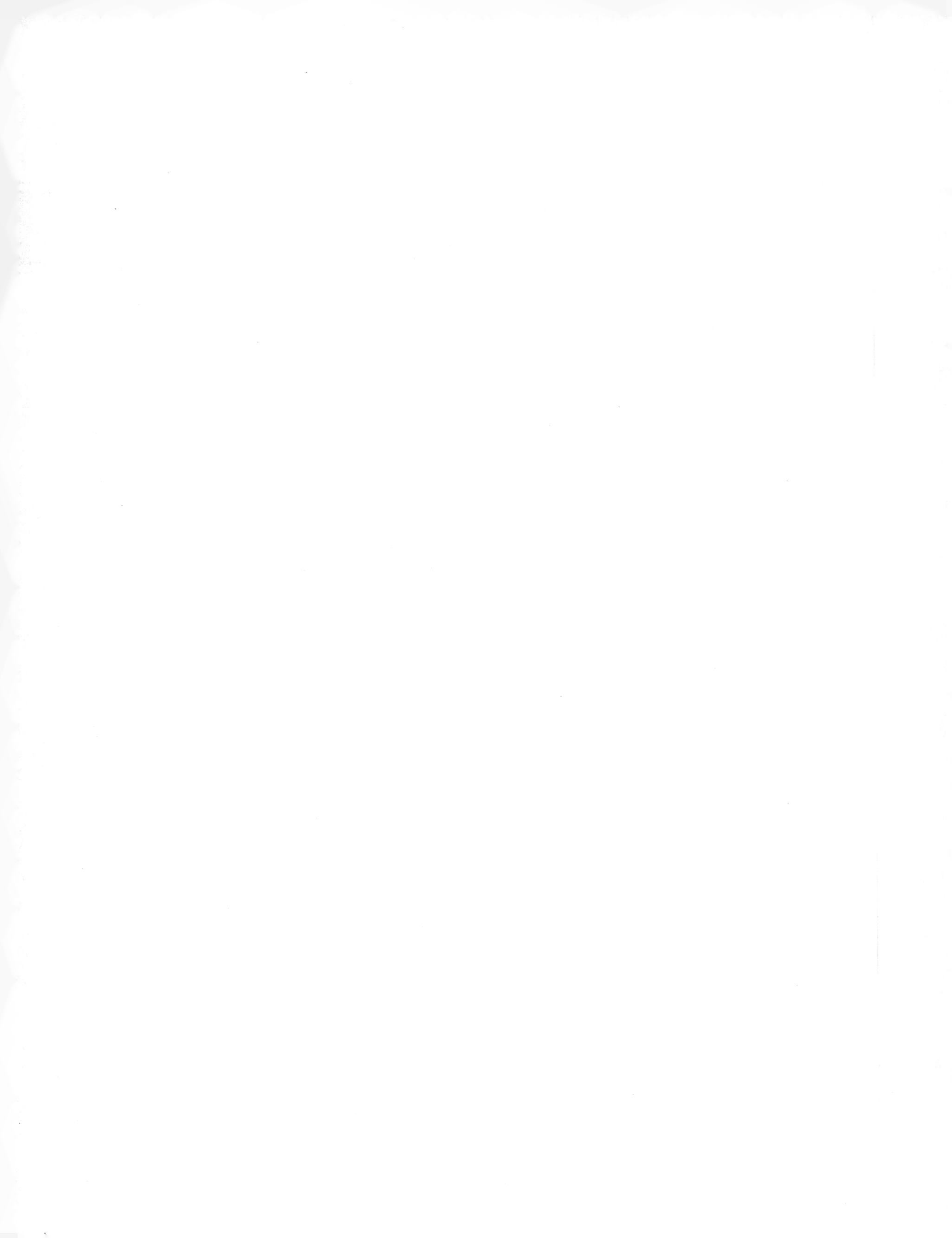

ACKNOWLEDGMENTS

WRITING A BOOK is always an intricate task. The writing itself is a solitary endeavor—each of us in turn focusing on crafting the narrative through numerous iterations to arrive at a text we hope you will find compelling, illuminating, and engaging. The preparation for writing and rewriting can also be an intensely social process. We three authors spent countless hours discussing ideas, refining concepts, and debating word choices. Doing all of this in the midst of the broadest and most contentious discussion of national health care that the United States has seen in decades made it all the more complex—and more interesting.

We also benefited from the insight, counsel, and education provided by many generous people. Among them are Margaret Anderson, of Faster Cures; Donald Berwick, MD, of the Institute for Healthcare Improvement; David Blumenthal, MD, of the U.S. Department of Health and Human Services; Mary Bylone, RN, of the William W. Backus Hospital; James Conway of the Institute for Healthcare Improvement; Kimberly Costa, RN; Christopher Crow, MD, of Village Health Partners; Martha Crowninshield O'Brien, RN; Richard Donahue, MD; Cindy Ehnes of the California Department of Managed Health Care; Eddie Erlandson, MD, of Work Ethic; John Halamka, MD, of the Harvard Medical School; George Halvorson of Kaiser Permanente; Richard Iseke, MD, of Winchester Hospital; Phillip Johnston of Johnston Associates; Patrick Jordan of Newton-Wellesley Hospital; Derik King, MD, of Emergency Consultants, Inc.; Gary Kushner, SPHR, of Kushner & Company; Lucian Leape, MD, of the Harvard School of Public Health; Paul Levy then of Beth Israel Deaconess Medical Center; L. Gordon Moore, MD, of Hello Health; Len Nichols, PhD, of the New America Foundation; Mitchell Rabkin, MD, of Beth Israel Deaconess Medical Center; Scott Ransom, DO, of the University of North Texas Health Science Center in Fort Worth; Glen Tullman, of All Scripts; Pamela Wible, MD; and Andy M. Wiesenthal, MD, of the Permanente Federation. You will meet many of these people in the text. They have introduced us to new ideas, practices, and people. They have enlarged our vistas and we are indebted and grateful.

This second edition carries with it in spirit the contributions to the first edition of this book by Phyllis B. Kritek, Velvet G. Miller, and Janice B. Wyatt. Although we have updated the text significantly to reflect the changing world of health care, much of the foundational wisdom from the original work still holds true.

We have also added to this second edition valuable insights from our colleagues Isaac Ashkenazi, MD, MSc, MPA, MNS, former surgeon general of the Home Front Command of the Israel Defense Forces, and Joseph M. Henderson, MPA, of the U.S. Centers for Disease Control and Prevention. They have been integral to the development of concept of the "basement" in Chapter Two and the meta-leadership framework and practice method in Chapter Ten. Our ongoing collaboration with them is one of the great pleasures in our work.

We are also thankful to the editorial team at Jossey-Bass for their inspiration, patience, encouragement, guidance, and editorial exactitude. Andy Pasternack, Seth Schwartz, and their colleagues have been integral to this revised second edition.

We must express our sincere appreciation to our friends and colleagues at the Harvard School of Public Health. They have supported our work and, most important, shared with us their personal experiences with the health care system as patients and caregivers. The experiences remind us that it is people the system is designed to serve, and it is people we all endeavor to keep healthy, to heal, and to comfort.

Our work would not be possible without the support of Regina Jungbluth, who manages our programs at the Harvard School of Public Health. Her diligent attention and masterful management of all of the facets of our professional endeavors affords us the freedom to research and write.

On our home fronts, the second edition of *Renegotiating Health Care* would not have been possible without the enduring support and patience of our dear families. They witnessed our late night and early morning writing forays and shared with us their life wisdom, experiences with the health system, and bountiful encouragement and confidence.

We dedicate this book to our teachers and students. Some we have met in the classroom and others in the field. This book reflects their collective wisdom, experience, and dedication to more humane health care and a healthier world.

And we offer our thanks to you, our readers, who allow us to do what we most value: to share these ideas so that they might find new homes, new uses, and new journeys. Our completion of this book is not the last step. It is the first.

THE AUTHORS

Leonard J. Marcus is founding director of the Program for Health Care Negotiation and Conflict Resolution at the Harvard School of Public Health (HSPH). He is also founding co-director of the National Preparedness Leadership Initiative (NPLI), a joint program of HSPH and the Kennedy School of Government. In collaboration with colleagues and through extensive research, he has pioneered development of the conceptual and pragmatic bases for the Walk in the Woods, meta-leadership, and applications of systematic dispute resolution to health care problem solving. He has consulted to, trained, and provided executive coaching to leading health care organizations and governmental agencies across the nation and around the world. He received his BA degree (concentrations in social work and Hebrew) and MSW degree (concentrations in administration and psychotherapy) from the University of Wisconsin and his PhD degree from Brandeis University.

Barry C. Dorn is associate director of the Program for Health Care Negotiation and Conflict Resolution at the Harvard School of Public Health. He is also clinical professor of orthopedic surgery at the Tufts University School of Medicine and has held the position of interim president and CEO of Winchester Hospital. Dorn is among the leaders in the development of negotiation and conflict resolution for health care. He received his BS degree from Muhlenberg College, his MD degree from Jefferson Medical College, and his MS degree from the Harvard School of Public Health. Previously, Dorn was a practicing orthopedic surgeon.

Eric J. McNulty is a seasoned business writer, speaker, and thought leadership strategist. He serves as senior editorial associate of the National Preparedness Leadership Initiative at the Harvard School of Public Health. Previously, he was editor at large and director of conferences for Harvard Business Publishing. McNulty has written for *Harvard Business Review*, *Harvard Management Update*, *Marketwatch*, *Strategy & Innovation*, the *Boston Business Journal*,

Worthwhile magazine, and other publications. His case studies written for *Harvard Business Review* have been used in numerous professional and academic settings. He received his BA degree in economics from the University of Massachusetts at Amherst and is completing his MA degree in leadership of meta-system-scale challenges at Lesley University.

RENEGOTIATING HEALTH CARE

PART ONE

CONFLICT

CHAPTER 1

WHY CONFLICT?

WHEN YOUR work is health care, your daily routine requires constant negotiation and involves some measure of conflict. Decisions affecting a number of people have to be made. Competing priorities have to be balanced. There is the pressure of time and the need for constant vigilance that the job is done correctly.

Health care work is accomplished via an intricately structured and constantly evolving set of relationships. Formal and informal rules determine who speaks to whom, who makes what decisions, who has and who does not have what information. People are organized and decisions are aligned in a cautiously defined order. The most important or momentous information, person, or decision gets the uppermost attention, and the rest trails behind. This sequence is intended to yield systematic and value-based decision making.

Most important, the work is done by people and for people. There is perhaps no endeavor more intimately tied to who you are, your identity, than the duties you perform or the care you receive through the health system. Health care is on the cusp of life and death and the quality of life. Whether you are in the role of patient, provider, or manager, your values, beliefs, and personality are exposed and interlocked with the values, beliefs, and personalities of others amid the interpersonal proximity of health care decision making, negotiation, and conflict. And if your role is in the realm of health policy, service regulation, or finance—far removed from the immediate point of care or population served—values, beliefs, and personality remain just as important even though the impact may appear far more abstract. What you do affects how—and sometimes even whether—others live.

What if this complex puzzle does not smoothly fit together? What if there are differences about what or who is more important? What if a mistake occurs? What if there is a clash of personalities among people who must closely interrelate? What if there is dissonance between the policies and procedures and the people who inhabit these relationships? What if various professionals are working under different incentives? How will this affect what you do and how you do it?

Consider the following scenario.

It is another hectic night in the emergency department of Oppidania Medical Center. A frenzy of activity centers at the desk, where nurses, residents, attending physicians, and emergency medical technicians gather to exchange information, tell stories, and take a rare break.

Nearby, Artie Ashwood, a twenty-four-year-old graduate student, moans in one of the beds. The monitors and machines surrounding him are beeping, flashing, and filling him with life-saving fluids. He has an enlarged heart, arrhythmia, and shortness of breath. It has been three hours since he came in, and it is time to decide where he should go next. In the visitor's room, his mother, Anna Ashwood, and girlfriend, Cindy Carrington, nervously await news of his condition.

The attending physician, Dr. Beatrice Benson, oversees the work of the medical residents. On crazy busy nights, she sometimes has to remind herself, "The emergency department is for triage—not treatment." She has to remember that their job is to assess the patient and decide the next step. If the problem is life threatening, they admit to intensive care. If the patient doesn't need to be in the hospital, they discharge with a treatment plan and instructions. If the problem is someplace in between, then they admit for observation and treatment. So, if it's an admission, the question is to which service?

A small cluster of staff have gathered to discuss Ashwood's condition. It defies a conclusive diagnosis: his young age is a concern. His symptoms could signal a dangerous situation. Hoping for more information, they hold him in the emergency department, waiting for stabilization. Nurses and residents are constantly monitoring his condition, but nothing changes.

Suddenly, Charlotte Chung, the triage nurse at the desk, announces the impending arrival of a patient with multiple gunshot wounds. The door to the specially equipped trauma room opens, and the staff move to their places around the gurney that will hold the seriously injured man.

Benson talks by telephone with the paramedics in the ambulance to assess the incoming patient's condition and prepare for briefing the staff. As she turns toward the trauma room, Chung suggests that the young man with the enlarged heart be admitted to one of the floors in the hospital, because it is looking like a busy night.

Preoccupied, Benson says, "Good idea," and walks off with no further instruction. Chung snaps a pencil in two as she watches Benson head toward the incoming patient.

There are, so far, three people in our story. Artie Ashwood's fate is in the hands of the people who surround him. He is in great pain. He is frightened. He does not know what is happening to him and what it might mean for the rest of his life. People are asking him questions, many of them repetitive. Some of those who speak to him seem genuinely concerned about how he is doing. Others seem to be asking rote questions from a prescribed list. He is afraid of being lost in this loud mass of people. He overhears that a gunshot victim is on the way. Might the hospital explode in shots if the attackers come here to finish the job? Even more frightening, might the nurses and doctors who have been at his side forget him once someone sicker arrives? He has been waiting for a long time. Can't they just fix him up and move him along already? He is intimately dependent on people who now seem otherwise occupied.

As the attending physician in the emergency department (ED), Dr. Benson oversees and has responsibility for the work of the ED medical residents and physicians. She simultaneously tends to many constituencies and concerns and is interdependent with many parts of the system. She is vigilant on behalf of the patients, watchful over the residents, and in touch with others in distant departments. When she asks, "Is intensive care backed up?" she hears a variety of answers: "Yes, we can accept a patient severely cut in an accident at work." "No, we are not taking a nine-months-pregnant, cocaine-addicted woman being dumped by a suburban hospital." By its very nature, her work is in the short term: her responsibility is to keep the flow of patients moving. She sees patients for a matter of hours before they disappear into the labyrinth of the hospital or out to discharge. She rarely sees them again. The long term is an abstraction. She has some power and influence, though others in the hospital understate the authority she believes is hers. There is, however, no underestimating when it comes to responsibility. For a miscalculation, the attorneys will chase Dr. Benson with their lawsuits, the administrators will challenge her wastefulness, and the patients will complain about their delayed or inadequate care. She is constantly negotiating and continually trying to keep the many parts of the system in balance.

Ostensibly, as the triage nurse in the ED, Charlotte Chung has the role of screening patients and determining the severity and urgency of their conditions. In fact her function is to create order among the unpredictable and sometimes chaotic flow of patients arriving at the ED. That order must align with the contingent of nurses, physicians, and other personnel staffing the shift. It is a matter of creating a fluid balance. Patients arrive at the hospital in pain or discomfort and are all anxious to be seen at once. Family or friends who accompany them advocate, question, and worry. It is up to her to decide who will be seen when, by whom, and where: she holds the criteria and judges each case accordingly. Physicians, nurses, technicians, and housekeeping personnel scurry to keep up the pace, caring for one patient and preparing for the next. They depend on Chung to make the right calls, to hold off patients who cannot yet be seen, and when the staff are overloaded, to focus on only the most severely ill. Her desk is like a lightning rod for conflict. She mediates among the needs of patients, the capacity of the staff, and the personalities who may explode under the pressure and stress of the decisions she is required to make. Her greatest sources of irritation are the obstacles erected by those, especially physicians, who hold greater authority but who carry far less perspective and understanding than she does.

Each of these people is part of the same reality, yet their perspectives are very different. The question is whether their distinct responsibilities, concerns, and decisions can combine in a congruent manner, allowing each to satisfactorily achieve his or her reason for being in the ED this night. If they can, the interaction will be productive and mutually beneficial. If they cannot, friction is inevitable. Conflict often has its roots in common experiences seen from different perspectives and with expectations that are seemingly at odds.

Different Purposes

The complexity of health care interaction and decision making can be illustrated by the simple analogy of the cone in the cube (Figure 1.1). Two people peer into different holes in an otherwise opaque cube. Their task is to determine what is inside. The person peering into peephole A, on the side of the cube, sees a circle. The person peering into peephole B, on the top of the cube, sees a triangle. They are both viewing the same shape but from very different perspectives.

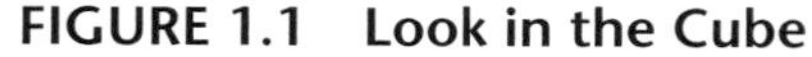

FIGURE 1.1 Look in the Cube

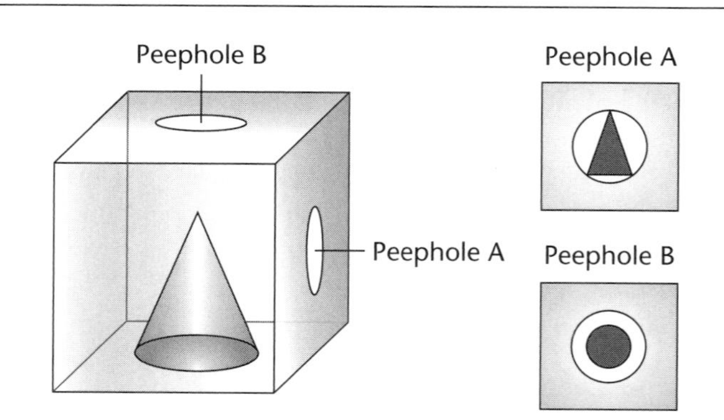

The person peering into peephole A points to his extensive education and expertise, declaring, "Do you realize how smart I am? If I say it's a triangle, then it's a triangle!" The person peering into peephole B counters, "I don't care how smart you think you are. I control the budget in this institution. If I say it's a circle, it's a circle!" Although this analogy is simple, it is emblematic of the failure to account for the multiple dimensions of a problem. Whether those involved are physician and nurse, patient and clinician, or administrator and payer, there are myriad ways for people to get mired in different perspectives and positions on the same problem. Achieving an integrated perspective is at the heart of the health care negotiation and conflict resolution process.

We often begin our health care negotiation and conflict resolution course with a classic game theory simulation exercise called *Prisoners' Dilemma*. (For a discussion of Prisoner's Dilemma and game theory, see Luce & Raiffa, 1957; Goldberg, Green, & Sander, 1987; Rahim, 1992.) This exercise demonstrates the difficulty of negotiating when people have little opportunity for direct or prolonged interaction, like prisoners in different cells trying to communicate. Each participant in the exercise is part of a foursome divided into two pairs. The two pairs sit with their backs to each other—which intentionally limits any direct interaction between the pairs—and an instructor moves messages on paper between them. In a series of transactions, they exchange *X*'s and *Y*'s, which when combined could translate into either gains or losses for each of the two sides.

To simulate conditions in real organizations, the directions for the exercise are purposefully ambiguous. One line in the directions encourages the participants to "do the best you can to achieve a high level of benefit from the transactions." The unspoken quandary is that the *high level of benefit* is intentionally left open to interpretation. Because they must begin negotiating immediately, the players often do not have a common definition for what they are trying to achieve. As a result, one of the four players may assume that *winning* means his pair receives more points than the other pair. Another player may conclude that winning requires collecting more points while also reducing the other side's points. A third may assume that winning means each team receives an equal score. And finally, the fourth may surmise that winning means both teams get a score close to zero.

The problem is readily apparent. If each player assumes a different interpretation of high level of benefit, there is certain to be conflict. In essence, one person is playing one game, *defeat the opponent*, while his or her partner is playing another game, *let's all win together*.

Even among the most subdued of players, the interchange becomes eagerly animated. At face value they are only exchanging *X*'s and *Y*'s—symbols with no inherent value. The heated exchanges emerge from the underlying belief systems, perspectives, and objectives that influence the players' actions during the game.

Each person is playing, in part, to advance and validate his or her own belief system. It is common for someone to say during the after-exercise debriefing, "It wasn't that I was going for points. I was trying to show that we can play to win together." It is also common to hear, "I love to win, no matter what I am doing." Each party strives to justify the principles that frame his or her behavior.

The cone in the cube problem and Prisoner's Dilemma parallel the situation in the ED: different perspectives on the same problem combined with differing objectives, a recipe for a high level of consequences and emotional conflict.

Artie Ashwood stares up at the tiles of the hospital ceiling. He is in a great deal of pain. He is frightened. He wants his computer. Then he could go online and get answers for himself about what is happening to his body. They won't even let him use his smart phone, which would let him turn to his online social networks for help. He hopes that the people around him will care for him well. His confidence in the system is flagging.

Ashwood's condition continues to defy a conclusive diagnosis. Hoping for more information, Dr. Dave Donley, the resident who has been following Ashwood, holds him in the emergency department, waiting for the stabilization. Nothing changes.

Her earlier suggestion to move Ashwood still unheeded, Charlotte Chung signals Dr. Benson over to the triage desk and asks if anyone might be ready to move along. The waiting room is full, and the gunshot wound is stretching everyone thin. Perhaps if Benson decides on her own, things will start happening. This is a nursing maneuver Chung learned a long time ago. Turn your problem into someone else's and then hand her your solution. When she chooses it, congratulate her wise decision. She dislikes having to play this game but smiles to herself every time it works.

Benson nods and shifts into command mode. She calls over to Dr. Donley, "We're too busy to hold this fellow any longer. Call cardiac intensive care and tell them we've got an admission. Tell them he needs to go up there right away."

It has been a busy shift on the cardiac intensive care unit (CICU) as well. Seven of the CICU's eight beds are filled. Six of these patients require heavy-duty care. The seventh patient had been sent up by the ED three hours ago, and once the CICU nurses and physicians completed the workup and admission, it was clear that the ED had misjudged that patient: it was not a case requiring intensive care. The CICU had had enough of the ED for one night. With three hours left in the shift, the CICU staff were hoping the night would calm down.

The chief resident of the CICU, Dr. Eli Ewing, knows that he is running an expensive unit. That misjudged patient not only consumed a great deal of unnecessary time and work, it also cost the hospital and some insurer a lot of money. Ewing believes he has a responsibility to screen out patients who do not require this most technical level of care. Ewing also has a responsibility to the staff. In the parlance of the teaching hospital, a *wall* is a resident who succeeds in keeping out admissions to the unit. A *sieve* is someone who doesn't know how to say no. Walls are heroic, sieves are not—and Ewing is clear about which he prefers to be.

Ewing takes the call from Donley. Still smarting from the last case, Ewing listens sardonically to the report on Ashwood's enlarged heart. Donley admits he is not certain that the patient is in a medical crisis. Ewing's reaction is terse: the patient doesn't need to be admitted to the CICU and the unit is not going to take him. He suggests calling one of the general medical floors, which can do a far better and far less expensive job of babysitting. Ending the call abruptly, Ewing turns to the CICU staff and smiles, "Another victory!"

Donley is perplexed. Is there something he is missing? He walks into the bustling trauma room, where Benson is now intently overseeing work on the patient with the gunshot wound. He explains the situation. Benson barks back, "Tell Ewing he is taking the patient. End of story."

The ensuing back-and-forth goes nowhere. Forty-five minutes later, Benson emerges from the trauma room to find Ashwood still in the bed. "They just won't take him," the frustrated resident explains in defeat.

Enraged, Benson grabs the phone and demands that the CICU chief resident get on the line. "I want you down here right now." It is now a battle of rank versus wall.

"Look," Ewing replies sharply, "this guy doesn't need to be admitted to the CICU. If you want him in for observation, send him to one of the medical floors. We've already had to sweat out one misread from you guys tonight."

"Fine, then let's see what Fisher thinks about this case." Dr. Fred Fisher is medical director for the medical center. This is now a power contest. Benson has no doubt that she will win.

The CICU resident pauses. "Fisher? You're going to run to Fisher over this?" Ewing decides that Benson wouldn't risk escalation unless she were sure of how Fisher will react. "All right, don't get too worked up. I'll be down."

The parties in this emergency department admission scenario are in a situation similar to Prisoner's Dilemma. They have little opportunity to meet. Yet they must engage in a series of transactions and reach a set of common decisions that are utterly interdependent. As with the cone in the cube, they are looking at the same patient but seeing very different images.

Although the parties share many common objectives, their definition of *high level of benefit* is heavily influenced by their immediate context, be it a crowded emergency department or an overworked CICU staff. The ED weighs the care required by each patient against that needed by other patients flowing into the hospital. Therefore, decisions are relative to ED conditions at the moment, as well as the patient's immediate medical needs. The CICU's decisions are based on far more standard criteria. An insurer will not reimburse the hospital for this expensive level of care if a patient's condition does not warrant it. Thus the emergency room staff have one set of criteria for admitting a patient to the CICU, and the CICU staff have a very different set.

When the ED attending physician ordered the CICU admission, the problem with the patient still wasn't clear. The possibilities ranged from minor to life threatening. So the admission decision was made with limited information and a great deal of ambiguity. However, once parties adopt a line of thinking, they can become allegiant to it. Each believes there is much at stake, be it the patient's life, the work of the staff, money, time, or professional prestige. The interchange then becomes passionate as the parties defend principles. "The emergency department decides who is admitted and to which department they are going," maintains Benson. "Without that authority, I can't make this place work."

Ewing counters, "Only the CICU can determine who needs its care. Without that authority, this hospital would turn into expensive chaos. With the threat of lawsuits hanging over us, no physician wants to take the risk of undertreating a patient. Before you know it, every patient will be sent through the CICU as a precaution."

Each of the parties, from his or her own perspective, was trying to wield the control necessary to satisfy his or her considerations. Nonetheless, given the different criteria that the parties brought to the task, it was likely that they would experience a great deal of conflict in the process. The CICU resident was trying to insulate the system as well as his staff from the issues he foresaw. The attending physician was trying to maintain a reasonable balance in the ED while doing what she felt was best for the patient. The ED resident was mediating between the two. And the patient was hoping that the people who would determine his fate could assure him the best possible level of care.

Bottom line, what binds the people, institutions, and activities that we call *health care* is the patient. Although the patient focus is a constant, there are so many different meanings and interpretations of what good patient care is that, ironically, it often becomes a fulcrum for passionate conflict.

The Complexity of Conflict

The first step in negotiating and resolving conflict is beginning to understand it. Even the effort to begin reflecting can mark a turning point, because polarized disputants are often more interested in winning than they are in understanding.

Many times it is difficult, even in retrospect, to fully comprehend the origins and manifestations of a conflict. (For a discussion of conflict analysis, see Likert & Likert, 1976; Potapchuk & Carlson, 1987; Kolb & Bartunek, 1992; Losa & Belton, 2006.)

We want to understand the causes of conflict so we can modify the ingredients that vary its presence and impact. Conflict itself is inevitable. Nevertheless, it does present us with choices. There is good conflict and bad conflict. Good conflict effectively exposes problems, it generates creativity, and it open possibilities that would otherwise not be found. It is conducted in a respectful manner, it is focused on the problem and not the people, and it follows a mutually accepted process. Bad conflict is a bitter distraction, is costly, and can be destructive, especially when negotiating high-stakes decisions regarding health care. Bad conflict is conducted in an adversarial manner in which defeating or even destroying the other side becomes more important than solving the presenting problem. As we begin to observe and understand conflict, we can make choices about both substance and process. We can learn from conflict. It is a vehicle to help us better perceive ourselves, the people we work with, and what we are trying to achieve together. If we truly comprehend it and intentionally choose how to work with it, conflict can uncover opportunities for institutional as well as personal improvement.

What are the ingredients of conflict? If you wanted to create it, what factors would you blend together?

To start with, formulate ambiguity. Take information that could be interpreted in different ways by different people, depending on their knowledge, values, and life experiences. Exclude some important elements of that information, and distribute what remains among different stakeholders. Introduce events that could be viewed and interpreted in disparate and contradictory ways. Create uncertainty about options and outcomes. Sprinkle a dash of vagueness over the mix.

By itself, ambiguity is inconsequential; that changes when it is baked in the heat of requisite decisions and actions. Artie Ashwood presented to the emergency department without a medical chart. The ED staff have no information about his baseline medical condition. In addition he is unclear about his medical history. It is impossible to unequivocally predict what is going to happen next. And who knows how his insurer will assess the appropriateness and necessity of care when his case is reviewed in retrospect? If the wrong decision is made, it could be unnecessarily fatal for Ashwood or unnecessarily expensive for the hospital. Yet a series of decisions must be made by a widely dispersed cast of characters.

Next, add complexity. The more people who are involved in or affected by a decision, the greater the potential for conflict. Some people are physically present in the scenario: physicians, nurses, and patients. Others are not actually on the scene but their presence is felt nonetheless. They are the people who devise health care policy, who construct the rules of reimbursement, who determine appropriate professional conduct, or who write hospital policy. Even though one person holds the responsibility for making a health care decision on the spot, that decision is colored by hundreds of people who allow or who constrain what can or cannot be done.

This complexity would not be so problematic if it weren't attached to stakes. Although there may be only one decision on the table, such as whether or not to admit, the stakes differ considerably for the many people involved. Those stakes may be measured in terms of professional responsibility, legal or financial liability, personal pride, or a tough night on the job. They may also be measured in terms of quality of life, time, pain, and stress.

Now, add to this mix competition and evaluation. There are competing departments, professions, and institutions at play. Each wields different amounts of power, prestige, and status. In the intricately hierarchical structure of health care, professionals ascend and descend based on both their own successes and failures and those of others. The CICU resident hopes to boast to his subordinates and his superiors that he has protected the unit from another unnecessary admission, and expects to rise another rung on the ladder of respect and admiration in the process. His conquest becomes someone else's conundrum. However, if his superior is later admonished for wrongful refusal of a patient, the penalty is a precipitous slide down that ladder. Likewise, the attending physician in the emergency department wonders what influence she has on the floors and departments above her. Can she keep patients flowing smoothly through the ED to appropriate destinations? She is dependent on the efficiency of the lab, the timeliness of medical record retrieval by the records department (a process that may or may not be electronic), and the cooperation of the medical services throughout the institution. What if her work and decisions are not respected? It could spell disaster for her, for her department, and for the patients dependent on her work. That conundrum is amplified for the triage nurse in the ED. She views and experiences the logjam first and most immediately, yet she has limited authority to dislodge it and often must fall back on her ability to wield persuasive influence over those in charge.

Like ambiguity, this competition and these hierarchical predicaments would not matter if they occurred in isolation, but here they are boiling up in a context of obligatory cooperation. Information must be exchanged. Care for ill patients must be uninterrupted as they move from one department to another. A heavy workload in one area of the hospital requires assistance from other areas. And the whole operation must be in conformity with the differing rules of reimbursement set by the many health care payers, the evolving standards for quality of care, and the unique needs and desires of patients and their families.

Combine all of the above with stress and pressure. Time is not an abstraction in health care. It is measured in moments when a life can be saved. It is measured in colossal dollar amounts when there is a delay in discharge for a patient who need not be in the hospital. There is little room for error or delay. With time so critical, it is imperative to synchronize actions and decisions. Given the extraordinary interdependence of health care services, procrastination on the part of one individual, department, or institution strains the entire system.

Stress and pressure are amplified by consequences. Whether measured in terms of the patient's quality of life or the institution's financial balance sheet, the implications of even routine decisions can be overwhelming when multiplied by hundreds of patients. Artie Ashwood prays that he will be able to return to a normal life after this horrible night. He hopes the people caring for him have the competence and compassion to make sure that happens. Charlotte Chung and Beatrice Benson both know they are juggling an acute set of choices: a misjudgment could cost them loss of professional prestige, a liability suit, or even their license to practice. Dave Donley knows that he is building the foundation for the rest of his medical career, and he hopes it to be a beginning that will serve him well for years to come. And Eli Ewing wants to show that he can handle the tough decisions required of physicians. That reputation could help win him a prestigious position once his residency is over.

When the most incendiary ingredients are flung into this mix, conflict can become ugly and frightening. Mistrust, lies, trickery, and malicious behaviors breed suspicion and aggression. Manipulation, fear, hostility, and counterstrategies insert a dynamic that can be near impossible to break. As emotions fuel thinking and behavior, each side assumes a battle position. The outrageous acts of one side justify and goad those of the other. Eventually, people lose sight of what the original issues were all about. The conflict assumes a life of its own.

Finally, incorporate all these ingredients into the near constant and evolving process of change. Health care "reform" initiatives cycle through the system regularly. With each wave, reimbursement formulas and incentives are recalculated and realigned, organizations are restructured, professional responsibilities shift, and social expectations adapt. In addition, at the heart of the health system are rapid changes in knowledge, research, and technology that enlarge what health professionals must know and do. Some people welcome these changes and eagerly pursue the opportunities they present. Others recoil from them because these shifts threaten their status, comfort, or influence. This clash between comfortable security and precarious, unknown opportunity magnifies every conflict. The health care system is akin to a colossal jigsaw puzzle in which the parts—money, organization, service, training, and people—are aligning themselves into a new order and a new fit all the time.

Choices About Conflict: Good or Bad?

Thomas Schelling (1960) distinguishes two fundamental approaches to the study and understanding of conflict. One approach views it as a problem, the other as an opportunity.

Those who view conflict as pathological believe it is best silenced or eliminated. Seen through this lens, conflict reflects negatively upon an organization or leader. Conflict is an annoyance in and of itself, as are those people who raise it. People who instigate conflict are labeled *troublemakers*, and the problems they raise are associated with them personally. When this perspective pervades a group, discussion usually descends to blaming, polarization, and nasty personalization of the issues.

This perspective shuns the disruptive implications of conflict and change. This is a conservative view that regards conflict as a challenge to the existing power arrangements. For example, the members of a long-standing management team would likely be intimidated by calls for change within their organization. The concerns and dissatisfactions of those who ignited the conflict are delegitimized, as they endanger the authority and influence of those in charge. The actual problem is lost in the struggle to determine who has the legitimate authority to raise concerns and make decisions. You might hear some version of "there is nothing wrong with what we are doing or how we go about doing it; the problem is with the people who are raising the problem."

From this point of view, conflict and contest are intertwined in their meaning. The only response to conflict is to end it with a quick and decisive victory. Conflict is viewed as a threat and a source of vulnerability by both sides. Going for a win is akin to fighting for survival. It is an instinctual, self-protective response that allows only an inherently limited set of options.

When conflict is regarded as intrinsically bad and the people who raise it are treated as troublemakers, then little can be learned or gained from the everyday problems an organization or group of people naturally encounters. Rather than considering what may be wrong or what might be fixed, attention is directed to silencing the dissenters and invalidating their concerns. The paradoxical outcome is that the original problem is then exacerbated. Not only does the source of the original dissatisfaction remain. The conflict itself becomes an annoying distraction, gobbling time, resources, and a wealth of missed opportunities. For those who raised the issues, the walls and silence imposed upon their concerns form yet another layer of frustration to endure.

The second approach to conflict views it as a naturally occurring social phenomenon. It is to be expected that people and organizations vacillate in their interests, priorities, concerns, and relationships. When seen from this perspective, conflict is acknowledged and handled as one measure of the problems or concerns that merit appropriate attention. To silence differing points of view by erecting concrete barriers between them and the established views is also to oppose the values of an open, resourceful, and intellectually entrepreneurial enterprise.

Those who view constructively framed conflict as a positive contribution encourage constructive expression of differences so they can be acknowledged, addressed, and, one hopes, remedied. Rather than discounting expression of dissatisfaction, these leaders solicit it as a way to move toward resolution. This perspective recognizes that the most successful organizations are those that can efficiently and accurately respond to internal as well as external contingencies. Effective solutions are devised by tapping into wide-ranging sources of credible information and then working to invent mutually acceptable solutions.

This approach does not imply that all expressions of conflict are inherently valid. Absolutely not. Not every issue and concern has merit. People may raise matters that are irrelevant to the purposes of an organization, are beyond reasonable expectations, or are without validity. Even so, such issues may still deserve some attention. You might question why the misinformed expectations arose in the first place, and you might want to improve information and communication as a result. That is to say, even when an issue is without merit, it may reveal something important about the conditions, people, or circumstances that spawned it.

Those who approach conflict in this way encourage its expression, endeavor to find its roots, learn from it, and when appropriate, modify conditions. Expressing, learning, engaging, exchanging, and changing form a recurring cycle of robust organizational practice. Often, finding the resolution is a matter of negotiation. The responsibility for enhancing the process by framing the issues constructively lies with all parties to the disagreement. If conflict is to be an opportunity to add value, the initial framing, the response, and the subsequent bargaining must be conducted in a manner that respects the legitimate concerns of all sides.

The approach of this book is to view constructively expressed conflict as an opportunity. It regards conflict as part and parcel of human endeavor and thus part and parcel of health care. It is to be expected. If we accept that differences of opinion, and sometimes even heated differences, are predictable occurrences in health care, then we can prepare for them. We then reframe conflict as opportunity. Conflict is a plus when used as one test for determining what is and what is not working about health care. It can serve as a gauge that points to what needs to be improved. This positively constructed method for attending to conflict can be one part of a continuous quality improvement strategy.

Charlotte Chung wonders aloud what can be done to change this nightly standoff between the emergency department and other units of the hospital. Sure, part of it goes with the territory. There will always be some creative tension between the unpredictability of what happens here and the orderliness of the routines in the rest of the hospital. Nonetheless, there has to be a better way to play out these decisions so that people, herself included, don't get caught in the cross fire.

Artie Ashwood's mother, Anna, and girlfriend, Cindy, have never been on the best of terms. Now, pacing impatiently in the ED waiting room with no information and no treatment decision, each has convinced herself that Artie is going to die. Their old animosities rise to the fore, as each is certain that Artie's death will be a greater tragedy for her than for the other. Anna mutters over and over, "My baby, my baby." Cindy grits her teeth and thinks to herself, "My lover, my lover. You screwed up Artie and now all you care about is 'my' baby." Together they approach the triage desk, pleading to be allowed to see Ashwood.

Chung explains that he is allowed only one visitor at a time. Anna and Cindy both explode, each arguing that she is the one Artie really wants to see. Chung stares them down and then patiently asks them to take a seat while she goes back to see what's happening.

Enough is enough. Chung darts up and heads right for Dr. Benson.

We prepare ourselves for conflict by better understanding it and better negotiating our differences. We prepare our organizations for it by anticipating it and by building mechanisms to resolve it in its early stages. And we incorporate a concern for it when we craft public policies that regulate work and interactions in health care settings in a manner that appreciates the very human and very intimate complexities found in these settings.

It is prudent to expect any nation to periodically readjust its health system, a process shouted out from the headlines as "health reform." New policies, procedures, expectations, and pressures will put their mark on the everyday negotiations and interactions of all parts of the system. These new policies will reframe professional, fiduciary, and organizational relationships between doctors and patients, patients and insurers, nurses and patients, doctors and businesses, and among the many others who are part of the health care system. If those relationships are reframed correctly, then the system will work to keep people healthy and, when they need care, to appropriately provide the service they need. However, if the relationships are not carefully designed, and if appropriate incentives, restrictions, and protections are not in place, people will face great disappointment when they need care for themselves or for a member of their family. The work of health professionals and the fates of those who depend upon these professionals' work and counsel will form a story of bitter disappointment (Thorne, 1993).

This book is a map to help you better understand conflict, negotiate choices, and build systems to improve the processes of decision making. The book is not intended as a blueprint for a better health care system, a more satisfying health care career, or improved health care experiences. Rather, it is a guide to the process for getting there.

CHAPTER 2

MOVING BEYOND CONFLICT

IMAGINE—FOR illustrative purposes—your brain divided into three layers. The uppermost layer is the neocortex, the new brain, where your creative thinking, learning, and most complex problem solving occur. It is the strength of this brain layer that distinguishes humans from other species. In the midbrain is your mental toolbox. This section directs activities that you have learned and mastered. For the experienced motorist, it is this section of the brain that drives the car, often with scant direction from the neocortex, which is otherwise occupied with thinking, daydreaming, or talking. It is the midbrain that directs the myriad personal and professional activities that you conduct in rote fashion. The bottom layer is the old brain, a section of your neuroanatomy shared with all other mammals, birds, and also reptiles. It is your old brain that regulates autonomic functions such as your breathing and heartbeat. It is here also that your protective instincts are ignited.

Resting in the middle of your brain is the amygdala. This almond-shaped structure acts like a filter, checking signals to ensure that nothing threatening or frightening is happening in your environment. When the amygdala perceives that you are safe, it remains, in effect, in an off position. However, when your senses detect an unknown or threatening signal, the amygdala is activated, triggering your old brain and its protective triple-F mechanisms of fight, flight, or freeze. We call this reaction *going to the basement*, where you are limited to this triple-*F* set of options (Ashkenazi, 2010). You have the sensation of being overcome with fear, anxiety, or panic.

Going to the basement is not a voluntary act. Once your amygdala takes over, you lose cognitive control of your brain. Just as you cannot stop your heart from beating, you cannot stop yourself from going to the basement. In more primitive times this function protected your ancestors from threatening predators, stimulating them to run as fast as possible or to adopt the fierce countenance of warriors. It was survival of the fittest. Those who could run the fastest or fight the hardest triumphed and dominated their environment.

The descent to the basement is a common, everyday experience. The parent whose child fails to come home at the appointed curfew goes to the basement. The husband who discovers as he heads to the airport that his spouse has emptied his wallet of money is in the basement. The child who loses at a board game descends to the basement and cries in disappointment. There is nothing wrong with going to the basement, especially given that you cannot constrain the triggers that send you there.

Even though you cannot control going to the basement, you can control how deep you fall and how quickly you rise up. The response to cardiac arrest in a hospital patient provides an example. An alarm is sounded indicating that a patient's heart has stopped beating. Everyone in range of the signal goes to the basement: someone is about to die! Even those with responsibility for responding go to the basement. Autonomic physical responses are triggered, including a faster heartbeat and, with it, more rapid breathing. However, the responders quickly recover by ascending into the midbrain toolbox, swinging into action with well-practiced routines and procedures that are deployed with almost automatic precision. Supplies are prepositioned on a cart, and the cart is moved into place. Everyone on the team has his or her station surrounding the patient. With extraordinary calculation and speed, predetermined steps are activated. Those close to the patient are out of the basement and functioning effectively. If the routines are not accomplishing their intended effect, an on-the-scene leader rises to neocortex thinking, considering options beyond the routine to help the patient. People on the sidelines watching this tumultuous choreography of activity remain in the basement, frightened, frozen, and with nothing they can do. As the patient's heart beat returns to normal, there is a sigh of relief. It was that small dip to the basement that got those responsible moving quickly, and it was their rapid recovery that allowed them to function successfully when every second counted.

Although this adrenaline rush and basement behavior protected your ancestors from threatening carnivorous adversaries, modern humans rarely need fear wild animals in their midst. And yet the instinctual mechanism that takes you to the basement remains in place. As a result, extraordinarily smart people can go to the basement, and stay there, over a clinical difference of opinion, a cut in a departmental budget, a personal or professional offense, or even whose name is listed first on a published paper. With people's options limited when in the basement, these differences then turn into emotional and nasty fights for dominance. Survival of the fittest becomes the theme, and combatants struggle to attain the dominance that ensures their good standing when the dust settles. The conflict assumes a life of its own, fueled more by impulse than rational thinking or insight.

Moving beyond conflict requires you first to recognize what sends you to the basement and then what happens when you get there. How far do you fall? How long do you stay there? What keeps you there, and what helps you to rise up from the basement? The methods, techniques, and skills presented in this book are designed to help you answer these questions for yourself, provide you with insight about answering these questions for and about others, and once you have that information, help you to get yourself out of the basement while you guide others out as well. Although we are wired to descend to the basement, we are not wired to rise up and out. That is something you can learn, practice, and master as part of your fine-tuned negotiation, conflict resolution, and leadership repertoire.

Conflict Escalation

The deeper you go into the basement and the longer you stay there, the more difficult it is to get out. As you rationalize how and why you got there, your logic only drives you deeper. It is sometimes remarkable just how far people will go despite the evidence. Why? Because they must start ascending out of the basement by using their midbrain before the evidence can be comprehended.

Among the simulation exercises we have used in our conflict resolution teaching is the *Arms Race*. In this exercise, we auction off a one-dollar bill. The bidding starts at ten cents and goes up in increments of at least five cents. Before the auction begins, we inform the participants that all proceeds will be donated to a worthy charity. (We have raised money for multiple sclerosis, shelters for the homeless, and a hospital in Haiti.) We also explain the unique rule of the game: you must pay whatever you last bid, whether or not you make the final offer that wins the dollar bill. If you bid ten cents, someone else bids fifteen cents, you raise your bid to twenty cents, and then the other person gets the dollar for a quarter, you still have to pay your last bid of twenty cents. (For a discussion of games and negotiation, see Brams, 2003.)

The game has a robust beginning. People are eager to participate in the auction and the bidding climbs rapidly in small increments toward a dollar. As it approaches the dollar point, the pace slows. Often bidding grinds to a halt at ninety-five cents. Usually ten or so people have been actively bidding, and they are now faced with a choice. Up to this point, they have been dealing with a relatively small risk for a potentially profitable outcome. "After all," they reason, "this guy is selling a dollar and I could get it for twenty-five cents."

We walk over to the person with the ninety-cent bid and suggest, "You might as well bid the dollar. This way, at least, you come out even. Otherwise, you'll pay ninety-five cents and have nothing to show for it." (Yes, we recognize that this is manipulation. It is done purposely to demonstrate a common phenomenon in conflict escalation. The game effectively portrays the dynamics of disputes, and most participants accept this function.) She decides to bid the dollar. The person with the ninety-five-cent bid realizes that he too may lose his bid with nothing to show for it, so he goes to one dollar and five cents. Usually at this point some participants drop out, although enough remain for active bidding to continue. The higher we go above the one-dollar bid, the greater are the increments between bids. We move from increasing in five-cent increments to making twenty-five-cent jumps, one-dollar jumps, and even three-dollar leaps.

At this point, of course, the game has become seemingly irrational. If someone were to enter the room and observe the exercise, they would marvel at a group of intelligent professionals yelling out bids of fifteen dollars and eighteen dollars for a mere one-dollar bill. At one seminar, two health care executives both decided they wanted the dollar. They became entangled in a bidding war that reached thirty-one dollars! Other participants sat in wonderment as the two nervously moved the bidding beyond the bounds of the conceivable. It finally stopped when the loser ran out of money: he had just thirty dollars in his wallet.

This exercise is designed to illustrate in stark terms what happens when one goes to the basement, losing sight of the value of what is at stake. The dollar bill itself starts and ends with a monetary value of one hundred cents. And yet it has assumed other value by the time the bidding is over, enough to warrant a thirty-one-dollar price tag. How might this insight help you in bringing disputants up and out of the basement?

Conflict Costs

Conflict consumes time and money, distracts attention from other critical activities, and overwhelms our ability to make rational decisions (see Blake & Mouton, 1984; Benderesky, 2003; Burkowski, 2009). When five workdays are devoted to doing battle, the time lost is irretrievable. Just as Arms Race players must pay their last bid in the simulation exercise, disputants must pay the $100,000 legal bill accumulated on a $25,000 dispute, even if they lose. And when a dispute plagues a health care practice, the toll on staff morale lingers well beyond the last salvo of the fight.

The bidding simulation is called "Arms Race" because it is analogous to the irrational pattern of competition that occurred during the Cold War arms race between the United States and the Soviet Union. Though each side could destroy the other several times over, when one nation developed a new weapons system, the other felt compelled to further up the ante. We now recall that perilous period with the hindsight and wisdom of history. The world was subjected to enormous risk, cost, and diversion to build and maintain an ultimately unusable armament that threatened human survival.

The problem is that once we have acted irrationally, we feel compelled to justify our madness. We do that by "winning": "You see, it made sense to pay twenty-two dollars because in the end I got the dollar!" The fear is of paying twenty-one dollars and *not* getting the payoff. One can just imagine the conversation with a spouse after a day in the classroom: "Honey, you see, there was an auction, and the instructor was selling a dollar. I paid twenty-one dollars, though in the end, I didn't get the dollar." Insult compounds injury.

Picture yourself and a colleague in this bidding war. The encounter can take you to the basement. What do you do if you learn that the price is likely to reach ten dollars? You both can still reduce your losses if you stop bidding at three, five, or even eight dollars. Even better, if you both had anticipated what was about to occur, you could have stopped the bidding very early, at the ten- or fifteen-cent level, gotten the dollar bill, split it, and both be ahead together. Stopping well before the one-dollar mark is reached allows other benefits as well, because the total time, money, and investment is less than the cost of the issue at hand. Let's translate this into a real-world example. If a difference over budgeting is settled before it becomes a time-consuming squabble, negotiators are more likely to find a creative solution that shares costs and perhaps even provides mutual benefit. It is harder to achieve a positive outcome after the investment in the process becomes a ridiculously expensive burden.

You build a motive for resolving conflict by identifying and fairly distributing the dividends derived from reaching a resolution. Those dividends may be tangible, such as money, space, or equipment, or intangible, such as time, reputation, or satisfaction. Money not used in the battle can be split among the parties involved. Office space, for example, needed by one group in the first shift can be shared with a different group in the second shift. Collaborators can share the kudos for resolving a dispute, combine the accomplishments of cooperation, and join in the benefits of good communication. If these benefits are known and mutually recognized, this potential itself may provide the motive to settle. You all must first, though, get out of the basement, by engaging in constructive and nonadversarial discussion, so that you can begin to ponder those dividends.

Turning the Obsession

Bidders who climb beyond the one-dollar mark are often caught by the obsession to win. The dollar has taken on new value. It assumes a much larger and symbolic meaning, enmeshing self-image, public position, and personal objectives. To obtain the dollar is to achieve status, recognition, and power. To lose it is to risk humiliation. Once the obsession to win prevails, jumping off the bidding bandwagon becomes unthinkable.

Bidders captured by the obsession are quick to formulate a rationale for their bidding. They later explain that they were doing it for a "cause." They talk about the wonderful charity to which the money is being donated. They express their admiration for the philanthropic import of the humanitarian mission and desire to make a contribution. This cause becomes a mask for their infatuation with getting the dollar.

This is a common human phenomenon. If we become convinced of the "rightness" of a purpose, there is little we are willing to withhold in its pursuit. The cause could be a moral principle, such as upholding a patient's right to determine the course of his or her care. It could be upholding your organization, especially if your professional survival depends on that organization surviving some plight. Or it could be acting on behalf of a profession or a larger affinity group, your country, ethnic group, or religion. If the cause is right, you might be willing to sacrifice your life, risk arrest, or ruin your career in the name of the mission. Once we have made the first irrational leap—bidding one dollar and five cents for a dollar bill—it is difficult to turn back. After all, how can you justify doing something that is clearly illogical? You march under the banner of your symbols—causes, professional prestige, or organizational purpose.

Anyone who opposes the cause is "the enemy." Overcoming the enemy assumes a virtue of its own, propelling the mission into a matter of personal standing or even survival. People are heard to say such things as: "If we don't shut them down first, our hospital and our jobs are gone." "It's a matter of professional pride. If everyone thinks they can do our work, soon there won't be a need for cardiologists." "We have to show the hospitals we can't be pushed around. Otherwise, why would the health commissioner want to keep our department funded?"

Conflict often is fueled by focusing on images of an "enemy." President Ronald Reagan referred to the Soviet Union as "the evil empire," and President George W. Bush later referred to Iraq and North Korea as the "axis of evil." In these evil places, there were no children in brightly colored clothes, no ballerinas or intellectuals. The predominant images presented were of missiles and weapons of mass destruction. This enemy image was intended to rally the nation and its allies and to justify increased spending for defense and weapons stockpiling. Once the parties to a conflict view each other as the enemy and see their battle as a struggle for survival, conflict escalation becomes boundless.

In this way the dollar in our arms race exercise assumes value well beyond its face value. During the exercise, we contribute to this inflation of value by noting several features of the bill: "It's printed on both sides. It has a genuine picture of the first president of the United States. And it is suitable for framing." These facetious remarks somehow only fuel the fiction that this is a special dollar bill that you very much want in your possession.

Imagine a shift: the obsession to win transformed into an urge to settle. The obsession to win was fueled by its own momentum: it swelled so quickly that it became seemingly unstoppable, with bidders falling further into the basement with each move. At that point the momentum itself was frightening for the disputants, as they lost control of the acceleration and their role in it. Recognizing that ominous quality of obsession, the parties can be motivated to stop, gain a moment of perspective, and then rise up to their midbrain functioning. Introducing systematic and tempered negotiation can motivate disputants to settle in order to avoid irreparable disaster and ruin. Cautiously moving together out of the basement in order to achieve settlement becomes as righteous a purpose as the arguments that started the conflict in the first place.

Changing the Game

After the arms race simulation, several people typically observe that they entered the bidding because it was fun. Conflict can be fun. There is the thrill of taking a risk and wondering what will happen on the other side. There is the sense of engagement and participation that comes with being part of the action. There is the rush of victory. Participants often do not appreciate how high the ultimate stakes could go: they launch the game by risking a few cents in an amusing exercise. Several end it having committed much more, both financially and emotionally.

The politics of health reform in this country often assume the carnival atmosphere akin to a sporting contest. The sides line up, the stakes are laid out, and the conflict begins. There are presumed winners and losers, and the media feed the frenzy with reports that recast the development of health policy as a field of battle. Although this sort of adversarial process may work for determining who wins a championship, it is doubtful that it is the best way to work out the intricate and intimate subtleties of making the health care system work well. Similarly, a conflict between two departments in a hospital can offer the same thrills as playing a game of ball. There is the sensation of belonging to a team with a common purpose and a common enemy. There is the challenge to outdo the other side. There is the anticipation of victory and the anticipated delight of watching the other side fall in defeat.

A technique sometimes used in mediation can help parties in a dispute transform the character of their interaction as they rise out of the basement. The parties enter the mediation room and, naturally, choose to sit on opposite sides of the table. The mediator opens the session, describes the process, and asks each side to offer a brief explanation of the problem. After assessing points of disagreement and agreement and pinpointing the key problems, the mediator rearranges the disputants at the table. Asking them all to sit together on one side, the mediator symbolically places the problems on the other side. The game of win-lose is then reframed: it is now between the problems on one side and the collective capacity to solve them on the other. If the disputants can develop a mutual desire to move up from the basement and beyond the conflict, this reframed conversation can help them turn the corner. It is no longer me against you. It is us against the shared problem.

Changing the Attitude About Conflict

Placed together, cost, obsession, purpose, entanglement, and the pursuit of victory evoke strong emotions: anger, fear, joy, anxiety, pain, elation, and distress. These emotions of conflict along with basement impulses and behaviors assume a momentum of their own. When individuals are gripped by rage, mistrust, or animosity, forging a clear balance between what makes sense and what feels right becomes difficult, if not impossible for them. These emotions and the fight, freeze, and flight compulsions cloud vision, inflame passions, and erect walls between one individual or group and another. Passion is neither right nor wrong: it is simply there, and so it must be factored in when you assess what is causing your own conflict to escalate and what might turn it toward resolution.

At the end of the arms race exercise, we pass a hat, and the people who participated deposit their last bid of the game. Someone counts the total sum of money collected. The exercise leader notes that the dollar did not simply cost this group the amount of the last bid—31 dollars in our example. In fact, the real aggregate cost to the group was the total sum collected—in this example, 196 dollars!

The actual cost of conflict is not merely your own legal bill, lost time, or frazzled emotions. For the managed care organization, nursing department, or medical practice, the real costs of conflict are the combined losses for each of the staff members in terms of time, morale, and the dispute's effect on the quality of patient care. For a community health project, the real price of infighting among coalition members is a loss of services and support for the people they intend to help. For the patient, a breakdown in communication with caregivers results in increased vulnerability and anxiety over interrupted care and then the negative impact that these emotions can have upon health status. Each of these examples has long-term implications that will have a negative impact on future interactions.

If you and your partners in conflict want to move toward resolution, someone must interrupt the process of escalation. It could be you, it could be another party to the dispute, or it could be someone not in the immediate fray, perhaps a colleague who has watched the costs of the disagreement accumulate. What can be done to forge the motive to settle? What is the change in attitude that will bring about a break in the antagonism?

Stage 1: Accept Conflict

Stage 1 in moving beyond conflict is to accept it as part of the terrain of your health care practice. If you acknowledge that in some form conflict is inevitable, then you can develop pragmatic strategies to survive and even thrive with it. Health care involves so many people with differing perspectives, so many complex decisions without easy answers, so many interrelated tasks, and so many problems that can bear life-or-death implications. With so much happening so quickly, chances are that you will bump up in conflict with others at some point along the way. Not every bump need be an overwhelming obstacle.

When professional disputes are expected as part of the lay of the land, they can be addressed as problems to be solved, a potentially creative aspect of the work. They can be anticipated, prevented, managed, assessed, and resolved.

They are a part of doing business.

Several years ago, one of the authors spoke with a physician who was planning an innovative service for AIDS patients. Engaging the necessary network of insurers, providers, and community agencies demanded a complex and consuming process of negotiation. When the author asked what would happen if a conflict emerged among these many groups once the service was in operation, the physician replied, "Well, then we'll just shut it down." Although that response seems extreme, it is not uncommon. If one can't work with conflict, then the only available option is to sacrifice one's enormous work, investment, and opportunity.

Conflict, when understood to have functional advantages, can even be a plus: a form of expression you want to encourage. The willingness to voice a concern or raise a problem provides an important check and balance on the work of health care. If a nurse believes an inappropriate medication is being prescribed, flagging the problem will benefit the patient, the physician who ordered the medication, and the health system in which the problem occurs. The interchange can be constructive only if the nurse knows how to raise it and is prepared to do so, and when the physician knows how to respond to it and is able to accept it. If this balance of give-and-get is not in place, a high-consequence piece of information will be lost or ignored. From a patient safety perspective, encouraging proactive expressions of concern provides another layer of protection.

The airline industry has recognized the importance of conflict as part of a system of checks and balances and considers the role of conflict when doing postcrash analyses of conversations between pilots and copilots recorded on cockpit voice recorders. One early investigation of this kind focused on the January 13, 1982, crash of Air Florida flight 90 in Washington, D.C. It was a snowy day at Washington National Airport, and flights were backed up for hours. After much delay the Air Florida 737 jet was finally deiced and allowed to head for the runway, where it sat for over thirty minutes. More snow and ice accumulated on the wings, forcing the pilot to return to the terminal for another deicing. Once again the plane headed for the runway, and after another delay it was cleared for takeoff. Just as the plane started to accelerate, the copilot observed a dangerous buildup of ice on the wings and mentioned it to the pilot. Impatient to finally get off the ground, the pilot ignored the warning and accelerated down the runway. Without proper lift, the plane could not fly, and it crashed into the 14th Street Bridge and the icy Potomac River. In reviewing the tragedy, investigators realized that the problem was not one of aerodynamics: it is known that airplanes cannot fly with ice on their wings. Rather, this was a problem of conflict and communication. If the pilot ignores the copilot, a vital source of information and balance is lost to crucial decision making. Commercial pilots are now required to attend cockpit resource management courses, during which they are trained to better express and work with their differences.

A conflict does not exist between two people if not given some form of expression. This expression can manifest itself in many ways: people can verbalize it; they can be silent about something they ought to contribute to or fail to attend a planned meeting; they can file a lawsuit. If a person is unhappy with someone and does not in some way reveal her displeasure or disagreement, then she has personal frustration and anxiety, but not conflict. The question becomes how the conflict is initially framed and presented. It could begin, "You jerk, you did it again!" or it could begin, "I think there is a problem here that negatively affects both of us and that we should discuss." These are two very different ways to express the very same predicament. The first breeds a climate of antagonism and the second opens a door to resolution.

Conflict is a social phenomenon. It exists between two or more people. Even if the disagreement is not acknowledged or understood by the recipient, once it is out in the open, the bidding has begun. The question is how to express disagreement—and how to hear it—so that the problem can receive some form of constructive attention. Without such an exchange, building progress toward a resolution is a formidable if not impossible task.

Stage 2: Recognize the Choices and the Consequences

The second stage in moving beyond conflict and in building a new and more collaborative set of motives comes in recognizing the costs of ignoring a shared problem. If two people work together closely and one becomes annoyed with the other, then both have a problem. If they are dodging fundamental issues, the risk that the matter will escalate grows. The tone of the conflict is shaped by initial expressions and reactions. Will it be a fight? Will it be a solution? What are the consequences?

Remember, the fact that one person disagrees with another, has identified an avoidable error, or is annoyed is not inherently bad. Whether or not the disagreement becomes a problem depends on how it is managed. If the problem is ignored, dismissed, or demeaned, then the person has a new problem on top of his original source of trouble. He has avoidable double trouble.

The dangers of a fight unresolved are especially acute in health care. Clinicians function in close quarters, exchanging information and assisting one another amid the busy pace of patient care. A standoff not only damages professional relationships but also invariably infects patient care, spreading the contamination well beyond the scope and cost of the original dispute. Similarly, an unyielding attitude agitates the balance necessary for effective health care management. It interferes with the stability of relationships necessary to guide a steady strategy and operational course for the organization. Certainly, combat over health policy and regulation sends providers and patients scurrying to keep one step ahead of the next obstacle. The cat-and-mouse game only distorts the cost and quality of care. Whatever the forum, the tasks of health care require extraordinary interdependence. Unresolved conflict is a formidable obstacle.

Forty-six-year-old Gail Gonzalez has spent the bulk of her nursing career in intensive care, most recently in the intensive care unit (ICU). She has always found ICU work to be the ultimate in nursing, helping the people who most need attention. It is exciting and challenging work, with something new to learn every day.

Heather Harriford, who is twenty-five, has been out of nursing school for three years and in the ICU for the past seven months. She is not sure she wants to stick with the ICU. The work is draining. Everyone is always in crisis mode. People seem to forget the basic courtesies of "please" and "thank you" when they are in the unit. She doesn't mind it from the patients—after all, they are quite ill. It's the families that really bother her. Families don't understand that the ICU staffers have a job to do and that they can't do it if family members are constantly bothering them.

The charge nurse has assigned Gonzalez and Harriford to set up Artie Ashwood in Room D of the unit. Ashwood has been moved up from the emergency department, his ailment still not fully understood.

"Ewing really wimped out with this one," Harriford complains as the two move around the bed, setting up the equipment surrounding Ashwood. "I thought we were going to have a quiet night after he put up such a stink about that last patient. If Walker were still chief resident, this never would have happened."

Before she can think, Gonzalez blurts out, "It's not a matter of wimpy. This patient needs to be here." She immediately stops herself. She hates it when a nurse or doctor talks about a patient while in the patient's room. Harriford set the trap once again and Gonzalez walked straight into it. She is furious at herself for responding. Each of them hurriedly finishes her tasks in stony silence.

Harriford is the first out the door and heads off to the nurses' station. Gonzalez marches out shortly after and catches up to her at the desk. Two other nurses and a physician are quietly working on patient charts. "Never do that again, Harriford. I've told you this a million times. If you've got a complaint, make it out here, not in the patient's room. Be a professional. And furthermore, Ewing wasn't a wimp! That patient is very sick. He's in the right place." She stomps off toward the hallway.

Harriford turns to the others, who had watched the exchange. It takes just one word to mount her defense: "Bitch."

Both Harriford and Gonzalez have a problem. Its expression poses dangers for both of them. It also poses dangers for their patients, the hospital administration, and the other people working on the unit. What if their hostility spreads? What if other members of the staff take sides: the older nurses against the younger nurses? What if their problem gets in the way of the vigilance and cooperation necessary to keep the ICU operating at necessary efficiency and effectiveness?

Stage 3: Understand What Motivates the Stakeholders

Stage 3 in shifting toward resolution is declaring the desire to settle. This desire eventually must be expressed and known to all parties to the dispute.

We periodically receive calls from health professionals who are caught in a conflict and interested in mediation. At times the call comes from a staff member concerned about an escalating conflict that threatens his or her viability. At other times it comes from an attorney prompted by a judge to find a settlement for a malpractice case without burdening the courtroom. Sometimes the call comes from a director wishing to resolve conflict among subordinates without a managerial dictate.

We ask the same question of all parties: "Are each of you interested in finding a settlement? If not, mediation is not appropriate."

The response is rarely an enthusiastic "Yes!" This hesitation stems from both pain and strategy. When we are speaking directly to one of the disputants, we find that he or she generally feels angry, vengeful, and bruised. The thought of settling is mixed with the vengeful desire to see the other side destroyed and in even greater pain. We acknowledge these feelings, given the expected nature of conflict and the emotions associated with it.

We also find that disputants are concerned about appearance; this is their strategic concern. They recognize that continuing the battle is costing them dearly. A total win is unlikely. Nevertheless, they do not want to give the appearance of capitulating. They want to distinguish the desire to settle from the acceptance of defeat. We assure them that settlement in mediation is voluntary. If they are not pleased with the process or outcome, they can walk out at any time. Throughout the process they remain in control of what they are or are not willing to accept as the settlement of the negotiation.

An attorney once told me that the insurance company she represented did not believe a settlement was warranted in the malpractice case we were discussing. I replied, "Fine, then we are not interested in mediating the case." She called back several weeks later to tell us that "the carrier reassessed the case and they are now ready to discuss settlement." After that, finding a resolution required little more than four hours of mediation. In another case the mediation discourse had descended into bitter feuding. Eventually, one party turned to the other and proclaimed, "Before we sat down here, you said you were looking for settlement. You are not acting like someone looking for settlement." The other party calmed down. The reminder was helpful to both.

Whether the effort to agree takes the shape of a formal mediation or an informal discussion, unless all parties share some motivation to resolve the conflict, it is unlikely to be settled. If only one party wants to find a resolution, the conflict is likely to continue. It may even escalate into a win-lose situation, with one party eventually falling to defeat. Or one party may give up, becoming resigned to a loss, abandoning employment, or surrendering the battle.

Between continuing to fight and deciding to settle, opting to settle is often the better of what the parties may see as two bad choices. Even when reluctant, the choice to move forward legitimates beginning to weigh the settlement options. Conflict is full of unpalatable choices. The key is whether all parties can begin to accept that none of them is likely to achieve an outright win. Once they recognize this, their motives in the conflict shift toward exploring resolution.

Stage 4: Seize the Learning Opportunity

Stage 4 in overcoming conflict is learning from it: not an easy task. The words sent each disputant's way are laden with emotion and accusation. Both sides descend to and lurk in the basement. They hear what is said through the filters of their own defensiveness and hurt feelings. Both sides are reactive.

Why should the parties struggle to learn? Why should they kindle a sense of curiosity about what envelops them both? Because beneath the rhetoric there is some measure of validity to what each of them is saying. Even though the slurs and accusations exchanged may not be valid, behind these aspersions are genuine feelings, concerns, convictions, and beliefs that lie at the heart of the dispute. In fact, each party has much in common with the other party, more than they imagine. There is much to be gained in understanding what are these points of commonality and difference. Both parties then discover that their different experiences, training, and beliefs have molded divergent approaches to everyday problems.

We often find this during a mediation. At the first mediation session we seat the parties around a table. Each disputant opens with a brief explanation of how he or she sees the conflict. While their adversaries listen, disputants recount the words and events that led to the standoff. The talk is usually solemn and measured. At this stage of the process, disputants begin to hear each other and everyone's very different story, and for the first time they are calmly listening. They are learning about shared differences and commonalities. They discover their regard for one another, their frustrations with one another, and their newfound yet common desire for settlement.

This learning process was key to the resolution of a dispute between two physicians that we mediated several years ago. In the course of the mediation, the two physicians were surprised to learn that they shared many of the same objectives for their joint practice. On the questions of money and management, the matters about which they battled, there was fundamental agreement. On the most important issue, whether they respected each other's clinical skills, there was complete congruence. What then were the problems? The most important turned out to be differences in age, attitudes, and personality. One of the physicians was nearly sixty years old, preferred a hierarchical approach to decision making and authority, and said so:. "When I was in his position, I paid my dues to my mentors. I've been paying my dues all my career, and now it's your turn to pay yours." The other physician, fifteen years his junior, was in college and medical school during a very different era. The younger doctor brought different expectations to the negotiation and had no patience for a hierarchical decision-making structure and certainly no interest in paying dues. He grew up learning to question authority, and he felt that there was no need to submit to the demands of his senior colleague. With better understanding, they found that they could accept their personality and attitudinal differences in exchange for maintaining an important common objective: keeping their joint medical practice alive.

Stage 5: Perceive the Misperceptions

Stage 5 is assessment. To listen and to agree are not the same. Is there some validity to what the other person is saying? Conflict is often accompanied by a story, a narrative. One person has a set of stories that line up with her version of the "facts." The other person has his own collection of stories that similarly pick and choose among the "facts" to create a logical array of explanations and a conclusion. What is the problem that underlies the words and stories? Is one person perhaps reacting to an experience separate from the immediate problem? Or instead of reacting to what the other person is actually saying, is one person perhaps reacting to the timing or the tone with which it is said? Something said in public may have a very different impact from the same words said in private.

Gail Gonzalez always finds a cup of blueberry yogurt to be her best source of relaxation and comfort. She sits alone in the nurses' lounge off the ICU. She pounds furiously at the yogurt cup as the white layer at the top turns blue. She needs to compose herself before she heads back onto the floor. She is boiling mad.

She reminds herself of why she hates Harriford. Harriford is arrogant, inexperienced, and behaves inappropriately. Gonzalez also hates the young nurse's popularity. Perhaps that mouth will finally be Harriford's undoing and create enough trouble that she is finally shown the door.

Despite those feelings, Gonzalez had to admit that she had the same reservations as Harriford about the patient. He needed to be in the ICU but not because of his condition. No, he needed to be in the ICU because sending him to a medical floor would have been dangerous. Everyone in the hospital knows that the medical floors are so understaffed they can barely make it through the night. One sick patient needing close observation would overwhelm them: they have other patients needing care. Sadly, it wasn't always that way. And it's true that the ICU isn't doing anything for this patient at the moment except watching him. If he was not here, though, and his condition changed for the worse, he would probably die before anyone on the medical floors could notice.

And then there are the crazy reimbursement incentives. What if he is a Medicaid patient? It's always easier for the hospital to collect when it's evident that the patient is really sick. That's the logic of the system: if he is not sick enough to go to the ICU, he is not sick enough for someone to pay the bill.

All these big questions are beside the point, though, when it comes to Harriford. You don't create more stress for the patient by mentioning your concerns at his bedside. It's just common sense. What she did in there was simply wrong. What she does most days is simply wrong. They should be teaching these young nurses good manners and what it means to be a nurse.

By its very nature, conflict is a process of polarization. When two people are in conflict, they characteristically move to opposite sides of the issue. They fortify their own positions by overstating their case and by ignoring information that does not conform with it. As the conflict escalates, they become more resolute in defending their position and destroying that of their opponent. Everything the other side does is woven into the story of what is right and what is wrong.

Conflict is also a process of simplification. We ignore the reasons, justifications, viewpoints, and concerns of the other side. We dismiss the texture of their statements, and we are blind to the weaknesses of our own. Our thinking is reduced to clear-cut terms. Their position is without merit; ours is valid.

Given this common tendency to polarize and simplify the issues, accomplishing a balanced assessment of both the other party's concerns and one's own concerns is no easy matter. Ury (1991) suggests that disputants "go to the balcony": that is, they need to get a view of the conflict from a distance. Each needs to understand the dispute from the vantage of the other party's experience: How might the responsibilities, training, and objectives of the hospital CEO affect her view of the staffing question? In light of the medical staff's experience and salary expectations, how might hospital leaders understand their unrelenting resistance to adoption of an electronic medical record system? How is the terminal illness of their child affecting the parents' ability to cope with the requests of the staff? All of this is not to say that each disputant must agree with those on the other side of the conflict. The CEO may be callous, the medical staff may be unreasonable, and the parents may be obnoxious. Yet, as we begin to grasp the other side's rationale, we transform the conflict from black and white to gray, from right and wrong to common ground, and we take the first step from conflict toward resolution.

Stage 6: Choose Beyond the Enemy Image

Often, people enveloped in a dispute assume there are only two choices: they can win or they can lose. Furthermore, they may think, "When I win, I want to inflict some multiple of the pain and expense I suffered upon my opponent." And then they may have this frightening thought: "If I lose, they win and are free to impose that same retribution on me." In these scenarios, even when there is a clear winner both sides suffer unrecoverable losses of time, money, and professional regard. The hours spent plotting, the opportunities lost in the process, and the discomfort shared among colleagues are endured by all sides in a win-lose scenario. The winner gets to lick his or her wounds in the comfort of victory. The loser is left to ponder what might be the next line of attack. We once witnessed a bitter win-lose battle among physicians in a major academic medical center. The outcome was an apparent win for one side and dismissal for the other. Years later, we happened upon the lead "winner" in that fight. He admitted sadly that viewed in retrospect, the damage caused by the conflict was so deep and long lasting that there really were no winners, just losers of various degrees.

Finding common ground is a process of joint discovery. Stage 6 requires disputants to embark together on that quest, to develop options for settlement. An option might be a compromise. It could be an exchange, or perhaps an acknowledgment or an apology. During this quest, the parties amplify their learning about one another. And even more important, they begin learning about themselves.

In portraying the other side as the villain, disputants have ignored their own contributions to the predicament. How have our behaviors or demands polarized the dispute? What changes might we consider? What do we really hope to achieve? What will satisfy those objectives? What concerns us about losing? What do we hope to retain? The answers to these questions gradually become evident as the parties consider, and accept or reject, newly discovered possibilities for agreement.

Stage 7: Ponder the Possibilities

Imagine this: what could you and your colleagues accomplish if you were able to systematically resolve routine conflicts and achieve a culture of collaboration? And also consider this: what are the consequences of continuing these battles? Contemplate too the possible rewards: money, professional satisfaction, and loads

Iris Inkwater dreads early-morning meetings such as the one she has today. As chief executive officer (CEO) of Oppidania Medical Center, she balances the competing demands of many departments. She sometimes feels her job is nearly impossible, especially now with all the health reform changes crisscrossing her desk. On one side she is negotiating with regulatory agencies, insurers, and a distant Congress in Washington, all of whom expect more service for less money: not as easy as they seem to think. On the other side she has to make the hospital deliver with fewer dollars to spread around: a painful process. And as each piece of new technology rolls out of an enthusiastic research and development enterprise, physicians and patients clamor for it, even though, as Inkwater knows, it will be outdated far sooner than it will be paid off.

Last week Dr. Fred Fisher, medical director for the Oppidania Medical Center, asked for this morning's meeting. He requested that three people be in the room: Inkwater; Janice Johnson, the vice president for nursing; and himself. He wants to discuss staffing for the night shift on the medical floors.

Fisher and Johnson exchange the usual niceties as they enter the office. The mood turns serious when Inkwater looks to Fisher and asks, "What's on your mind?"

Fisher is ready to explain: "I've been talking with a number of the residents and chiefs. We have a major problem with staffing on the medical floors, especially at night. The nursing coverage is so thin that residents are reluctant to admit onto those floors." He explains that there is an unspoken assumption that if patients are sick enough to be in the hospital, they're too sick to be on a medical floor. If there was confidence that there would be better coverage, they could reduce the number of people going into the ICU, and save a bundle of money in the long run. "As it stands now, I think this is a dangerous and wasteful situation," he says. "I did mention this to Janice a while ago, but there has been no improvement."

Johnson is seething. This looks to her like a setup, and she doesn't like this accusation being made in front of her boss. She looks at Inkwater, makes eye contact, and then turns to Fisher. She wants to signal that she is taking the high ground in this discussion. And she ultimately needs Iris to be on her side, or at least not against her.

"Fred," she says, "I recognize that this is a problem. I share many of your concerns. Each of our departments is working with a bare-bones staff. You only brought this to my attention two weeks ago. Since then, I have been meeting with my supervisors to see how we might shift people around and resolve this problem. It's not only a matter of head count; it's also a question of who has the experience and the desire to go where. I know that you have people putting pressure on you. But you have to understand, this is a complicated problem that can't be solved overnight."

Johnson looks back at Inkwater. Inkwater is impressed. There is a lingering silence. Fisher is caught off guard and feels a rare moment of speechlessness.

Inkwater redirects the conversation. "There seem to be a number of issues here. Beside the general problems of staffing and money, there is also the question of timing. Fred, I don't hear Janice saying that she doesn't want to respond to your request. It's just a matter of when."

"It's not that simple," Fisher responds. "We have patients coming in here every day. We can't tell them to hold off while the nursing department decides to do a reshuffle. I have the medical staff down my back. These guys are worried about liability. What if something happens to one of their patients while we're waiting to fix this mess? And this is not a new problem. It has been in the making for more than just two weeks."

"Fred, I do want to fix this problem, though I'm going to need your help," Janice offers. "Unless Iris tells me differently, I cannot look forward to any expansion in the number of nursing positions in the department. The only department that is overstaffed right now is the ICU. I might be able to move someone from that unit down to the medical floors, and to do so, I'm going to need your support. They've gotten accustomed to a large staff up there and they're going to squawk. I'll still be up to code, so we don't have to worry about legal problems. It's more a matter of political problems and pressures from the medical staff there."

Fisher is unprepared for this line of reasoning. He had hoped that Inkwater would submit to his argument and offer Johnson some room to maneuver in the budget. That's what had always happened in the past. Why wasn't Johnson getting it? She should be appreciating his help.

Inkwater backs Johnson. "I am afraid Janice is right. We're going to need your assistance on this one."

Johnson adds, "One of the young nurses on the ICU, Heather Harriford, has been talking about a transfer to another unit. She is only reluctant about a cut in pay. I think I could keep her at the same scale as a way to encourage her to move."

Fisher has heard of Harriford. Ken Kavanaugh, chief of the ICU, has mentioned her. He feels she is a good nurse, yet he's heard she doesn't fit in well with the other ICU nurses, many of whom have been with the unit for many years. If Kavanaugh were to lose anyone, he would put up the least fuss about Harriford, especially if her move were accompanied by a real effort from the rest of the medical staff to go easy on ICU admissions.

Fisher turns to Johnson with a half smile. He ultimately wants to find a solution and he realizes that this time, hardball will not work. He also does not want to come across as too easy. He hesitates and then softly offers, "OK, it's not ideal, but let's give it a try."

of recognition may be waiting on the other side. These are the benefits of making the system work intentionally as a whole. There is the peace of mind of having the dispute behind you. And there is the intellectual satisfaction of solving a challenging puzzle.

These possibilities breed a sense of hope and resourcefulness that can motivate disputants toward resolution. If unpleasant consequences are the sticks, then the possibilities of shared overriding values and professional achievements are the carrots.

Finding these opportunities, however, can be elusive in a large, complex, and sometimes impersonal organization. The immediate parties to the conflict may not have the authority to change the operant variables.

Stage 8: Discover Common Purpose

Fisher had a turning point. It came when he realized that he was in the same game as Johnson. He was even on the same side of the table. He too wanted a solution.

> As he walks back from the meeting to the sanctuary of his office, Dr. Fisher ponders the conversation. Things are not as simple and straightforward as they used to be. It's not merely clinical interests against the administration or even nurses against doctors. It used to be like that. You fought for what you wanted and kept the spoils of your battles.
>
> Fisher reflects back to his days as a young doc in training. Those were the days when doctors ruled the roost. Ask, or demand, and it eventually was yours. He had spent time practicing in the military and had adapted well to its command-and-control structure. Back in the civilian world, things were becoming tighter and tougher. "Politicians think they can be better doctors than those of us who made it through medical school," he concludes. "The game has changed. Now it's different. If you are going to get anything, you're going to have to give something up. It's just no fun. No fun at all."

Stage 8 in moving beyond conflict is finding a common purpose and the related common solutions or opportunities. No problem is simply about what one department wants versus what another department wants. Rather, if the parties view the hospital as a whole, then they can find that they share a combined interest in making the system work. Yes, that does sometimes mean that through negotiation one has to give something to get something in return. It is a perspective that implicitly acknowledges that all people and units of the institution are interdependent, are parts of a system. Once people view health care as an interconnected mechanism, then they can see that if one of the parts malfunctions, the whole machine ultimately becomes less efficient and effective. Common and shared responsibility makes for common and shared remedies.

Stage 9: Anticipate Conflict and Plan for Its Resolution

If conflict is a known and anticipated phenomenon in health care organizations and relations, then you can prepare for it intentionally. As you plan a program, establish an organization, or reorganize your institution, you can ask a series of questions to help prepare for the possibility of conflict:

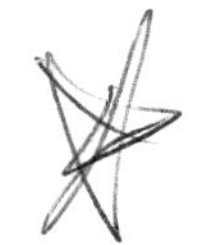

- What is our overall strategy, and what are the potential differences that we may encounter as we further develop and implement that strategy?
- What will we do to negotiate those differences so they cause minimal operational disruption and distraction?
- What can we do to constructively frame the conflicts that do occur and resolve them productively?
- How can we change or rearrange decision making, communications, and organizational structures to reduce the likelihood of conflict?
- What will we do to learn from conflict and then to translate that learning into change that will reduce the likelihood that problems will recur?

With these questions on hand early in your strategic planning and in place every day in your operational processes, it is far less likely that debilitating conflict will distract your work.

Stage 10: Lead Beyond Conflict

We call the stage 10 attitude shift that moves people beyond conflict *whole image negotiation*.

The *whole* is the big picture in health care. It is what you, your colleagues, and your institution are trying to accomplish together in your work. It is an enlarged sum of the parts, one that equates to far more than the combined value of the distinct parts on their own. Moreover, the word *whole* is closely linked to the word *heal*, which means to make healthy or restore to health as well as to resolve a conflict, settle, and reconcile.

Once people have the whole in mind, they can seek that expansive picture in their exchanges, finding common purpose and otherwise unavailable opportunities in collaboration with others in their system. If they are looking only after their own departments, their own institution, or their own professions, the chances of making the system work as a whole will be greatly diminished. Building solutions based on common interests and objectives will create outcomes that will better succeed in the long run for all of an institution's interdependent units. That is the nature of health care.

In addition, the word *image* encourages people to envision possibilities, and also avenues to reach those possibilities, that are not readily apparent. The health care system, by its very nature, is in constant change. What emerges on the other side of each phase of transformation—whether from innovative technology, new reimbursement formulas, or mysterious afflictions of the body—challenges the imagination. Our greatest discoveries emerge from that willingness to peer beyond current reality to find innovative solutions. When we find those opportunities and construct systems that best meet the wide range of common needs and interests—fairly balancing resources, services, and costs—our chances for constructing a health system that is robust and responsive are greatly enhanced.

The best negotiators are those who bring imagination to the table. They can find solutions where solutions are not readily apparent. They can artfully introduce processes that are otherwise unknown to the other parties. And they can achieve outcomes that would otherwise be elusive.

Whole image negotiation (W.I.N.) provides a shared win, a triumph that all those who are part of the process can share.

CHAPTER 3

SETTING THE STAGE FOR NEGOTIATION

NEGOTIATION IS a multidimensional process. Your understanding of the dimensions, the dynamics, and the steps in the process improves your negotiation strategies, style, and outcomes.

Negotiation is a social process. When you do not have absolute control of your circumstances, when you are interdependent with other people, and when decisions or actions are taken that involve those other people, you negotiate. To negotiate implicitly means that you cannot have it all.

Negotiation is therefore about exchange. Its purpose is to produce an action, outcome, or decision. You negotiate in order to gain something from someone else. In return the other person will likely want to receive something of value. To get what you want, you must be willing to give that something or be certain the other person is somewhat satisfied. This premise applies to business negotiations, international relations, and interpersonal interactions just as it does to many different negotiation platforms in health care. It even applies to the interaction between a clinician and patient when discussing a care plan. The patient must understand the clinical choices that are available, his or her responsibilities, and the result of these choices and responsibilities. When viewed as a negotiation rather than simply "doctor's orders" the question of *patient compliance* is reframed.

Negotiation is about discovery. It is how you learn what other people want to receive and are willing to give. It is how you inform them of the same considerations about yourself. It is what happens when you explore a new business possibility with another practice group, opening opportunities that you might not otherwise have recognized.

Negotiation occurs in stages, over time. It begins with this learning and discovery. Negotiators define what they want or what they perceive. Information is exchanged. Through that exchange, the parties determine whether they can find an agreement to satisfy their different desires. In so doing, they determine the outcomes of the exchange. For people with an ongoing relationship, the outcome of one exchange influences what happens in the next round. Robust and respectful negotiation can set the tone for a constructive organizational culture.

Negotiation is shaped by power. In the give-and-take of negotiation, power is an often invisible yet palpable force at the table. The more power a stakeholder has, the less he or she must give. Conversely, the less power someone has, the more he or she must give to accomplish a deal. Because those with less power generally have less to give, they often find themselves dependent and vulnerable during negotiation. As a result, at times the process of negotiation becomes focused on the accumulation and display of power as precursor to the actual exchange of gives and gets. This power is circumstance contingent and is related to but somewhat different from formal authority, wealth, or other standard symbols of power. For example, the humble homeowner who possesses the last lot in a parcel of land desired by a hospital for expansion wields great power in the negotiation of a sale price even though he has far fewer resources than a large medical institution.

These negotiation dimensions are dynamic: they constantly shift and change. As they change they engender new balances and imbalances. The changes define and redefine relationships and actions.

Health care is shifting rapidly in many ways. These shifts may affect each of these negotiation dimensions. To assume that these dimensions are static is to significantly limit your negotiation effectiveness. When you understand the dynamics at work you are better able to influence the course of their evolution.

Negotiation as Exchange

Negotiation may be thought of as explicit or implicit. While related, and at times even overlapping, these two variations have distinct characteristics and dynamics that are important to distinguish. Discerning the subtle nuances helps you discover patterns and dimensions that expand your problem-solving capacity. It is important for you to understand both variations and on which plane you are operating during a negotiation.

Explicit Negotiation

Negotiation is often thought of as the bargaining that occurs when purchasing an item or service whose price is not fixed. For example, in bargaining for an automobile, there is a back-and-forth about perceived value, in which the condition of the car, how many extras it has, and the state of the market are all factors. A deal is either struck or not. Likewise, negotiation describes what is done to reach or influence a decision about which there is a choice. There is negotiation about who gets what office space, for example, or when someone will be on call or on duty. When you ask, "Is it negotiable?" you are asking whether there are options to influence the ultimate decision or action.

Negotiation also refers to the process used to settle a disagreement. Parties negotiate until a resolution is achieved or a stalemate blocks progress. When there is a deadlock that requires that a decision be finalized, as in a legal suit or a personnel action, someone else will likely be asked to decide for the disputants. This third party could be a judge or an organizational superior.

Negotiating a purchase and sale agreement, determining a work schedule, and settling a dispute are examples of *explicit negotiation.* The terms of agreement are observable. The parties have a clear understanding of the nature of the process and the criteria for making the decision.

Implicit Negotiation

By contrast, *implicit negotiation* involves unspoken assumptions about the motivations and inducements that frame the exchange. These assumptions are rarely discussed in the midst of a negotiation. Implicit negotiation relies upon social convention to govern relationships and purposes. It is as if the parties have an invisible script that defines their behaviors, relationship, and expectations. The script establishes the rules of exchange and the roles and status of the people involved. Both social convention and health policy are embedded in this script.

For example, when Leonard ("Lenny") Marcus's son Jeremy was eight years old, he was fascinated during a trip to the Middle East by the back-and-forth of bargaining in Arab marketplaces. A copper tea set that was originally offered for $120 was eventually purchased for $50 after a session of dramatic haggling. Upon the family's return to Boston, Jeremy tagged along to the grocery store to replenish the food pantry. At the checkout counter, he asked, "Dad, so how much do they want for that spaghetti?" "Ninety-nine cents," Lenny responded. "Ninety-nine cents?" Jeremy piped up, "you can do a lot better than ninety-nine cents for that spaghetti." When Lenny explained that this sort of explicit dealing is unheard of for grocery items, Jeremy was disappointed. In the United States, haggling at a supermarket would violate the common script of appropriate social convention and supermarket behavior. In the Middle East and some other cultures, haggling over the price of any item is much more widely accepted.

Though open bartering over the price of spaghetti is considered inappropriate, implicit negotiation does occur when you buy groceries. As long as you have the choice of shopping at another supermarket, you can go elsewhere to get a better price. Knowing this, the store is motivated to offer high-quality goods at competitive prices. This sort of implicit negotiation works only when there is more than one source of the desired goods. If social convention marked spaghetti as a negotiable item but there was no other source of spaghetti, your negotiation leverage works only if you are willing to forego pasta, or if you are so large a purchaser or important a customer that the store owner wants to keep your business.

Implicit negotiation is at the heart of the development and implementation of health policy. Although arduous debates swirl about the bottom-line costs of each legislative bill, the specific rules and regulations embedded within a policy effectively establish the assumptions and motivators for implicit negotiation. For example, if individuals are required by law to purchase health insurance or pay a fine, the choice is effectively framed. If the fine is not sufficiently hefty, chances are that many individuals will weigh the cost of insurance and care against the fine and chose not to buy insurance. Similarly, if legislators mandate the transparency that allows consumers to openly compare the quality and cost of care between alternative providers, the dynamics of implicit negotiation are explicitly changed. Assumptions about what will sway thinking, behaviors, or actions among insurers, providers, manufacturers, and patients underlie the dynamic debates among policymakers and their intentions for health reform. Unintended consequences on the road to high-quality, cost-effective care occur when policymakers wrongly assume what will motivate people and how actions and interactions will affect one another.

Implicit negotiation is also the process by which people exchange intangibles such as information and social status. Intangibles are constantly being traded in clinics and between health care institutions. These intangibles determine the substance and process of decision making and action. They are possessed by one person and desired by another and can often be more important than the actual exchange of goods and services.

Information Exchange. Information is the most commonly exchanged intangible. Information includes the knowledge, expertise, and data necessary for sound decision making, along with the ability to make sense of it. Knowledge encompasses everything from the psychosocial status of a patient to the clinical options for a particular disease category. Expertise incorporates the proficiency to apply knowledge to particular decisions and actions. Whereas knowledge and expertise are cognitive capabilities resting with people, data are those dispassionate facts and figures that predict the likelihood of a particular medical outcome or trends affecting market share. When combined with experience, knowledge, and expertise, data can spawn wisdom.

Given the scope of information necessary for good decision making, it is unlikely that one person alone can possess the necessary acumen. That is why health care has been so social an enterprise: essential information must be gathered, exchanged, and circulated among numerous people involved in a case. This information is held by health professionals, researchers, administrators, and, most important, by the patient himself or herself.

We now live in the information age. The value and possession of information is changing rapidly as the Internet, electronic medical records (EMRs), and the secrets of our DNA are becoming more openly available and then more readily processed and analyzed by ever cheaper and more powerful computers. The proprietary and exclusive grasp on knowledge and information is therefore eroding as it becomes more readily available and comprehensible. This democratization of the heretofore secrets of medicine is revolutionizing the medical balance of power and therefore the dynamics of negotiation throughout the system. One's negotiation leverage is diminished when there are other, cheaper ways to get the same benefit.

It is noteworthy that in the United States, the adoption of EMRs has been remarkably slower than the pace of acceptance in other developed countries. As we write this, the penetration of EMRs, while increasing, is still slow. According to a recent CDC survey, about 20.4 percent of office-based physicians reported using a "minimally functioning" system, and only 38.4 percent reported using a full or partial EMR system (not including billing system; Hsiao et al., 2008). Among the factors explaining the resistance has been a reluctance on the part of clinicians and insurers to lose control. What happens as information and its integration shift more and more from clinician to patient? The rapid emergence of information technology will increasingly alter the balance of these long-held implicit negotiations.

Exchanging Social Authority, Responsibility, and Recognition. The second and more perplexing category of intangible exchange lies in the balance of authority and responsibility that typifies health care systems. This factor is further complicated by the subtle dynamics of recognition and status. Within an organization or among professional colleagues, your relative position is embedded in a hierarchy of relationships. These relationships in turn frame and shape your self-perception and affect your personal satisfaction, engagement, and motivation as you work.

Authority is about who decides. *Responsibility* is about who is accountable for results. Who has the authority to order medications? Who is responsible for the patient's welfare? Who draws up the budget? Who is responsible for the cost of ordered procedures? Who determines whether a patient will be resuscitated?

What is the system legally allowed or obligated to decide for the patient? What set of decisions rests solely with the patient? Where do the moral obligations of each player lie? It is easy to see how authority and responsibility can come into conflict, especially when legal responsibility is not tied to a clear demarcation of medical authority.

Who has the authority is determined by the social framework of decision making. Authority is assigned and delineated in job descriptions, laws, social mores, and other signals and structures that affect behavior. As the health system is reshaped by legislative, market, social, and technological forces, the question of who decides is a moving target. This problem of shifting decision authority and responsibility is aggravated by already complex and overlapping domains of jurisdiction, blurring the lines between what is in one person's or group's complete control, what is in the realm of no control, and what is negotiable (Figure 3.1). In perhaps the most stark illustration of the split between authority and responsibility, a patient may have the authority to demand expensive end-of-life care though it is the insurer who has responsibility to pay the bill. Or the insurer may decide not to authorize expensive care, and it is the patient who assumes the burden of pain and loss that results.

The complexities of decision making for health matters can be exemplified by the process of choosing among insurance plans. In choosing an insurance option, an individual balances choice and cost. Some plans, usually the more expensive, place few if any restrictions on which participating providers, including specialists, one may see. Others, generally less expensive, restrict access to a specific network of providers and require a referral from a primary care physician before a visit to a specialist will be covered. Lower-cost plans may also have a higher deductible,

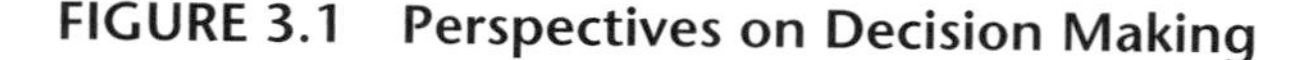

FIGURE 3.1 Perspectives on Decision Making

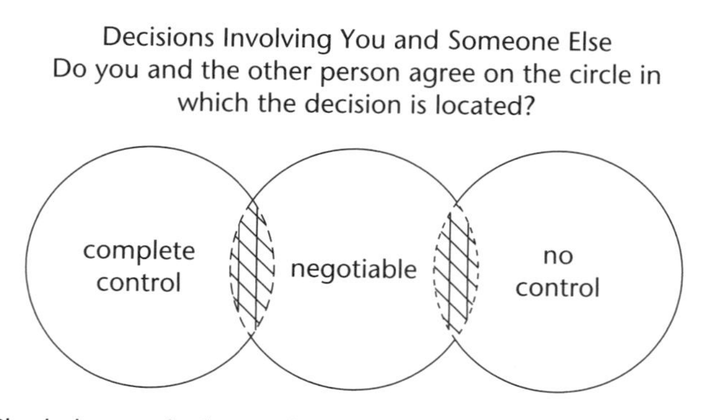

Shaded areas depict conflict in the decision-making process.

cover fewer procedures or treatment options, or place a cap on the dollar amount covered in a given period. The first option provides relatively greater freedom in choosing physicians and hospitals along with greater peace of mind that most contingencies will be covered. Those who select a managed care option limit their decision-making authority and options in exchange for lower health insurance costs. The point is that one decision frames a cascade of subsequent options, decisions, and negotiations.

Likewise, in the past clinicians were able to order procedures with little interference from an insurance company review manager or other third party. Now many procedures must routinely be approved through a process of negotiation, with the clinician making the case for the necessity of care while an administrator pushes back about cost or efficacy. The clinician bears responsibility for the patient's care and wants the authority to order the tests, procedures, and medications she deems necessary. The administrator bears responsibility for ensuring that his firm pays only for care that has been shown to be both medically necessary and cost effective. He too wants the patient cared for, but he also wants his firm to be financially viable in order to cover this and other patients fairly. He wants the authority to refuse to pay for tests, procedures, or medications he deems to be excessive or unproven or for which there is a lower-cost substitute. The administrator may feel that the clinician has little concern for his responsibility—financial prudence—and the clinician may feel that the administrator has little concern for her responsibility—medical prudence. In the middle is the patient. Let us assume that each of these two people has benign intentions: the doctor is not padding her fees with treatments she knows to be superfluous; the administrator is not participating in a bonus program that rewards him for denying necessary care. Each takes his or her responsibility seriously. And yet, because each looks at responsibility through a different lens, each wants to claim the authority to fulfill his or her responsibility as he or she perceives it (remember the challenge presented by the two views of a cone in a cube, discussed in Chapter One).

Further complicating this situation is a third party—the patient. If the procedure is disapproved, the patient must choose whether to appeal to the insurer, pay for the treatment out of pocket, or forego the treatment altogether.

The most rancorous negotiations and difficult challenges for the health system are about the shifts in where these lines of responsibility and authority are drawn. What decisions are placed in what sphere? Who has the authority to determine the cost of drugs? Who can and cannot prescribe medications? And who is obligated to pick up the bill if the patient cannot pay? If regulatory and insurance companies rule that reimbursement rates are nonnegotiable, then providers find their compensation package in the zone of no control. The resulting frustration generates conflict and often creates antagonism that is a barrier to effectively negotiating strategies to provide the best care possible (see Figure 3.1). The impasse itself becomes another complexity in the effort to improve care quality while managing costs.

Indeed, during a period of rapid change, many decisions that were at either end of the spectrum—no control or complete control—may shift to the middle circle, to the arena that is negotiable. Health care administrators, concerned about balancing their books, want to sway decisions, such as clinical decisions, to the point where they can exert more direct control. Patients are apprehensive about weakened leverage, especially if they lose control over when and from whom they receive care. Private practice physicians, accustomed to entrepreneurial independence, fear lost control of their earning capacity.

The script of health care decision making is continually being rewritten, especially when the health system is in one of its periodic cycles of reform. During a time of change, it is common for different people to read from dissimilar draft scripts, drafts that represent what they presume will be the final version. Some, especially those who did well in the "good old days," cling to the old scripts. Others shift to the anticipated script and the new opportunities presented by the change, certain that their associates will follow. And many are simply caught in the confusion, adjusting to the prevailing expectations for the day or occasion. Patients may have one set of new expectations, insurers another, policymakers still another, and those at the front lines of care may have little say in how their jobs have been recast. These differences are a source of perplexing conflict and, in very real terms, are at the heart of what renegotiating health care is all about.

The very drawing of these lines is a matter of implicit negotiation. What do *you* decide? What do *I* decide? What do *we* decide? How do these decisions affect the things for which each of us is held accountable? As it pertains to policy, the negotiation occurs in Washington, D.C., and state capitals around the country. As it relates to patient care decisions, it occurs in administrative offices, hospital hallways, and clinics every day, all the time. The pace and flavor of these negotiations are indicators of the system's evolution. There will be escalating conflict if clarity and consensus are not reached on what decision is in which sphere.

These dynamics are intimately connected: authority is to control what responsibility is to consequences. In health care as we have said, both authority and responsibility are in constant motion. And as they shift, so too do consequences. The evolution of capitated payment arrangements, for example, has brought new transparency to the relationship of these dynamics: primary care physicians realize immediate financial effects of the care decisions they make for their patients. If they are able to render care inexpensively, they reap monetary gain. If their choices represent substandard care, they risk legal and professional liability or the flight of patients to other providers. The option is theirs to shape the balance.

Responsibility is often interpreted in a limited way to mean institutional or legal repercussions. When a budgetary decision flops, we point to the administrators responsible and expect them to bear the consequences. Likewise, if the outcome of surgery disappoints, the patient may turn to the legal system to hold the surgeon and hospital accountable. Our society's obsession with litigation has turned finger-pointing into a profitable industry.

Though we impose consequences on the administrator or surgeon whose decision or action is most directly connected with a poor outcome, the real burden is endured by a broader network of people. If the new sports medicine clinic fails, the consequences are felt not only by the administrators: the repercussions are felt even more directly by the physical therapists and others who lose their jobs. Similarly, in spite of the elaborate system of compensation for victims of malpractice, ultimately it is the patient who bears the most awful consequences of an unfortunate surgical outcome.

In health care there is a daunting quality-of-life, and at times life-or-death, dimension to decision making. And responsibility for the quality of health care is itself very expensive. However, the question of who owns the responsibility can also be somewhat ambiguous, so it is bartered and shifted to enhance protection, or at least perceived protection, for the many people who participate in or are affected by a decision.

Especially as they pertain to fiduciary obligations or legal liability, responsibility and risk are constantly negotiated and exchanged. Nurse practitioners seeking greater authority to prescribe medication also bear an increased responsibility and liability for malpractice. Solo practice physicians recruited by managed care plans exchange some of their independent authority for the opportunity to have access to a larger pool of potential patients and to have more order in their lives. The elements of this exchange are formalized in insurance premiums, professional contracts, and business deals. Autonomy, as a bargaining chip, has great professional significance for those who work in the system and great personal meaning for those served by it.

Of course the problem with so linking decision-making authority to responsibility is that it allows the misperception that those at work in the health system are acting as individuals and thus are solely responsible for their successes and errors, rather than working within a much larger network of interconnected decisions and actions. The patient safety movement in recent decades has made a compelling case for viewing errors and failures as system problems and not simply matters of individual culpability. According to this reasoning, a robust routine of checks and balances should catch mistakes before they have a negative effect on patient care. Viewing errors and their elimination in system terms has shifted the culture of blame to an emphasis on correction and improvement. This movement, in subtle yet very real terms, has recast the implicit negotiations that contribute to safe patient care.

A third element of social status exchange, and certainly the most perplexing, is recognition. For those who work in the health system, *recognition* is the professional acknowledgment, appreciation, and fulfillment they derive from their work. For patients, it is the dignity and satisfaction experienced when receiving care from others. In his analysis of human needs, Abraham Maslow (1970) defined the highest meaning and accomplishment derived through social interaction as *self-actualization*. Self-actualization is experienced both in the acknowledgment we receive from others and from our own inner sense of meaning and purpose.

For health care professionals, there is particular significance to recognition. Their career choice is not intended only as a source of income. More important, a health care career offers the opportunity to intelligently and constructively help other people, a valued status in our society. Saving a life, improving the lot of an ill person, and preventing disease are valued as exceptionally meaningful and prestigious social endeavors. The value of this work is either validated or invalidated by colleagues, patients, and the system that pays the bill.

Validation, therefore, is a particularly important currency of exchange for those involved in health care: we give it to others; we get it from others. Validation and its rewards are derived from an appreciative comment, acknowledgment of important information, and the granting of decision-making authority. For example, a nurse might implicitly say to a physician, "I am giving you an important piece of information about the patient." The implicit negotiation that goes with this is, "I do hope you will recognize its significance and therefore my value and contribution in sharing it with you." The feeling of validation that comes from such recognition bears value: people are willing to work for less monetary compensation when they derive a sense of social meaning and satisfaction from their employment.

Invalidation results from ignoring a remark, negating a piece of information, or excluding a colleague's participation on the basis of prejudice, hierarchical standing, or interpersonal relations. People are invalidated when the observations they make are ignored but the same observations are recognized when someone with higher status restates them and grabs the credit. Those who invalidate are often blind to what they are doing and its impact on others. This sort of invalidation is common in intergender, interracial, interprofessional, and patient-provider relations. Sometimes it is explicit and intentional. More often it is unspoken, but it nevertheless has the effect of one person saying to the other, "I purposely invalidate what you say to reinforce the fact that I am superior to you, and you must concede your place." This attitude is based on deep-seated assumptions and beliefs—elements of implicit negotiation—about relative value and relationships. Sexist remarks, even those made inadvertently by well-intentioned men, fall into this category. The resentment, alienation, and desire for retribution resulting from invalidation are costly when they compromise the interdependent negotiations and work of health care. They also lay the groundwork for deeply personal and emotional conflict

Exchange and Whole Image Negotiation

How does the premise of negotiation as exchange pertain to health care? When you negotiate the purchase of a car, the terms and nature of the exchange are explicit. You give the dealer money and the dealer gives you a car.

In health care the exchange is not as direct. One person receives the service, another pays for it, someone else regulates it, and a complex web of people deliver it. Moreover, these pieces are circuitously connected, so that one person's action is not immediately reciprocated by another's reaction. When your colleagues are unhappy with their salaries, even though they may not have negotiated these amounts with you, their dissatisfaction will affect you. Similarly, if one unit of the hospital is not working well—the pharmacy, for example—that will have ramifications throughout the institution. Even though you may not have the authority to change how the pharmacy operates, its delays could directly affect your work and responsibilities. Little control with full responsibility is a scenario for increased tension, which will usually result in conflict. Therefore it is in your genuine interest to have all the pieces of the system function in balance so that your piece itself can thrive. When you work among interdependent people and professionals, your win against another department's loss eventually will ricochet back to you. The resentment of this department's members will provoke them to go for a win over you in the next round. Moreover, their weakness only diminishes your own vitality. If the whole system does not work well, it is unlikely that any of the pieces will be able to excel. Given the closely linked nature of health care work, all the parts of the system ultimately rise and fall together.

Whole image negotiation is based on the premise of interdependent systems and interdependent work. If the aggregate is balanced—the big picture—then your work is more likely to be efficient and effective at the individual level—the pragmatic picture. These two pictures are intrinsically related. Therefore, by negotiating on the assumption of shared objectives, you also better your own lot.

Using whole image negotiation, you bargain for the shared balance just as vigorously as you promote your individual portion. When this premise permeates the culture of your institution, the system as a whole works better. W.I.N. implies that all the parts integrate so that each will benefit from the others' actions. This integrated whole will deliver better care than will the individual parts in competition with one other. Each stakeholder achieves greater benefit by negotiating successfully the shared interests that offer mutual advantage.

Katherine Knight has been nurse manager of the intensive care unit (ICU) for more than five years, gaining the reputation as one of the best nurse managers in the hospital. The award she received for leading integration of innovative new ideas resulting from the total quality management program implemented three years ago sits prominently on her desk. Despite ups and downs in the nursing staff on other units, the ICU has maintained high morale and low turnover. The loyalty and support she shows her staff are repaid in hard work and low absenteeism.

Knight is disappointed when Janice Johnson, the vice president for nursing, approaches her about cutting one position on the ICU night shift. It feels as if she is being penalized for her very success. Up to this point, she has been able to hold off the staff cutbacks that have plagued other units. Johnson patiently explains that the move is part of a much larger strategy across the hospital: to remain competitive in the eyes of insurers, the hospital is seeking ways to responsibly reduce patient care costs. A review of ICU patients over a period of time has found that many could have been transferred to one of the general medical floors had proper staffing and expertise been available there. Cost-conscious insurers could become reluctant to reimburse for admissions to the ICU when it appears to them that adequate care could be delivered on properly staffed medical floors. Johnson explains the reasoning: if the hospital places a better-trained nurse on the general medical floor at night, hospital physicians would be more willing to move patients onto the less expensive general medical floors. Knight has to admit that it all makes sense on paper.

As she listens to this story of outside pressures and the proposed changes, Knight purposefully expresses her disappointment but does not resist the move. "Frankly, I have my doubts, Janice," Knight says, "but I'm willing to give it a try if you'll agree that we can review the situation again in three months." Johnson agrees. The next step is for Knight to talk with Heather Harriford. If Harriford accepts the move, Knight will meet with the entire staff to explain what is happening and why. At the end of the day, Knight wants to be and be known as a team player.

Later that day Knight calls Harriford to her office. Just as she was intentional in handling the meeting with her boss, she is very deliberate in directing the discussion with her supervisee. She opens the dialogue by reflecting on prior conversations with Harriford. "Heather, I know that you have several times expressed your desire to transfer out of the ICU. I have been asked to recommend someone for transfer to the general medical floors." Knight wants Harriford to know that this is neither a test of loyalty nor a reprimand for her sometimes explosive behavior. Knight wants Harriford to view the transfer as an acceptable and attractive option. It is important to Knight that Harriford is aware that this is not Knight's call and that it is not being done specifically to single out Harriford. "What are your thoughts about making the move?"

Harriford pauses. She knows her answer is yes, though before jumping to respond she wants to clarify and secure several perks. She reminds herself of the advantages of being clever when negotiating. It is to her benefit to appear as if she needs some gentle persuasion.

"Before I answer, may I ask a few questions?" Knight nods, and Harriford asks about salary, a future possible promotion to supervisor, and flexibility of hours. Knight has already checked with the nurse manager on the general medical floors and is able to answer affirmatively on all counts.

Knight clarifies the reasons for the move. "You are a young, bright, and energetic member of this staff. If the hospital is to reduce utilization of the ICU, we are going to need someone up on general medical who can receive patients transferred from the ICU and the emergency department. Your knowledge and expertise will be an invaluable asset for the general medical staff. Your smarts and your talent have been recognized here at the ICU and in other parts of the hospital as well." Knight also wants to give her some words of warning, words that could come in handy later. "The only thing in your way, Heather, is your temper. Get control of your flare-ups and there's no limit to where you might go in your career."

Harriford smiles and holds out her hand, ready to shake on the agreement. "It's a deal. When do I start?" And after a moment of hesitation, she adds, "Thanks for that heads up, Katherine. I hear you." Knight asks her to hold off telling anyone about the assignment change until that night's staff meeting.

Health care is a highly social enterprise. It demands many people working closely together engaged in numerous and frequent transactions. The success of the enterprise depends on its capacity to enhance the fluidity of those exchanges.

Negotiation as Discovery

Your most effective negotiation tool is a good question.

People often enter negotiation focused on what they want to get. They expend great effort pushing their case. They concentrate attention on what they are going to say next rather than on what is being said. They listen but do not hear. They ignore as distractions the concerns and desires of the other people at the table.

When Dr. Larry Lumberg spots Fred Fisher racing down the hallway toward him, he doesn't know what to expect. Lumberg is the forty-one-year-old medical director of the emergency department. Fisher, medical director of Oppidania, is nearly a generation older—in both years and attitude. Lumberg despises the paternalistic relationship he must endure as a cost of the supervising and mentoring that Fisher bestows.

Fisher bypasses social niceties and gets right to the point. "Walk with me," he says pulling Lumberg into his wake. He speaks in a low, almost conspiratorial tone. "Larry. I want you to open the tap on ICU admissions at night. Don't hold back. Inkwater is giving me a hard time about boning up the nursing staff for general medical. Until things change, we up the pressure on the ICU. That'll get some action. I'm off to a meeting at the medical school. Call me if there are problems. Carry on!" Fisher waves over his shoulder as he turns right into the busy corridor that leads to the parking garage.

Lumberg is left standing trying to digest Fisher's directive. That's classic Fred Fisher, he thinks. Fred may have left the military but his mind-set is still in uniform. No questions, no reasons, no options. This command-and-control way of going about business is still rattling to Lumberg. He mutters out loud, "Of course, his 'solution' will create more problems and make me look bad in the process."

Lumberg is a good friend of Melanie McKenzie, the chief of the surgical intensive care unit. He places a call to her. "Look, this is off the record, but Fred Fisher just dumped an order to go heavy on ICU night admissions on me. Do you know what's going on?"

McKenzie chuckles, "Yeah, Fisher's nose is out of joint. He just had a meeting with Inkwater and Johnson. He's as impatient as anyone with the problems the nursing staff's been having on the night shift in general medical. But I heard that Johnson is asking Knight to try to get one of her nurses to make the move. The problem for Fisher is more one of who is running the ship. He doesn't like the fact that Johnson didn't jump immediately. This is probably his little revenge."

"His revenge, and I'm going to be seen as the villain," Lumberg replied. "Does Fisher know about the change on the nursing staff?"

"I assume so but I don't know how soon Johnson will get someone to make the switch. I tell you, I'm not wild about this whole thing myself, though in the long run I'm sure it's for the better. These aren't the good old days anymore, and we're going to have to reduce the CICU head count if we hope to keep our payers happy and doing business with us. We've got to look as good as we can in the public reporting on comparative quality and price."

"Right, I know. I feel like I'm practicing medicine in a glass house," Lumberg sighs. "Who do you think Johnson is going to try to move?"

"Heather Harriford would be my guess. She is a very good nurse but I don't think she's been a great cultural fit in the ICU. She's smart, very smart. She has a lot of energy and that will make her a good addition over there."

Lumberg contemplates what he's learned. He has to assume that if Melanie knows about Harriford's possible move that Fisher does as well. Why hadn't he shared that? What is Fisher's real agenda?

This phenomenon is particularly evident when a person's relative self-perception is one of superiority. It is evident in the way men relate to women, doctors to nurses, administrators to clinicians, nurses to family members, and older people to younger people. This behavior reinforces the hierarchical nature of social ordering by demeaning the concerns and contributions of those considered less important. It frustrates those being silenced. And it wastes valuable knowledge and expertise. As significant information is lost to the process of negotiation, the options at the table are reduced.

Enter negotiation with the intention of learning. Be curious. Learn about the other side. Learn about your options. And learn about yourself: what do you want, why do you want it, and what options have you not considered? Be sufficiently open to let others learn about you. Allow for the possibility that in the process of learning about one another, all those at the table might discover options not imagined at the outset.

By making negotiation a learning opportunity, you build the foundation for the next round.

Negotiation as Steps in a Process

There are those who regard negotiation as a direct linear process, with beginning, middle, and end, and a definitive objective. Each transaction is a separate event, disconnected from what happens before and after.

Another view of negotiation is that it has a beginning, middle, and end, though not necessarily in that order. The middle of one round may be the beginning of the next. The end of one negotiation may affect what occurs in the midst of a negotiation in the next room. Even the ultimate objectives for the negotiation may be changed by new information learned during the process. This fluid and evolving process, rather than the linear process, best describes health care negotiation.

Iris Inkwater considers her work with outside entities to be one of the most important parts of her job as CEO of Oppidania Medical Center (OMC). In particular, it is her contractual negotiations with insurers and managed care organizations that are most vital to the financial welfare of the hospital. She likes to get to know the people with whom she will be working and usually lunches with the chief representative of the other organization before serious numbers are placed on the table. In her mind, good relationship building is the first step in knowledgeable strategic planning. Today she is having lunch with Nathaniel Norquist, chief financial officer (CFO) for Community Health Plan (CHP), the third-largest managed care organization in the state. Because of a concentration of CHP customers in the geographical area OMC serves, CHP holds the hospital's largest managed care contract, accounting for 19.5 percent of OMC's business.

Midway through her Caesar salad, Inkwater places the critical question on the table: "Well, Nathaniel, how are we looking for next year?"

Norquist leans back and pauses. "Iris, I'll tell you the truth; things are going to be tough. You know we're working in an aggressively competitive market. There's a lot of pressure from our big customers: controlling health care costs is a top priority for them. We have to keep our pencils pretty sharp. Your shop is 14 percent above the costs coming in from other hospitals. We've always had a good relationship, Iris, and our customers tell us their employees are satisfied with services they get from OMC. But I have to be honest with you. If you can't come in line for us with the other hospitals in town, we'll just have to direct our business elsewhere." His last words hang in the air. "Iris, I know this is not what you want to hear but we're in a different world now."

Inkwater feels like she's just been punched. She had expected a hard line from Norquist but not an ultimatum. She speaks softly and carefully, "Nathaniel, what exactly do you see as the problem?"

"It's a matter of timing and then dollars, Iris," he responds. "Our data show that Oppidania simply moves more slowly than the other hospitals. It takes you longer to get people in and out of your facility and it costs you more. When in doubt, you tend to opt for the more expensive course of care. I know there is a lot of pressure concerning liability and your quality standards are high. Nevertheless, other places seem to keep themselves covered without piling up the dollars. I'll be sending you a report from our new analytics system that breaks things down by department, procedure, patient demographics, and more. You'll see that the numbers don't paint a pretty picture."

Inkwater swallows deeply, realizing she is in for rough sailing when she brings this bombshell back to OMC. "Nathaniel, we've worked well together for a long time. If you stick with us, I know we can work this out."

As Inkwater drives back to the hospital, she plans her next step. The hospital will have to offer CHP concrete proof that serious efforts are being made to trim costs. And it will have to show some quick successes. "We'll impress them with what we can do to turn this around," she thinks to herself. "And if we can't, I'm sunk."

With information and tasks so closely intertwined through professional systems, reimbursement, oversight, and regulation, each negotiation in a health care system is implicitly connected to others. This is true not only of negotiations that proceed across a system, involving various sets of groups such as nurses with doctors and patients with insurers, it also describes a series of negotiations with a particular individual or group over time. In each round in which you are a party you gain information, experience, and an emotional response to others at the table. These acquisitions influence your attitude and approach to the next round. Likewise, others create impressions of you. If the previous round went smoothly, the parties return anticipating a repeat of that satisfactory experience and outcome. If it was a battle with winner and loser, the former comes hoping to regain victory and the latter comes to reap revenge.

With a long-term view of negotiation, you can launch into each round as an investment in the future and a payoff from the past. Each transaction fortifies the foundation upon which your professional relationships are constructed.

A systems view of negotiation acknowledges the interdependence of interaction. When you negotiate in a vacuum, nothing is connected. When you negotiate in a system, everything is interwoven. A change in one place demands an adjustment in the next. A solution in one section generates a reaction in another. The decision reached at your table affects negotiation tables far removed from your scene of action.

The best negotiators view negotiation as a fluid process. With each round, they adjust style and strategy to accommodate unforeseen contingencies and information. Flexibility, resilience, and tenacity accommodate these shifts and can turn them into a plus.

Negotiation and Power

When it comes to negotiation and power, there are three types of negotiators. The first are those who don't have power and want to get it. In their minds, their negotiation problems stem from a lack of power. The question they most frequently ask themselves is, "How do I negotiate if I don't have power?" The underlying assumption is that without power, they may not even get to the negotiation table, and if they do get there, they will be paid little attention. As long as this assumption persists, their underlying question really is, "How do I get the power so I can dictate and not have to negotiate?"

Second are the negotiators with power. They too wonder about power, though in a far more circumspect way. Their concern is, "How do I negotiate to keep the power?" They know that power is far more ephemeral a thing than it appears. You can have it one day and then see it slip away the next. One can create the perception that one has it, while in fact, any number of culprits can steal it away in a moment. Once you've negotiated from a position of power, there is nothing more terrifying than having to live without it. It creates a sense of vulnerability that horrifies.

Third are the negotiators who recognize that if power is the only currency of a negotiation, then everyone's options and actions are severely limited. Why? When people have so much energy invested in getting power and maintaining their power base, they can reject good options and decisions, not because these are wrong but because they do not fortify the base of power for those in charge. Fortifying that base becomes an obsession. It has been so in health care for many years. If this is not changed, significant progress will remain elusive. Power wars are significant distractions. They get in the way of what the health system presumes to accomplish: delivering high-quality health care for patients while providing a fulfilling set of career opportunities for those who work in the system.

Wise leaders are changing their exercise of power and their processes of decision making. They recognize that by involving and incorporating a spectrum of ideas and people, their decisions and their support are strengthened. In so doing, they do not give power away. Empowerment, when done from a base of mutual respect and recognition, adds to the total sum of power. It does not mean giving in when there is disagreement, though it does mean extending acknowledgment. It does not necessarily mean sacrifice, though it does require sharing both the spoils and the struggles of collaboration. "Who is holding the power?" becomes less important than "what are we trying to accomplish?"

Can this third negotiator type emerge in health care? Is it possible for people to negotiate based on their common purpose rather than based merely on their comparative level of power? This book is based on the premise that such a breakthrough can be achieved in health care and we have seen through our experience that it is possible.

This third model does not naively suggest that power will go away or that it won't be an important currency in our negotiations. Rather, it proposes that power not be the central currency of good decision making. In its place there can emerge common interests, which better frame our endeavors. The uneven table at which we sat for so many years can be rebalanced so that robust ideas and resourceful options find room for sensible consideration.

There are many sources of power available to you in your work. There is certainly the power of position, based on your formal organizational status. And there is also the influence that comes from knowledge, expertise, and the capacity for discovering new ways to frame and conduct the business of your institution.

Fisher's secretary hands him a rare telephone message when he returns to his office: "URGENT! Inkwater wants you in her office 8:00 A.M. tomorrow for an important hospital leadership meeting!" Fisher smiles. His plan has worked before it has even gotten off the ground. Inkwater finally realizes that she is going to have to shift things around for him if this place is going to work. Victory!

When Fisher arrives the next morning, Inkwater, Johnson (the nursing VP), the chief operating officer, and the chief financial officer are already huddled in Inkwater's office. Fisher likes to show up a few moments late to avoid the chitchat and the wait for others to arrive.

"Thank you for coming on such short notice," Inkwater opens. "I know that some of you had to change your schedules, and it is appreciated. I got some bad news yesterday. I met with Nathaniel Norquist, the CFO at Community Health Plan. This shouldn't be a surprise but they are under some very strong pressure from purchasers to hold down costs. It's a buyer's market out there and Norquist knows that only the competitive health plans are going to survive. What was a surprise was that we stick out like a sore thumb on the expense side—we run significantly higher expenses than other hospitals. CHP is able to run more detailed analyses of our performance than we can ourselves—and our numbers don't look good. CHP is threatening to take its business from us."

This is not what Fisher expected. He looks around. There is silence. The others have shocked ghostlike expressions on their faces. This is not good news.

Inkwater continues, "We all know that CHP could pull out of here and get away with it. Unfortunately, it is our largest and most steady source of income." She explains that OMC can't depend on federal and state money—they are getting squeezed there as well. She shares her concern that other managed care organizations may follow if CHP leaves. She knows that previous belt tightening has been a pretty bloody exercise, with every department out to protect its turf and keep the pain in someone else's territory. "I need everyone to work together on this. If we can't pull together and come up with some imaginative ways to solve this problem, we could all find ourselves closing this place down. We've seen it happen elsewhere, and there is no reason why it can't happen here."

The meeting continues for another half hour. The CFO and COO report on their preliminary evaluations of the financial impact of losing CHP's business. The chief information officer bemoans the lack of investment in back-office technology that would have made it easier to spot these trends themselves—and earlier. Inkwater talks about new premises and new assumptions for framing the work of the hospital—a heightened culture of cooperation. She purposefully ends the meeting on an upbeat note. "If we really pull together, we can make this a win for the OMC and the patients we serve. It's up to each of you to communicate this attitude to your staff. It has to pervade the way you think and act professionally. If it doesn't, you won't be able to make it work effectively for those you lead."

The problem with running your organization and your career from the basis of crude power is that it has the capacity to become an obsession. Moreover, because of power's ephemeral quality, you have to continually reinforce power to be certain it is there for you.

There are other ingredients of effectiveness that can guide the efforts of people who work closely together. Interest-based negotiation offers a common framework and language for building a collaborative context for those endeavors. What is interest-based negotiation, and how can you make it intrinsic to your style and strategy? The next chapter answers these questions.

PART TWO

NEGOTIATION

CHAPTER 4

INTEREST-BASED NEGOTIATION

WE BRING a storehouse of hope to our negotiations. There are the ostensible tangibles we aim to acquire: for example, money, space, or equipment. Beneath those concrete acquisitions, there is that sense of purpose that motivates our very reason for being at the table: a breadth of intangible needs, concerns, ambitions, and fears. *Interest-based negotiation* evokes that range of human response. The intent is to engage in problem solving that elevates and responds to the breadth of those interests and in the process to invent added options for settlement. By attending to interests, parties are able to resolve a broader spectrum of desires, out of which can be woven a greater range of choices and a more fulfilling reach of mutual benefit (Fisher, Ury, & Patton, 1991).

Interest-based negotiation defines an approach to the process of expanding and exchanging both tangibles and intangibles. Rather than regarding each other as contestants, interest-based negotiators associate as collaborators, seeking overlapping objectives. Recognizing their interdependence, they discover that they both advance by enhancing the advancement of one another. Out of the process of building trust and opening communication, they derive genuine confidence that extends well beyond any particular transaction.

Interest-based negotiation is particularly compelling when parties are engaged in tasks that elicit their underlying objectives—their sense of purpose—as is typical in the work of health care. It is especially pragmatic when there are limited resources to divide, as is also often the case in health care settings, because those limited assets can be most cleverly extended through collaborative strategies.

In spite of this model's inherent utility for health care, there are those who shun it, preferring win-lose, competitive practices instead. This chapter compares two approaches: the first being the interest-based, or integrative, approach intended to coalesce the parties, and the second being the positional, or distributional, models that view each party's interests as exclusive of the other's. Then this and the next two chapters focus on methods and techniques of interest-based negotiation and how they can be integrated into your professional health care routines. Chapter Eight considers circumstances in which a positional approach is in fact your wiser choice, and it offers recommendations on how to succeed when that is your best option.

Setting the Negotiation Tone

By using integrative approaches, you will enhance your long-term negotiation effectiveness. In contrast, using distributional methods not only reduces your immediate negotiation credibility, it also erodes the reputation and trust necessary for constructive bargaining.

Although some may relegate interest-based negotiation to the *kumbaya* school—Why can't we just all get along?—there is in fact a wealth of both theoretical and mathematical evidence for the advantages of this model. First, the adversarial method results in significant distraction from ongoing work as stakeholders invest time and resources in defeating the other side. Second, this approach limits the scope of possibilities to a dyadic set of choices: we either win or we lose, and given that choice, winning is better. Third, the win-lose option greatly inhibits the sharing of information and allocation of resources, limiting what could be known or discovered and imposing strain on the little that may be available in the way of time, goodwill, goods, or services. Conversely, reduce the distractions of the contest and expand the options beyond simple victory and defeat, and with that a range of otherwise unlikely and potentially mutually beneficial options are suddenly on the horizon. Interest-based negotiators choose to put themselves in a place where opportunities come their way, and more often than not, they achieve more in doing so.

When you are using positional bargaining, your primary concern is to satisfy your desires and those of your constituency. Meeting the needs of the other side is unimportant. You want to take as big a slice of the pie as possible. In your mind the size of the pie is fixed. Through negotiation, the bounty is distributed. The more others get, the less you get. You want to control the process to ensure that you get the portion you want. You yearn to win.

In contrast, when using integrative negotiation, you seek an arrangement that ensures both sides a fair measure of satisfaction. You want to achieve your own negotiation objectives. You likewise have an investment in the other side's accomplishing theirs. You want to explain your interests, learn theirs, and in the process generate options to accommodate both sets of constituents. You view negotiation as an inventive process for integrating interests and generating new opportunities. When it comes time to slice the pie, you and the other party want to hold the knife together to affirm mutual trust and good faith. You both want to achieve a gain-gain outcome.

Is the distinction one of selfishness and altruism? Is the distributional bargainer greedy and the integrative bargainer socially responsible? The answers do not easily fit into one category or the other.

Subtleties emerge through understanding the different purviews of the stakeholders (this is another illustration of the cone in the cube analogy discussed in Chapter One). The integrative bargainer understands that his or her lot is enhanced when the integrity of others is maintained. Especially when your survival is closely related to that of your partner, integrative bargaining is a strategy for self-preservation just as much as it is a method for staying out of the basement. Your viability is linked to the viability of your department, and the viability of your department ultimately depends on the viability of the organization as a whole. The effectiveness of any health system relies on the functioning of its many interdependent parts. Each component depends on the others' achievements. Negotiation with this understanding is a method for adjusting the balance to ensure both fairness and mutual security.

The distributional bargainer demands immediate gratification. Oblivious to the fate he or she might share with negotiating partners, the distributional bargainer measures achievement by the standard of current advantage. The distributional bargainer believes success rests on the failure, or at least the submission, of others. Negotiating partners are competitors, ready to snatch the goods. What another department takes only diminishes the bargainer's bounty. This negotiator's own success depends on his or her own bottom line, not that of adjacent departments. To claim triumph, the distributional bargainer intimidates, controls, and conquers.

For the distributional bargainer, the purpose is to win. The context is one of adversaries: the activity on the playing field distinguishes the winners from the losers. Truth is lost in the divisive process: a dangerous prescription for health care decision making.

The problem is that in many health care circles, distributional bargaining is the predominant mode of negotiation. Whether negotiation concerns professional, patient care, or organizational matters, the culture and inclination is to advance one's cause through a distributional approach. A nursing colleague of the authors recently recounted an example of this perspective as it occurred at a national nursing conference. In a frenzy of "doctor bashing," the tone of discourse turned into one of overcoming the rival force. The mood was "now it's our turn, and we're going to walk all over them." My colleague countered that as long as nursing adopts and reinforces distributional bargaining and does not use its emerging status to transform the rules of the game, then really nothing will have improved.

Similarly, rather than asking, "How can I adjust to better fit into a new health care reality?" doctors often huddle on how to negotiate to defend what little power and turf they have left. Health managers cling to corporate thinking, amplifying the importance of the bottom line as the singular measure of their success. Community health advocates can get into such a frenzy in advancing their cause that they don't remember to lay down their weapons against one another. And patients are convinced that the only way to secure service from their managed care plan or when hospitalized is through belligerent pressure.

Another colleague recounted a meeting of engineers pondering a new model design at a major American automobile manufacturer. The electrical systems department reported that new components proposed for the forthcoming car drew too much current from the system, threatening to shut down the battery. Each division had proposed innovations requiring more electrical draw than in previous models: the air conditioning had a more powerful cooling mechanism; the dashboard had a more splendid array of indicators and the capability to graphically display turn-by-turn directions; and a video feed of the area just behind the car now automatically started as soon as the car was put in reverse. Adding to the car's electrical capacity would considerably and unacceptably boost its weight and gasoline consumption. Yet there was no compromise at the table. Each representative took a stand, advocating single-mindedly for the best air conditioner, dashboard display, or video capability. No one was there plugging for the car as a whole. My colleague lamented, "*That* attitude is the problem with the domestic auto industry. It is not an engineering problem. It is a human systems problem. We aren't building a car. We are building components. We aren't aspiring to synchronize the whole machine to operate smoothly. No wonder the cars break down."

That attitude pervades our health system. The assumption that professional and organizational work and behavior can be better directed through competition illustrates the misconception.

The real question is not how can we control the parts to reduce spending. As long as that remains the primary consideration, the health system will not function effectively and efficiently to improve aggregate health status and costs.

Rather, two basic questions ought to frame the approach to health care negotiation that probes for answers:

1. *What are we trying to accomplish?* This question applies to all health care negotiations, from matters of national health policy to decisions regarding the operation of a clinic and care of a patient.
2. *How do we work together to achieve those ends?* This question directs everyone's attention to shared objectives and how to best achieve them together.

The aim here is not to postulate specific answers to these questions. Rather, the purpose is to present them as opening points and a strategy for everyday negotiation, whether about health policy, health administration, or patient care.

By this time Artie Ashwood has finally been settled into room 624. He knows he is feeling pain like he has never experienced before. The doctors still can't tell what is going on inside him and he is a tangle of fear, frustration, and confusion. They say they need to run more tests. They tell him not to worry too much, but their words are not reassuring. He can't fathom why, with all the high-tech machinery and well-paid doctors in this place, they cannot come up with a diagnosis.

The other thing he doesn't like is the way this hospital is being run. From his bed-level perspective it appears that the staff is terribly overworked. All of them seem to be nagging at one another. He heard it two nights ago, when they first brought him in. The doctor in the emergency room lost her patience. Then the nurses in the CICU started bickering about one of the doctors. And the more he asked questions, the less information he got. This is how they heal people?

He had read about this in his public policy course at the university—there was a section on health care and current issues. He was fascinated by the politics of health reform and the impact on the health care system. He knew about costs rising faster than inflation, about the millions of people without insurance, and about universal access and insurance. The section on policy implementation described the battles about whether to extend traditional fee-for-service insurance and set a per patient spending cap to encourage cost consciousness. The prof got the class into a discussion about whether all these changes would improve population health while it fulfilled the mandate to make the system leaner. The course made him feel fortunate to have reasonably priced health insurance through the university. But he was still worried. He's never been this sick before, and he had never paid much attention to what his policy covered and what it didn't.

What if they scrimp on his care? What if they kick him out before they know what is really going on? Maybe the reason they can't figure out his problem is because they are trying to save a few bucks. Will he wind up having to file a lawsuit?

He feels vulnerable and dependent. He has been depersonalized and then labeled with a bracelet wrapped around his wrist. The woman who took his blood had barely said hello before she removed four vials from his arm. Had she changed her gloves before she inserted the needle? He couldn't remember. Might he get even sicker in the hospital? What could all this mean for his dream of becoming an architect?

His gaze out the window is interrupted by footsteps coming around the old man in the bed next to him. A smiling man in royal-blue scrubs introduces himself. "Hi, I'm Oscar Ortiz and I'll be your primary nurse."

Oscar looks Artie in the eye. "I'm sorry I wasn't here earlier to give you the formal welcome to Six West. I was tied up with another patient. Let me know if you have any questions or concerns. I'll be with you through your stay here." The conversation continues on about Artie's anxieties, his questions, and their mutual interest in basketball. For the first time since he arrived at the hospital, Artie is starting to feel connected. Maybe he is a human being and not just a few bits and bytes somewhere in an electronic medical record after all.

Artie is beginning to feel that there is hope of getting better again. Somebody cares.

Among health care colleagues working together, common ground does not emerge by blithely dividing the spoils among those who win and denying them to those who lose. It emerges from a congruence of shared objectives and interdependent activity. By engaging that mutual purpose, we achieve a system that can evolve beyond its current predicaments.

On the one hand, there are those who will accuse this approach of being naive. It does not account for greed and avarice. One can point to the huge profits of pharmaceutical companies, the large salaries of physicians and executives, the malevolent workings of Medicaid fraud, or the dominance of certain professionals as evidence that social accountability is extinct. One could build a health system based on apprehension of the worst of human traits.

On the other hand, remember that health care intends to improve upon the most fundamental aspects of the human condition: the quality of life and, further, whether one lives or dies. This common purpose can inspire shared objectives that extend beyond merely balancing greed with innocence, or exploitation with plunder. Rather, this shared purpose can be the premise on which fair standards and socially acceptable outcomes are negotiated. Such a mind-set is a better fit for what it is we do in health care.

Integrative Negotiation: Finding Interests

You embark upon integrative negotiation by exploring interests: your interests, their interests, and your and their shared interests. The difference between distributive and integrative negotiation is this concern for shared interests. Distributive bargainers are concerned about their own interests. They show little concern for the other side, and therefore they are unlikely to find shared interests and solutions to satisfy both sides.

Interests portray what you care about. What is of value to you? What do you hope to accomplish? And what do you hope to get? You are a unique combination of experience, values, and ambitions. You bring a distinct profile of interests to the negotiation table. The challenge is not only to understand your own interests and how they affect what you do but also to learn the unique interests of the other people involved. Just as what you do emerges from your interests, so too does what they do. Using interest-based negotiation, you build agreement responsive to the needs, aspirations, and expectations of all the parties at the table. It is akin to assembling a puzzle. It demands discovery to find the pieces, ingenuity to put them together, and diplomacy to make them cohere. And of course, it requires patience, curiosity, imagination, and endurance.

Your starting point for interest-based negotiation is ascertaining those interests. This is detective work. Ask questions. Read. Observe. Find leads and follow them. And do not complacently assume that what you find is what it appears to be.

In the previous chapter, *a good question* was proposed as your most effective negotiation tool. The utility of this tool, though, is measured by what you do with the answer. It opens the door to a wealth of information, some explicit and some implicit. Your objective is to sift through that information and learn the real interests of your negotiating partners. Survey not only what they say: assess also what they do, their body language, their attitudes, and their anxieties. These are all important indicators of what you can offer to satisfy their interests.

When you enter a negotiation, you shoulder a profusion of expectations. On the surface there is something of substance you want to get. It could be money or information, a piece of equipment, a promotion, or a new office. Less apparent are the underlying gains you desire: such as recognition, professional fulfillment, and personal meaning. These hidden expectations play a vital role in the outcome of the negotiation. It is possible to achieve your substantive expectations yet still feel unsatisfied because something was missing. Conversely, you may not realize all your substantive expectations yet still leave the table feeling the outcome was a success. What is the hidden variable, and how can you discover and integrate it?

The first and most valuable interests to understand are your own. For example, is your interest *really* working out an arrangement to better handle patients? Or do you want to exploit the issue to get back at that administrator who was giving you a hard time last year? Revenge! Are you *really* worried about your patient's welfare upon discharge? Or are you advocating the superiority of your own skills over others? One-upmanship! Are you *really* concerned about supporting community-based care? Or are you demonstrating your authority and claiming turf? Control! At times, the easiest one to fool is yourself. When your real interest is blatant, everyone in the room is likely to know it—except for you.

Beneath your substantive expectations and those of others are a multitude of process preferences and emotional needs that prompt negotiation thinking and behavior. How do you discern them?

Process Preferences

A decision or settlement is reached through a *process*. There are numerous parameters that describe and define a process, and many of these parameters can be arrayed across a spectrum. This spectrum spans a range from formal decision making, with prescribed lines of authority, to informal decision making, which is driven largely by interpersonal influence and consensus building. The process for formal decision making is often set out in organizational bylaws and structures that delineate the people who are at the table, their relative authority, and the limits of their powers. However, even when a formal structure operates, informal influence can sway what occurs at the table and who is included. Process also denotes the scope of decision making and the criteria for decisions, which may range from narrow and limited to wide and far-reaching. The who, what, when, where, why, and how of a decision, taken altogether, describe the process.

Why are process preferences important? Each party brings expectations to the negotiation table, and not everyone present necessarily has the same vision. For example, if the subject of the negotiation is of vital concern to you, you would resent being excluded from the decision making even if the actual outcome of the negotiation were acceptable. You would think, "Why was I excluded? Are my views not respected? Might I be losing my job? If I was excluded this time, what could happen in the future?" The process by which any deal is made is imbued with meaning, in part because it affects the decision at hand and in part because it predicts what may happen when future decisions are made.

Consider the following illustration:

> A husband and wife fall in love with an antique clock they see in a catalogue. At $1,000 though, they decide the cost is too steep and they forget about it.
>
> Two weeks later, on an excursion through Maine, they stop at an antique store in a small town and to their surprise, in the far back corner, they find that very clock. The clock is in mint condition and perfect working order. It has no price tag. The husband boldly whispers to his wife, "I'm going to get this clock for $500."
>
> He goes to the front of the store and says to the owner, "See that antique clock in the back of the store?" The store owner replies, "Ee-yup." The husband says, "I'll give you $100 for it." The owner says, "It's yours."

When we tell the story in class, we stop at this point to ask our students, "How does the husband feel?" After a moment of silence, someone says, "Great." Then someone else volunteers, "Lousy, he regrets not offering $50." Another counters, "No, he feels guilty about cheating the store owner." Someone else suggests, "Yeah, but he got a great deal on that clock."

We then say to the class, "Let's say the story went a bit differently."

> The husband goes up to the store owner and says, "I'll give you $100 for that clock back there." The owner replies, "$900." The husband counters, "$200." The owner says, "$800" "How about $300?" the husband asks.

"$700," replies the owner. "$400," says the husband. The owner responds, "$600." The husband tries again, "$500." "Sold!" declares the owner.

Again we ask the class, "How does the husband feel?" This time, the class exclaims together, "Great!" Rarely does anyone disagree.

What does the story teach us?

It is counterintuitive for the class to view the $100 price with such mixed reviews and the $500 price with such unanimous preference. After all, in the second ending of the story the husband paid five times more for the same clock. What does this discrepancy reveal about process preferences?

The husband had expectations that he brought to his bid. In the first version of the story, he expected the store owner to counter his opening offer. The back-and-forth would help him assess the true value of the clock and provide assurance that he was getting a good deal. That this did not happen as anticipated leaves the husband wondering. Is his assumption of the clock's value amiss? Is there something wrong with the clock? Could he have gotten it for less? Or is he shamelessly guilty of cheating the owner? The negotiation process did not give him the answers he wanted. Poor guy. Every time he passes the clock in his hallway, these doubts haunt him.

In the second version of the story, his process preferences were fulfilled. His questions were answered. And he was satisfied that he got a good deal, half of what the clock was listed for in the catalogue.

Apply this simple story to the more complex negotiations typical of health care. You want to participate in decisions that affect you. You must be included when matters about which you have authority or expertise are decided. And you expect to be included when a decision is made about something for which you have responsibility. Others have the same expectations.

When process preferences are ignored, it is common to hear a version of this reaction: "Hey, great decision. I would have gone along with it if I had been a party to making it. Why was I excluded? Is someone trying to tell me something? Don't expect my cooperation in carrying it out!" Such complaints are not about the substantive outcome of the negotiations. Rather, they speak to people's dissatisfaction that their process preferences—their anticipated inclusion, in this case—were not taken into account.

You incorporate process preferences into your negotiation by planning the decision-making strategy. In other words, you explicitly negotiate how you are going to negotiate. You not only decide what you are hoping to accomplish, you also know how you might go about achieving it. Who should be involved? How should the question be presented? When should the discussions begin? And what might be the criteria that could sway the decision in one direction or the other?

Iris Inkwater calls them "think sessions." She and Perry Pudolski, the chief operating officer for the medical center, sit in her office on comfortable chairs, kick off their shoes, put their feet up, and with pads of paper on their laps, they think. Iris and Perry trust one another. Long moments of silence sometimes punctuate their free association and creative brain storming.

Inkwater muses, "I don't think this is merely a dollars-and-cents exercise, Perry. We are already very lean. I think this is a matter of how we go about doing our business. This could be—I hate to say it—a paradigm shift."

Pudolski chuckles at the overused term. "Perhaps, but Norquist is certainly focused on dollars and cents. He's made it very clear: we cost too much."

"I know that," Inkwater counters, "though in the long run, this crisis is about more than just cutting costs. There is a difference between doing things better and doing things cheaper."

"I think Norquist was pretty clear about cheaper."

"Oh, I know that Norquist is concerned about money. He's a go-between, and his only currency is money. He's a salesman. The difference is that we're running a hospital here. We have to question assumptions and challenge orthodoxies."

Pudolski remains silent. His way of thinking is to sort every problem into neat piles and then figure out each pile of issues methodically. Inkwater is different. She likes to mush things around and see what comes out of the mix. Maybe that's why they're so good together. They're different.

"For a whole lot of reasons, we've been willing to tolerate a surplus of inefficiencies in this place." Inkwater's thoughts appear to form as she speaks. She doesn't seem certain herself what is coming next. "Take the problem with the ICU and internal medicine. That's become a standoff, and we've let it continue because there was no good reason to fix it. We've had problems in our billing department because we've been reluctant to spend the money to upgrade the system. And I think all these dangling problems eventually filter down to patients. I'm sure they don't inspire confidence. In the long run that hurts us at our most vulnerable point, our volume."

"You're going to have to disturb a lot of concrete cobwebs if you want to tackle all of those problems."

"Oh, I know, and I may not be around to tell the tale. Nevertheless, I really don't think we have a choice. We can't overlook efficiencies that others have obviously found. And if we're going to do things differently, we have to have a clear and justifiable reason why. It's really a matter of survival."

"Well," Pudolski challenged, "how do you intend to go about creating this metamorphosis? I mean, I don't care what the politicos think they're doing in Washington. This is where the rubber meets the road. *This* is where the cost savings and quality improvements have to be found. Bottom line, Iris, what do you propose to do?"

"That's a good question. I can easily think of a whole slew of things *not* to do. That's the easier answer." She inhales and then continues slowly. "I think there are two key principles: attitude and involvement. If the staff approach this whole thing with the attitude that they want to make the hospital work better, and if they're all on board, I think we can do it. The key is that they have to be involved. They have to be a part of understanding the problems and a part of formulating the changes. They have to understand that if this boat sinks, we all go down together."

"So, to change the metaphor a bit, you're going to take them to the basement and then lead them out. Clever. I think though that you'll have an easier time getting some people to go along than others. Some of the characters around here are basement dwellers. They'll turn you into the enemy."

"Yes, you're right. Our biggest downside risk though is doing nothing. And there will be some who will simply stay away in the misconception that if they lie low they won't be affected. They'll want to control by withholding their participation. You know, Perry, sometimes passive-aggressive is harder to deal with than just plain old aggressive. In the long run, though, they'll have to see that the do-nothing strategy can't work here anymore. Fighting it internally won't work either. Everybody has to be part of the give-and-take. That's the attitude we'll need to nurture."

Beyond the matter of *what* is decided during your negotiations, there is the question of *how* it is decided. Even if there is consensus on the correctness of the substance, when there is disagreement on the process by which the decision was reached, concurrence on the decision itself vanishes—just as the husband found out when he got the antique clock for $100. This discrepancy between a fair outcome and an unsatisfying process can turn a negotiation into a bitter conflict. The evolution of process conflict can be confounding, because one party may assume that the decision itself is fine and meets acceptable criteria, whereas others may also agree with the substance yet be protesting the process. Process unhappiness can trump substantive satisfaction.

Attending to this question of process is vital to negotiation based on interests, because it speaks so visibly to the underlying concerns that people bring to the table.

What is said and done during the negotiation process, what can be seen, may in fact evoke a spectrum of emotions and needs that also affect what may or may not occur. When smart people go to the basement because they see themselves excluded from the process, they can say some very dumb things. Though not directly related to the substance of the discussions, these personal factors too influence the process and its outcome. These factors are all intimately connected to one another.

Emotions: Negotiation Is Imbued with Meaning

When you negotiate your salary, the outcome is about more than pay alone. More significantly, the negotiation reflects something to you about your value to the organization and, more generally, your worth and status within society. The bargaining implicitly accounts for what you have done beforehand. It is a benchmark that can either make you feel good or fill you with self-doubt, anger, and remorse. Similarly, when you negotiate for office space, the outcome is not only a matter of square footage. The location of your office situates you on the social map of the organization. The size, the number of windows, and the proximity to other people of influence publicly marks your own importance and prestige. And when you are included or excluded from an important policy meeting, the significance is not only a matter of scheduling convenience. Your participation or lack of it also reveals something about the value of your expertise and contributions among your colleagues.

If you view negotiation as simply about money, space, and scheduling, then you ignore the vital emotional significance of the process. This hidden dynamic prompts what you say and what you do. It motivates your reaction to viable proposals. It is the bag of feelings you bring to the table: fears, anxieties, mistrust, hope, anticipation, anger, and aspiration. Some of these sentiments are on the surface: they are known to you and to others. Others are known only to you. And lurking in your subconscious are a myriad of impenetrable feelings and constraints unknown even to you. They reflect your vulnerabilities and suspicions just as much as they do your dreams and aspirations. They are an expression of what motivates and what satisfies you. They emanate from the core of who you are: your values and what you believe to be true.

Just as your underlying emotions pull on your behavior and the choices you make during negotiation, so too do they pull in different ways for others at your negotiation table. What is totally logical to you may be rejected by the people across from you. Or they might offer a proposal that to you makes no sense at all. When your deliberations abandon the realm of the reasonable, you know that something else, other factors, have come heavily into play. These signals may not make sense to you and may make even less sense to them.

When this gulf of understanding opens, ask such questions as, "What concerns does this plan raise for you?" Listen carefully. Be empathic: "This must be very disappointing for you." Remember, you can acknowledge others' feelings without agreeing with them, saying, for example, "I appreciate why you might feel that way." Reflect on what they are saying. Do not tell them what they are feeling. Give them permission and safety to reveal what is bubbling inside: "Please know that I will keep this discussion in confidence." Validate their expression by disclosing that you also have feelings on the matter: "I know this is a tough issue for you. It surfaces many concerns for me as well." In so doing you demonstrate your empathy and desire to understand.

When emotional needs counter to the central purposes of the negotiation enter the process, you will often find yourself in a reactive mode. You may descend to the emotional basement, accompanied by others at the table. Negotiating when everyone at the table is in the basement is an undertaking fraught with danger.

If, however, you can anticipate the emotional topics—both those seen as accepting and those seen as opposing—that will affect the negotiations, you can then offer a proactive opening. Be explicit about the invitation, suggesting the topic early in the negotiation process. For example, "Before we get into the specifics about the merger proposal, I think it is fair to acknowledge that after being here so many years, this is a tough issue for all of us." If the issues are sensitive, use an implicit approach, gently touching on and acknowledging the subject, such as, "I imagine this must be difficult for you." Yes, you may open a floodgate. If it is done sensitively, however, this gesture could offer opportunities to find solutions responsive to both others' emotional reactions and yours. You are not sidestepping the issues. You are handling them directly (see Fisher, Kopelman, & Schneider, 1994; Gelfand & Brett, 2004; Druckman & Olekalns, 2008).

In fact, emotional apprehensions are often formidable, unseen obstacles impeding negotiation progress. Even when they can't be resolved, merely acknowledging the feelings can be significant for those affected.

Beyond acknowledgment, identifying emotional issues can guide your negotiation strategy. Learn what motivates the people on the other side. Can you offer them something to satisfy their interests? What incentives can you create to respond to their needs? What could be done to turn the emotions into excitement, enthusiasm, and with that, support and motivation for what you hope to accomplish? Even though the overt discussion may be about something as concrete as money or space, the underlying desires, anxieties, and impulses may be about professional recognition, job security, or resentment about a past humiliation. By addressing these underlying concerns, you enhance the prospect of finding agreement.

This avenue is particularly valuable when what you have to divide is clearly limited or shrinking: money, space, or time. Attention to emotional interests will give you more to divide. If the topic on the table is assignment of office space, and the real, underlying issue is respect within the organization, then offer the needed assurances about value and appreciation. In fact, if you tender added importance

Larry Lumberg (director of the emergency department) hears Fred Fisher growl "Enter" after his knock and cautiously makes his way into the spacious office of the medical director of the Oppidania Medical Center (OMC). Fisher is staring out the window and does not turn around to acknowledge his young colleague's arrival. Something's up, thinks Lumberg.

"Fred, is something wrong?" There is silence, and Lumberg prepares himself to hear of some personal or professional tragedy that has suddenly befallen his mentor. "What's happened?"

"Nothing's happened, Larry. Nothing's happened and everything's happened. I tell you, medicine is not what it was when I entered this profession. I think maybe it's time I get out before this whole thing falls apart."

"Fred, what are you talking about?"

Fisher turns and focuses on Lumberg for the first time. "Have you heard about this thing with the Community Health Plan? They are threatening to pull out of OMC. I tell you, Larry, there is only so much blood to squeeze out of this hospital and out of this physician. It just doesn't seem worth it anymore."

"What are you saying?"

"I chose to go into medicine forty years ago. It was a noble profession back then. We did good work for people, and we were treated with respect. We worked hard and we deserved every penny we got. We took pride and pleasure in what we did. It's not like that anymore. They are trying to manage us, squeeze us, and control us. It's becoming paint-by-numbers medicine, where a lifetime of experience is subsumed in favor of checklists and standard protocols. They want to replace us with machines, computers, and technicians. It's simply not worth it anymore. I think it's time for me to pack it up and call it quits."

Lumberg speaks slowly as he answers. He senses that Fisher is in the basement. "Fred, there is no doubt about it. Medicine is not what it used to be. It doesn't even resemble what I got into some twenty years ago."

Lumberg knows that Fisher doesn't need a lecture now about health care economics or management. This is a man whose professional pride and authority are being abducted. In Fisher's mind, there is something sacred about the practice of medicine. The inviolable profession is being destroyed by far-off Washington policy wonks, greedy insurance executives, and cumbersome Oppidania efficiency engineers. Lumberg grew up in a different generation. He can put what is happening into its larger political and economic context. He had struggled through those courses never imagining how much they would inform his career. These insights are beyond Fisher and his sometimes old-school tendencies.

"Fred, I know these are trying times. We are all being tested. You've made an enormous contribution over your career. Your ingenuity has pulled patients through tough times. There are countless people in this community who are alive now because of the care you gave them or because of the knowledge and professionalism you transferred to and instilled in your residents. Now the medical staff needs your leadership to pull this hospital through what may be our hardest test yet."

Fisher smiles inwardly. It feels odd to hear Larry giving him a reassuring lecture. It's usually the other way around. Larry, though, did a good job, he thought. As Fisher ponders Lumberg's words, he recalls his own Navy days and knows that he can't ask someone else to fight this battle. He reminisces briefly about patients, medical students, colleagues. "Yes, Fisher, old boy, you are still needed here," he says to himself.

Out loud he says, "Perhaps you're right, Larry." He brightens a bit. "But I don't think it is ever going to be as much fun as it used to be."

"Maybe it'll just be a different kind of fun," Lumberg counters with a smile.

and influence in recognition of the person who takes the office without a window, you may find everyone on your staff requesting the undesirable space. You have created new currency for exchange, and the more you have to trade, the easier it is to achieve settlement.

Emotional interests are of particular importance in health care because of the nature of the work. The characteristic social purpose and concern for quality of life that typify the field and give it particular meaning also accentuate the inherently weighty nature of negotiation. Staff working in particular sections, such as the oncology department, AIDS unit, or women's clinic, are particularly committed to defending the causes of their patients. An action or decision is particularly upsetting if perceived to compromise the quality of patient care or respect for patients. Addressing these interests by building safeguards or assurances into a discussion facilitates the process of generating a constructive agreement, especially when there are tough trade-offs to be negotiated.

Identifying Substantive Expectations

When you enter a negotiation, you likely have viewpoints on your process preferences, how you want the decision to be made. You are less likely to be conscious of your emotional inclinations and those of others. You most likely are clearest about one thing: what you want to get out of the negotiation—your substantive expectations.

The balance of substantive expectations among the parties is really a many-sided question. On the one hand, what is it that you want to get, and what is it that others want to get? On the other hand, what is it that you are willing to give, and what are they willing to give? This is the get-and-give of negotiation. From a strategic perspective you want to attend to all sides of this balance. Those who go to the table concerned only for what they want to get miss important opportunities to leverage larger, mutually beneficial advantages from the process.

You negotiate because you don't have it all. You don't control it all. You need something from someone else. You and your negotiation partners balance narcissism (one of you gets it all) with social interdependence (you both share it) to reach agreement on the terms of the deal. If you and the others cannot find a balance, the negotiation collapses and the transaction does not occur.

How do you and the others reach agreement? And how do you conclude the negotiation so that your partner—perhaps a colleague, a patient, or a representative from another health care organization—will choose to negotiate with you again?

To accomplish a gain-gain outcome, calibrate a standard of fairness to guide your negotiation. Construct that standard by assessing what is valuable to the negotiation at hand; time, expertise, money, effort, and outcome are examples. Agree on the value of what you propose to exchange by comparing what is on the table to similar commodities of established worth. For example, when setting salaries for a particular professional group, ask whether there are community or national standards that can provide a basis of comparison. When setting fees, ask how this locale compares or contrasts with other areas? This stage of the negotiation is arduous because the appraisal process is highly subjective. Your interpretation of merit and value may not be shared by others.

This practice of determining value is particularly arduous in health care. Real estate agents assess one property against *comparables* in the neighborhood. Car dealers pull out their Blue Book. There are no such golden standards in health care. Time is relative: what is the value of a physician's hour versus a nurse's? Outcome is relative: what is the value of a certain sum of money spent on an infant nutrition program serving thousands versus the same sum spent for a sole baby cared for in a neonatal intensive care unit? Opinion is relative: what is the value of a specialist's opinion versus that of a primary care practitioner? And given that the health care system is in transformation, an assessment of value made one week may be altered by the next week.

For this reason you should give careful attention to the appraisal phase of the negotiation process. If someone's or something's relative value is diminished, that will likely seriously offend some at the table. This offense can assume great professional, ethical, or personal meaning. When the opinion of one professional is weighed differently from the identical opinion of another, it can fuel bitter

Before leaving for home at the end of this long day, Larry Lumberg takes a detour to the front of the emergency room. He wants to touch base with Beatrice Benson, the attending physician on call for the night. Fortunately, she is standing at the cluttered triage desk looking over a chart with Charlotte Chung, the triage nurse. After exchanging greetings, he gets to the point.

"You know they have added a nurse to the night shift on general medical. The intent is to shift as many admissions as possible away from the ICU."

"I know, I heard about it. Look, we'll give it a shot. It depends on what kind of traffic we get here tonight," Benson replies noncommittally.

"With all these capitated plans, there's a lot of pressure to reduce expenses when possible," Lumberg explains. "As long as we're not putting anyone in danger, we should try to get in line."

Chung chimes in, "Actually, general medical is in better shape. One of the star ICU nurses has been transferred to Six West. They're much better able to handle questionable cases now."

"I can't disagree," Benson adds, "though quite honestly, I view this whole push as a matter of risk. I know one nurse is not going to change everything overnight. It is an important step, though, in giving us a better alternative we can live with. It still raises all sorts of possibilities that we will shortchange a patient who comes through here."

Three hours later, Benson is on the phone to Eli Ewing, the chief resident in the ICU.

"I was hoping not to hear from you tonight," Ewing sarcastically greets Benson's call.

"Well, nothing personal, Eli. I was hoping not to talk to you, either. Actually, I think you might like this call."

"OK, try me," Ewing replies.

"We have a fifty-six-year-old male here. He came in complaining of chest pains. We've pretty much ruled out a myocardial infarction. In any case, I think it wise to keep him here overnight for observation. A few weeks ago I would have sent him your way. I really don't think it's necessary, though. I ask just one favor."

"You got it," Ewing replies.

"Would you be willing to come down and look over the charts? It's been a busy night, and I just want to be certain we didn't miss anything. If everything looks in order to you, we'll move him up to Six West, and save you an admission."

"Sure thing! Oh, and by the way, Beatrice," Ewing hesitates, "I think this whole arrangement may work out in the end."

"Well, we'll give it a shot. If we can slow down on sending people to you guys, it's in all our best interests."

indignation. If the life of one person is placed above the life of another, it provokes moral outrage. And if the legitimate concerns of a woman are belittled to elevate the equivalent concerns of a man, it sparks gender animosity. In health care, you negotiate in these highly sensitive domains all the time.

If you and the others are able to agree on a standard of fairness, your next step is to propose an exchange. Compare what you are offering to what the other sides are offering. Determine if there is a workable balance among the interests of the many sides. Inherent in the negotiation process is that you are giving one thing and getting something different in return. That is why relative value is so important.

Once you have determined that the scale is in balance, you are better prepared to consummate the exchange. You now have in your reach something different from what you had before. You assess and reassess the prospects. Are you still satisfied? Are the other sides still satisfied? If the answer is a mutual yes, conclude the transaction. You all shake hands. If you all are pleased, you anticipate favorably your future transactions.

The utility of interest-based negotiation is its adaptability to these inherently subjective, emotional, and fluid circumstances. The starting point is exploration: questions, information, perceptions, and desires. This is a learning process that goes in both directions. It is through this strategy that you assemble the information necessary to assess value equitably, just as you teach the other side about what you require from the negotiation. It is a method particularly appropriate to the types of negotiation that occur daily in health care.

Forging a Common Language

Distributional bargaining positions negotiators against one another. When you negotiate on the basis of positions, you are rigid, uncompromising, and uninterested in other points of view. You are a contender, seeking conquest rather than congruence. You draw a line in the sand and hold firm on your demands.

In health care numerous lines divide who we are and what we do. Different professional groups sometimes interact as if they were speaking different languages and thinking and communicating with different priorities, sensitivities, and risk quotients. Nurses speak "nurse." Doctors speak "doctor." Health administrators speak "administrator," and so on through the other disciplines. These "languages" are defined not only by the distinct vocabulary of each specialty. They also reflect the unique cognitive framework used in each specialty to analyze information, make decisions, and assess value. Each profession has its own set of criteria. When presented with the same information, each deliberates differently. Each department, division, and discipline has carved a place for itself in the institution, promoting its members' perspective on what they do and the way they go about doing it.

That these differences exist is not a bad thing. In fact these very differences invigorate what can be accomplished in health care. Different perspectives can inspire creativity, serve as checks and balances on the work, and provide avenues for integrating the vast bounty of health care knowledge and skills.

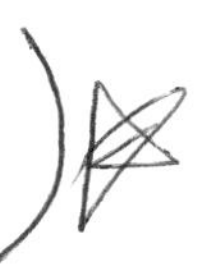

Those who work in health care are bound by the shared interests and values that frame what can be accomplished on behalf of the health of a patient, a community, or a population. Common ground can be achieved in the pursuit of these overlapping interests and expectations. As a tool, interest-based negotiation offers the integrative framework and common language necessary to tie the pieces together. By generating inventive options and new solutions, it affords a potent resource for overcoming the most stubborn of obstacles.

CHAPTER 5

FRAMING TO GENERATE OPTIONS

NEGOTIATION IS replete with conscious and subconscious decisions, trade-offs, experiences, people, and repercussions. There are facts and emotions to integrate. To elicit useful negotiation criteria, you must arrange this information into logical cognitive patterns: frames and templates.

The *frame* helps you understand and organize information so it is useful to you. The frame is your subjective lens, employed to direct your specific negotiation choices and decisions. It emerges out of your *template:* the unique and consistent blend of philosophy, attitude, and belief that is you and your character. If someone bears enduring prejudice, bias, or intolerance, that part of their template colors their specific frame each time they negotiate, even if those sentiments are subconscious and buried deep inside. If your template contains openness, compassion, and a willingness to learn, these principles will likewise characterize your every negotiation (see Bazerman & Lewicki, 1983; Strauss, 1994).

Assessing Your Template

Who are you? What are your values? What are your priorities? These are important questions that rarely offer simple or straightforward answers. Beneath these questions reside the many experiences, people, and influences that shape who you are. It is this unique set of causal factors that combine to mold your template. Like a filter through which you sift all decisions, interactions, and problems, your template embodies the character you bring to the negotiation table.

You might think your template to be as solid as the ground on which you walk. In fact it undergoes constant evolution over time. Just as terra firma shifts with periodic jolting earthquakes that reveal dramatic underground transformation, so too does your template adjust slightly each time you negotiate.

If a deeply personal experience, for example, reinforces your preconceptions about the stubbornness of surgeons, then that piece of your template becomes more rigid. So too are your attitudes about race, gender, and professional competence swayed by your particularly calamitous or uniquely positive interactions. Experiences that are memorable introduce new sentiments that shift your preconceptions. The surgeon who spends time to talk with you and then warmly pays attention to what you have to say could reset your notions about the possibilities and limitations of the profession.

You consciously challenge and change your template when you incorporate new ideas into your persona. Through what you read, experience, and contemplate, you cautiously shift your underlying premises. Often these shifts are in response to changing mores and attitudes in your surroundings. Evolving social sentiments about gender, racial, and sexual-orientation relations; professional interactions; and hierarchical ordering seep into your mind-set, causing you to consider and reconsider your approaches to everyday decision making. Rapid changes in the health system prompted by changes in health care financing and regulation demand significant alterations in the templates that many health professionals possessed when they graduated their advanced training. Some innovations and ideas you welcome, and some you abhor. Some fit easily into who you are, and others seem to contradict your basic values and nature.

Active introspection is a constant companion of good negotiation. At the conclusion of a recent intensive negotiation training seminar, a hospital human relations vice president commented, "I came here thinking I was going to learn how to change other people. What I learned is that before I can hope to do that, I have to be willing to change myself." He had discovered much about his attitudes on gender relations, his preconceived notions about clinicians, and his blind spots, all of which had been hampering his negotiation capabilities. He now recognized that by ignoring the information his template and core values deemed unimportant but that was in fact essential, he had offended women with casual remarks, ignored useful suggestions from subordinates, and discounted worthy options just because they were outside his field of experience. His blinders wouldn't let him see.

When you learn to be a carpenter, you become skilled in using a hammer and saw, the tools of the trade. When you endeavor to be a better negotiator, the tool you learn to better wield is yourself. You are the negotiator, and your effectiveness results from what you think, say, and do. Taking inventory of your template and frame is a first and ongoing endeavor in that process.

Understanding Your Frame

Your template describes your general beliefs and attitudes. Your negotiation frame is specific to a particular negotiation, problem, or dispute.

Your frame is the perspective you bring into the deliberations. It is your blueprint for assimilating information and taking action. To guide your negotiation strategy and choices, you want to understand your own frame and those of other negotiators. That understanding opens the door to generating creative options for resolution.

What are the building blocks of your frame? The key variables are people, problems, history, strategy, outcomes, priorities, and stakes.

People

Health care decisions typically involve many people. There are those who make the decision. There are those who are affected by it. A supervisor decides that one member of the staff must be assigned to the night shift. A resident decides that a patient is ready to be discharged to a nursing home. An insurance company executive determines that the company will no longer reimburse for care at one of the hospitals in town. The question is, which people should participate in reaching the decision, and what role should each person have?

There are three categories of people involved in a negotiation. They are distinguished by their proximity to the negotiation table. The *primary players* are the people sitting directly at the table, participating in the give-and-take. They have an immediate interest in the decision, and they are visibly involved in the process of reaching it. The *secondary players* are, metaphorically, standing just outside the door; they are the individuals being informed, consulted, and advised by the primary players. They are knowledgeable recipients of the decision more than they are involved players. Even though their opinions may sway the outcome, their influence is indirect. The *tertiary players* are not in the room. They are often unaware that the deliberations are occurring. They are the anonymous people affected by decisions: patients, staff, or the community. Although they bear the consequences of what is decided, they have little role in shaping the outcomes.

Your negotiation template generally and your negotiation frame specifically assign those involved in the issue to primary, secondary, and tertiary roles. This judgment derives from your opinion about how the people and process should be ordered. Not everyone involved will necessarily concur: problems arise when there are disputes about who is assigned to which role. Consider the examples at the beginning of this section. In the mind of the supervisor, she and her assistant are the primary players, other supervisors are secondary players, and the staff member assigned to the night shift is a tertiary player. What if the staff member expects to be a primary player? After all, it is her schedule and her life. The resident making the discharge assessment may consider the medical director a primary player. The medical director, however, may want to encourage the young trainee to assume greater independent responsibility. She prefers a secondary role in the decision. The insurance executive who wants to terminate the hospital contract considers the state's insurance commissioner a nonparticipant in the decision. Responding to consumer complaints, the commissioner nevertheless assumes his prerogative to become an active, primary player in the conflict.

If one of the involved parties has decision-making authority and adopts a unilateral command-and-control attitude, then in his or her mind there is only one primary player. Staff members, colleagues, or patients affected by the dictate are excluded from the process. If those relegated to secondary player status believe valid sentiments, information, and experience are being ignored, they naturally will resent the process, especially if it redounds negatively upon them.

Though often subtle, differences among parties about participation at the table are a common source of negotiation conflict. It is advantageous to clarify this matter before negotiation begins in earnest. Who is involved, and who has what authority at the table? If participation issues are ignored or not made explicit, on top of the disagreement about the issues at hand you will also be hindered by lack of consensus about the process preferences and assumptions about the authority and purview of those involved.

Problems

The second variable in your frame is your definition of the problem. What is it that you want resolved, settled, or changed? In what ways is the current situation unacceptable to you? What caused the current impasse or situation, and how can conditions be changed to alleviate the problem? The other negotiators with whom you are meeting will assess the same set of questions.

It is to be expected that people will bring different views of problem and purpose to the table. When not recognized and understood, however, these differences act as fundamental obstacles to negotiation progress. The process is then stalled until the negotiators acknowledge these differences in attitude and frame. This is another example of the cone in the cube impasse. If both sides adamantly stick to their different perspectives, they won't find the integrated understanding that is within their grasp.

A case mediated at a community health center illustrates the phenomenon. The center faced major budgetary reductions and operational constraints that were about to cripple its capacity to provide responsive and quality patient care. The conflict was portrayed as an irreconcilable standoff between clinical and administrative personnel. The administrators blamed the clinicians for being aloof and unconcerned about the well-being of the community and survival of the organization. The clinicians accused the administrators of being unashamedly incompetent. The flash point was the matter of clinical supplies. Clinicians reported that teenage girls were coming, as would be hoped, to the community health center for pregnancy tests. When the clinicians went to the supply cabinet, however, the necessary test supplies were often absent. The girls who had to be sent away without a test were reluctant to return at another time, having lost their confidence in the clinic. The administrators complained that the clinicians were to blame for the shortages because they were rigidly unwilling to properly complete insurance forms and forward them to the billing office. As a result the center was denied its rightful payments from insurers. Without money, suppliers were unwilling to deliver their goods. In the administrators' view, it was a budget crisis not an ordering crisis. The clinic had fallen into rampant finger-pointing. And again the most acutely affected tertiary party was the patient.

The mediation provided an important learning, reframing, and template-changing opportunity. It was discovered during the mediation that the clinicians were genuinely unaware that "completing the form" meant ensuring that it was sent promptly to the administrative floor. The clinicians had assumed that was someone else's responsibility. The administrators had assumed the clinicians were aware of the required procedures. The clinicians did not grasp the administrators' frustration. During the deliberations the problem was reframed from a personal blame issue ("it's his fault") to a correctable systems issue ("something is not working here and it can be corrected"). It was discovered that in fact there was no mechanism to transfer and trace income from appointment to reimbursement. The necessary organizational adjustments were made, and the possibility of new collaboration between the two groups opened up. What had happened?

Beyond the immediate problem, it also became clear that there were fundamental differences in the templates that the two sides brought to the workplace. The administrators perceived the clinicians as rich suburbanites who drove their fancy cars to the inner city, made themselves feel good, took a lot of money, and then returned to their cushy homes with little concern for the troubled community they left behind. The clinicians saw the administrators as local yokels whose performance was so substandard that they had to work at the community health center because no one else would offer them a job. Once the immediate problems in the clinic were resolved, the negotiation setting provided the opportunity for the clinicians to express their deep commitment to the community and the work of the health center. They explained that they could work for far more money, in a better space, and with all the supplies they needed in the medical centers not far away. They chose this work because they wanted to make a tangible difference for people in this community. The administrators likewise expressed their deep commitment to the community, their arduous task they faced in keeping the center financially viable despite budgetary obstacles, and the difficulties they encountered in negotiating with impatient payers and suppliers. They explained that given the difficulties in keeping the bills paid, they saw it as a miracle every time they flipped the light switch and the lights actually came on. The administrators worked in a condition of constant uncertainty, and vilification from clinicians only made it more difficult. Solving the presenting problem allowed each side to explore and resolve the underlying attitudes that had inflamed the conflict.

This accord was achieved in part by pursuing the question, What is the real problem? The two groups had to ascend beyond petty blaming. Without developing a common understanding, they would have persistently clashed. How could they solve "the problem" when they were in essence trying to solve different problems? But once they had established consensus on the fundamental issues, it was possible for them to move together toward an integrative solution and a plan for implementing and cementing their agreement.

History

There is a pragmatic, rational side to negotiation and conflict resolution. Simply put, you discern the problem and reach consensus on options. In the process you find good choices and lousy choices. The parties logically select the former.

In fact, real conflict and negotiation is rarely that straightforward. People bring an abundance of memory to the table. That memory is the collection of good experiences and bad that influence their attitudes about others: their "baggage." When experiences have been positive and productive, this good baggage enhances the negotiation. The resulting goodwill is like currency, appreciated and leveraged to enrich negotiation outcomes. When experiences have been negative, this bad baggage constitutes a formidable obstacle to progress.

When parties are negatively predisposed to one another, their negotiation choices may be motivated more by seeking retribution than by solving the immediate problem that is on the table. They are more concerned with dumping their trunkful of stories on the table than they are in talking about workable options. They are there to get even or score points. That motive takes on greater meaning than their immediate, best self-interest.

Old scores intermingle shades of fact with layers of illusion. What really happened is of secondary importance to what the parties believe happened. They go to their emotional basement just by virtue of being in the presence of one another. Words and actions assume meanings that supersede their intent. Emotions blur objective assessments. The parties are in "survival" mode, compelled by perception and misperception.

Several years ago we mediated a dispute between two high-ranking hospital administrators, "Alan" and "John." After hours of exploring the issues and options, we finally reached a tentative agreement on a plan that would allow both to continue their employment at the medical center. Noticing Alan's ambivalence, we decided it was time for a private caucus with him. We asked him to remain in the room, and we asked John to wait outside until we called him back for his own private conversation.

Once we were alone with Alan, one of us remarked about the outcome, "Alan, it seems that you got what you said you were looking for: the money, the quality, and the autonomy." Clenching his fists, gritting his teeth, and becoming red in the face, he seethed, "Yes, but I didn't get revenge." There was an intense pause and he continued, "I can't let him get out of this room and go back to his job unscathed by this whole fiasco." He felt the other administrator had maliciously undermined his career and in the process injured his personal life. Both Alan and John had brought great antipathy into their negotiations, and during the meetings they had reveled in recounting their stories of woe. Our job as mediators was to help them get beyond their bad history.

Alan's objective was to get even with his perceived "enemy" by inflicting pain on him. This type of basement behavior is associated more with street gang violence than it is with the intricacies of intelligent health care professional relationships. However, even though actual physical violence is rare in such relationships, the penchant for intergroup warfare is not. The result is decision making that offers the taste of revenge and yet only fleeting satisfaction.

Beware when "getting even" is a central ingredient of your frame or those of other negotiators. It is a warning: finding a mutually acceptable resolution will be difficult. Even when one of the parties is willing to acknowledge guilt and accept some pain—whether it be in the form of financial penalty, a public apology, or a professional sanction—it is unlikely to satisfy the other's appetite for revenge. If you are the one motivated by a desire for retribution, carefully assess the reasons, review your *primary* motives and objectives, and determine whether revenge alone will suffice. Though you might revel in the fantasy, a totally wholesome diversion, you want to be careful about transforming your rage into reality. What sacrifice might you suffer for the short-term pleasure of seeing your counterpart writhe? Conversely, if others at the table are determined to occasion your demise, be cognizant of the limitations of the negotiation process. There is only so much you want to give in order for them to get even. (Techniques for handling these situations are discussed in Chapter Eight.)

Strategy

There are three broad categories of negotiation strategy, spanning a spectrum running from cooperate to collaborate to contend. These categories are distinct in their means—the negotiation process—and their ends—what is hoped to be achieved. Some negotiators are persistent in the strategy they bring to the table. Some are always die-hard fighters. Others are forever in pursuit of *kumbaya*. Wise negotiators adjust their style and strategy to the situation at hand. How do you characterize your general working strategy? (This will be affected by your template.) How does your general strategy translate into behavior during a specific negotiation? (This will become your frame.)

Cooperators seek fair outcomes with clear parameters defining separate identities. When negotiating, cooperators emphasize the individual benefits that will accrue to each participant. They engage with others in order to achieve distinct gains: "I want to get mine; and because I want you to come back to the table in the future, I want you to get yours, too." Cooperators assess a decision or settlement based on balance: did everyone get his or her deserved slice of the pie? They are looking for a *gain-gain* outcome.

Collaborators are more concerned with common purpose and process than they are with dividing the pie. They emphasize overlapping interests and rewards. To them, the very act of joining in a common effort offers important satisfaction in and of itself. They favor melding work, credit, and participation so the parties can evolve from separate entities into an aggregate unit sharing a common destiny. From the perspective of collaborators, your gain is our gain. They put jealousy, suspicion, and one-upmanship to the side. They are looking to achieve a collective, mutual gain.

Contenders view others as discrete competitors, even others perceived to be on the same side. They emphasize conquest. For the contender, winning has meaning in and of itself. They strive for as large a portion of the pie as possible, and they justify their methods by reason of their higher purposes: triumph and dominance. The contender's concern for others is premised on how other parties' attitudes affect the potential for future wins. They give little in order to get more. Contenders crave to be on top in a *win-lose* outcome.

There are pure versions of these categories—for example, the contender who is always in a contest, even with a spouse. (We once heard a wife say to her husband, "Just because you are a surgeon does not mean that you can treat the whole world as if it is your operating room." And he retorted, "Why not?") For the most part, however, people's proclivities shift among collaborator, cooperator, and contender, according to the situation. The determining strategic consideration may be the circumstances of a particular negotiation. A contender might assume a collaborative strategy when impressed with the common purpose and the amiable nature of other negotiators. (This is a variant on "my enemy's enemy is my friend.") Or someone might be influenced by experience; a cooperator may become more contentious if recently burned in a negotiation. General social events may change attitudes. A collaborator is likely to become contentious when survival of a common mission is threatened. Your style adapts to your circumstances as you understand them.

Understanding your own and others' strategic template and frame will help you plan your stance at the negotiation table. What approach do you generally employ, and what approach do you favor in a particular negotiation? What approach are others using? How might their strategy affect the way you plan your own? Is yours adjustable? Is theirs?

A negotiation's outcome can only be as good as the strategy used in its pursuit. Early discussion and agreement on the strategic process, the form, and the format together shape the size of the field in which agreement can be found: the further you move toward collaboration, the wider your possibilities. The more contentious you are, the fewer are your options. Though the parties may open with one frame, conceived from their template, that frame is adjustable. Reframing the strategic process for conducting the negotiation creates new options for reaching settlement.

Iris Inkwater considers Dr. Fred Fisher to be "old school": white male, respected physician, early sixties, and in her opinion accustomed to being coddled.

Fred Fisher refers to Iris Inkwater as a "young upstart": white female, well-educated, mid-forties, and in his opinion overcompensated and not willing to pay her dues.

Inkwater thinks of herself as being somewhere between a cooperator and a collaborator. When necessary she can be a contender, though she feels that the costs of battle outweigh the benefits in the long run. In her mind the board of trustees pays her to have the smarts and the guts to use the strategy necessary to get the job done.

Fisher doesn't like touchy-feely conversations, and he doesn't like mucking around with a decision when he knows what needs to be done. He believes a bit of contention makes for creative tension: it keeps people on their toes. It turns the humdrum of work into sport. He finds meetings and group decision making boring. He is paid, and has been around here long enough, to *know* what needs to be done.

Inkwater has asked Fisher to meet with her. She feels it is important to reframe their working relationship, given the predicament facing the hospital. He is impatient with the discussion before they have even begun talking. In his mind, he can't be part of a solution to a problem he didn't create.

Inkwater has walked around her desk and taken a side chair so that she and the head of the medical staff can sit face to face without a piece of furniture between them. "Fred," she begins, "this hospital is facing a real threat to its survival. I want to be certain that you and I are working together. And just as important, I want to be certain that people who work here see the two of us working together."

Fisher looks askance. "Are you accusing me of wanting this institution to fail, Iris? Because nothing could be farther from the truth. But I am just a simple doctor."

"I am saying that our working relationship could be a lot better, and in fact has to be a lot better if we are going to pull through this."

"Look, Iris, you are paid to solve problems and to make sure those problems don't damage our capacity to take care of patients. If you have a problem, or if you have created a problem, don't expect us to solve it for you."

"That is just what I think we need to correct, Fred. I did not create this problem. You read the news. You know all the pressure the health system is under. This problem was not invented by me or even by Community Health Plan. The medical staff cannot simply retreat into its silo and pretend that the rest of the world doesn't exist. We'll get nowhere if we go around blaming one another."

Fisher sits in resigned silence. Inkwater does make sense, and he doesn't know what to do with it. "What are you suggesting, Iris?" He puts just enough condescension in the way he pronounces her name to make sure she knows who's on top here. Inkwater drops momentarily into the basement and then reminds herself of what she wanted to accomplish with this meeting. She gets back into gear.

Hoping to reframe their working relationship, Inkwater decides on a metaphor that Fisher cannot ignore and perhaps will even understand. "I suggest that we start acting as if we are fellow officers on the same ship. I may be in the engine room and you may be tending the big guns, but we both depend on the same hull to keep us dry."

Inkwater senses Fisher's discomfort at being caught off guard. Her metaphor has worked. She is playing his game and succeeding. She recognizes also the need to help him save face. "Fred, you have more experience than anyone in this institution. The problem is, they are changing the rules of engagement out there." Seeking to add a touch of humor, she adds, "It's time to get our battle rhythm." She looks straight into Fisher's eyes and smiles.

Fisher surprises himself. He smiles back. He begins to appreciate, oddly enough, that he and Iris in fact share a common problem. She is not the "enemy administrator." He begins to see her as just the opposite: she has the potential to rescue the ship. If she—no, we—can't come up with a solution, the whole medical center might sink. Her analogy is resonating for him. "Iris, I am just a simple sailor and I understand you can't sail a battleship alone." He pauses with a sigh. "You're right. I do believe we have to be working together. But it's going to take some adjustment on all our parts." Fisher does not want to retreat from his tried-and-true stance too quickly.

Outcomes

People enter negotiation anticipating what they will get. Indeed, the emphasis on *getting* is seen in the literature and marketing of negotiation: Roger Fisher of the Program on Negotiation at Harvard Law School coauthored *Getting Together* (with Scott Brown, 1988) and then teamed up with William Ury and Bruce Patton to write the landmark book *Getting to Yes* (1991—and still appearing first in search results for "negotiation skills" in best-selling books at Amazon.com in 2009) and then *Getting Ready to Negotiate* (with Danny Ertel, 1995). Ury published *Getting Past No* (1991) and *Getting to Peace* (1999). In his airline seat-pocket advertising, Chester Karrass (1970) and his company, claiming to have designed the most successful negotiation seminar in the United States, pronounce, "In business, you don't get what you deserve, you get what you negotiate." Negotiation is achievement oriented, and such slogans appeal to people's appetite for tangible and intangible dividends.

Your frame delineates what you expect to get, as do the frames of other negotiators. This is obviously an important accomplishment, as it defines your very motive for being at the table. It becomes problematic, however, when getting is the only dynamic at the table. If you are negotiating with someone whose sole objective is getting, it is unlikely that your own wishes will be satisfied. You and your counterpart are likely to reach an impasse.

Determining what you and what other parties want to get is essential for understanding your frame and the frames of others in the negotiation. Just as important is identifying what you are each prepared to give. This is a critical question for those involved in the process of health policy debates. Most of the rhetoric for change focuses on what each constituency wants to get. The key to resolution emerges as physicians, insurers, payers, consumers, legislators, and others articulate what they are willing to give or give up to adjust the health system so it can better provide high-quality, cost-effective, preventive, health-promoting policies and practices.

Limiting what parties give and get simply to an exchange of what they already have is a lackluster approach that provides only marginal substantive gain. Creative negotiation embraces the cultivation of new currency. You then get more because you have created more to share and exchange. This process of inventing new and more advantageous options is termed *expanding the pie*. How does expanding the pie work?

Imagine that you are bargaining to purchase a used car from a private individual. The discussion focuses on the cost, condition, and value of the automobile. You are at a stalemate on the price. You won't buy it for his asking price and he won't sell it for what you offer. Then you find an opportunity to expand the pie. You learn that the owner needs to use the car for two more weeks, at the end of which time he is leaving the country. He cannot wait until the last minute to complete the sale. This adds a new currency to the exchange: time. Because you do not need the car immediately, you offer to complete the sale but to postpone the delivery, if the owner comes closer to your price. Recognizing that he has saved himself the cost of a rental car for two weeks, the owner agrees, and you and he consummate the deal.

To think of negotiation only in terms of getting is to limit it to a unidimensional endeavor. Yes, you may harbor the fantasy of getting everything you want. Yet that is neither a constructive description nor a productive frame for achieving the best possible outcome from the negotiation.

It is far better to think of negotiation as multidimensional. On one side there is getting what you want the other party to give. On another side there is giving what the other side wants to get from you. By adding multiple dimensions, you build a process for achieving an exchange that resourcefully and productively links the getting and giving. *Giving to Yes* may not be a catchy proposition, but face it: what you are willing to give is the enticement that ultimately consummates the deal.

Priorities

Negotiation is a process of relativity; there are no absolutes. Issues and concerns that are of paramount importance to one participant may be irrelevant to another. Values, emphases, and consequences are perceived and experienced quite differently by each party. Making an appraisal of these distinctions is essential for crafting a settlement.

Consider the car negotiation described in the previous section. For the seller, gaining two more weeks with the car and concluding the sale was a higher priority than getting the top dollar price. For the buyer, using the car for the next two weeks was a lower priority than getting a better price. The parties were able to consummate the deal by creating an exchange that meshed their two, relatively different yet ultimately complementary priorities.

To analyze the parties' frames, list the relative importance of each of their measured objectives. For example, the car seller's list would read (1) agreement on a sale, (2) use of the car, and (3) a sufficient price. The buyer's list would read (1) a better price, (2) the condition of the car, and (3) time of delivery. In this case the parties' different priorities could be combined to create a fit.

Similarities in priorities can also be used to craft a settlement. When negotiating parties agree on top priorities, such as the importance of continued operation of an AIDS clinic in a community, the significance of institutional efforts to improve patient safety, or their mutual desire to settle a conflict, the identification and acknowledgment of this consensus provides critical dispute resolution leverage and thereby increases the likelihood of bringing the parties to agreement. Completing the deal requires you to line up the points where priorities are shared and the points where they are different in order to accomplish a fit and, with it, a deal. By making a business case for improved quality of care, clinicians and managers are able to coordinate improvement activities even though they are primarily motivated by different objectives.

Each party to a negotiation naturally brings to the table different purposes and priorities. Balancing the relative importance of these priorities is what the negotiation process is all about. Discerning the different templates and frames guides the parties toward crafting a match that allows each to better achieve his or her different yet complementary negotiation objectives.

Stakes

There are negotiation preferences: the rewards and benefits you hope to acquire. These represent your fantasies of what will be achieved. Anticipating these benefits, you negotiate. And then—good or bad, like it or not—there are negotiation fears: what it is that you desperately want to avoid.

Stakes are the tangible outcomes facing the parties. Stakeholders arrive at a decision point when they seriously weigh these outcomes, asking, What will be the costs if I hold off? What can I get if we settle? What will I be required to give? Do I want to remain in this unresolved limbo? The answers to these questions can reveal an incentive when they reflect an expectation of rewards. They can reveal a threat when they signal fear of objectionable consequences, causing one or more parties to delay settlement in order to avoid a greater loss.

There are three kinds of stakes: good stakes, bad stakes, and opportunity stakes.

Good stakes are the bounty you reap from the deal: a well-priced piece of medical equipment, a few extra days of vacation, or a lucrative contract. Agree to the terms of the offer, and these splendid prizes are yours. Other parties have placed inducements on the table to persuade you to agree, making it unappealing to walk from the table. Likewise, to encourage others to accept your offer, you sweeten it with inducements that are hard for them to refuse.

Bad stakes are the adversities that befall you when a deal goes sour: the loss of your job, the imposition of a fine, the closing of your program or department. Depending on what you do at the table, these objectionable fates could be in store for you. In view of these circumstances, staying at the table when threatened with bad stakes can be as painful as walking away. You confront the personal dilemma of choosing between bad options. One choice is to accept your lousy consequences. Another is to retreat to your negotiation hopes and wishes, believing there is some way to forestall the bad outcome, defeat the opponent, and achieve a triumph. Yet this move could propel the negotiation into another spiral of conflict escalation.

Opportunity stakes are the undefined possibilities, for gain or for loss, that could result from the deal. They are revealed to negotiators by questions about what could be or what could have been. Rather than offering direct outcomes, such as "I'll give you $2,000 right now," or, "Here is your program," an opportunity stake is conditional: "If we can develop the program, there is the likelihood that it will generate $2,000." Opportunity stakes are the calculated contingencies and risks that you choose to accept or reject through the negotiation process. These options mature with time, accruing value or disfavor as they evolve. You assess an opportunity stake for perceived risk and reward, asking, what is the likelihood that this transaction will generate the hoped for value, and what will it cost me or how will it distract me in the process?

Opportunity stakes have two sides: the *upside* is improvement and the *downside* is loss. Creation of the program you hoped for is an upside opportunity. The demise of your existing program is a downside loss. An opportunity stake, whether its outcome is up or down, often can only be judged in retrospect and only with a taste of the hypothetical: "If only we had begun the program, we could have been holding $2,000 right now." Or, "We took a risk on the program, and it worked to benefit us all."

Stakes come packaged in mixed blends: a combination of good, bad, and opportunity stakes. You may be required to swallow bad stakes in order to secure the good ones you desire. Upside and downside opportunities mix into the brew, barely seen though always influencing the willingness or reluctance of the parties to swallow the stakes. Seldom are the choices all good or all bad. Often they are arranged to form a combination that is only relatively better or relatively worse for each of the parties.

During the negotiation process, stakes are created, assessed, and exchanged. Creation might take this general form: "If your department extends its hours, we will allot you additional office space." Assessment balances costs and benefits: "The stakes are the gain of added space, along with responsibility for a longer workday." And exchange establishes the deal: "Our department will extend its hours if you will also allot the department a new staff position." The other party balances the combined cost of the square footage and the staff position against the increased revenues from evening hours to decide whether the exchange is reasonable.

How might appreciation for and deliberate calculation of stakes move the negotiation process forward? Stakes become real at the negotiation decision point. They are a spur to settlement. "Before the end of the week, we will either give your department the extra space or give it to someone else. Reject the extra hours, and you lose the space." That is the choice. You accept or you reject the stakes on the table, good and bad. You assess the risks of the opportunity stakes: what are the odds that they will land in your favor, and what are the odds they won't?

Whether good or bad, there can be a reluctance to accept stakes. Especially when the stakes are lousy, negotiators may deny the actual choices in their effort to avoid what may be less than hoped for or bad consequences. They may need time to concede what they do not want to give up, while they test the limits to determine if the stakes are real. There is an acceptance period, sometimes of seconds and sometimes of years, while the parties learn to live with the facts of the outcome. The deal is consummated when both parties accept the stakes for what they are.

Negotiation, then, is a process of learning, molding, and accepting the stakes.

It was not a good meeting.

Iris Inkwater, Perry Pudolski (Oppidania Medical Center's chief operating officer), and Rajeev Rao (its chief financial officer) walk to the Rosebud restaurant across the street from the Community Health Plan (CHP) offices to grab a cup of coffee and debrief themselves. They have just finished their first round of negotiations with Nathaniel Norquist and his crew at CHP. They settle into the protective seclusion of a booth before they let go.

Rao is steaming. "They've got us against the wall. I don't see any room to maneuver with what they've put on the table."

Inkwater is subdued, staring blankly at her cup. "There is no way we're going to come out of this looking anything like what we look like now."

Pudolski echoes her tone. "Yes, call it 'reorganization,' 'right-sizing,' or whatever—they are all euphemisms for layoffs."

"The problem is that we're at a competitive disadvantage," Rao offers. "Because of our location and our patient mix, our costs are simply higher than our competition's. Putting us on the same scale with the suburban outfits is simply comparing apples and oranges."

"Well, unfortunately," Inkwater counters, "community responsibility doesn't carry much weight these days, guys. If our rivals can do it for less, then they're going to get the business."

"What's your sense of where we need to go, Iris?" Pudolski asks, with resignation.

Inkwater tries to summon optimism. "We have to rethink the hospital. Obviously we're going to have to look at some major budget reductions. And nothing can be off-limits anymore. We have to have the guts to face up to personnel cuts, and I mean a serious assessment of each department. And we're going to have to look into cooperative options or maybe even a merger with other hospitals as well. Wow, I thought we dodged that bullet fifteen years ago." Inkwater stares down at her coffee cup. It is a stunning realization.

She continues, with measured determination, "The problem is that, as an expensive, inner-city hospital, we don't have much leverage. That means that we're probably looking more at a takeover than a consolidation. In that case the three of us can expect to pack our bags and say good-bye. They'll have no need for us. After all, how many CEOs, COOs, and CFOs do you need in one organization? But ultimately that option will be up to our board—and the board of whichever organization finds us attractive."

Pudolski sees his career, his aspirations, and his mortgage payments flash before his eyes. He had been on the hospital administration fast track. The move to Oppidania Medical Center (OMC) had been a big career leap for him. He knew at the time that it might be risky joining a facility like OMC, but he also knew that the risk came with a substantial upside. Now it looks like his worst fears may be realized. Still, he isn't ready to give up hope. "I don't think we should throw in the towel yet, Iris." He is not sure whether his optimism is just wishful thinking.

"Oh, Perry, don't get me wrong. I'm not giving up." The implicit support of her friend and colleague is cheering. "I'm just saying that this is serious business. OMC has to survive for a whole list of good reasons. And if we begin this process by excluding a set of reasonable options, then we're not going to find the key to the puzzle. That's scary. It's scary for the hospital, it's scary for our staff and the people we serve, and it's scary for us. It's going to take a lot of courage and a lot of leadership on our part. In the long run, I believe that is how we are going to be judged—for our courage. I just don't think we have any choice. We have to consider all the options."

"Such as?" Rao asks.

"Such as, we come out 'leaner and greener,'" Inkwater counters, with building confidence. "Rajeev, in principle we have to turn around some of the numbers—even if it is only to be attractive for a merger or takeover. We have to look at real costs and real production." New possibilities make their way into her thinking. "That means we may have to become something less than a full-service hospital in order to be of service at all. We have to reconsider what we do and how we go about doing it. We can contract out more services to reduce expenses: moving to vendors may help us stretch the budget. We'll have to renegotiate our fiduciary relationship with some of the physician groups. And if we are to have any credibility, we'll have to tighten things up administratively."

Pudolski joins in. "Fred's not going to like it, but we will also have to seriously look at some of the medical departments in terms of volume, real costs, and income. Our mission to be a comprehensive medical center may have outlived its utility. We are not the only show in town. It may make sense to explore joint arrangements for high-tech procedures. We are dropping a ton of money into machines that get outmoded well before we pay down their cost."

"Yes, although you don't want to throw away our big moneymakers," Rao says. "Several of those high-tech and high-profile procedures can keep us profitable for a long time. And the medical school won't like us tinkering with their tidy little playhouse."

"Rajeev, that's why we need your in-depth interpretation of the numbers and their implications. Many of the departments have survived on illusions about their income and expenses. And the medical school is going to have to live with a big chunk of us, which is much better than no chunk at all. They have to realize that they are a partner in this with us and not an adversary. The game has new rules now."

"Iris, what do you realistically see as the odds of our pulling out of this?" Pudolski asks.

"If we buckle down, I actually think they're pretty good. If we don't, we can turn the building into artist lofts, and we'll all take up painting," she jokes as they leave the restaurant and head back to the hospital.

Negotiation Claimers and Creators

One way to think about negotiators is to divide them into these two types: claimers and creators (Raiffa, 1982).

Claimers engage in the negotiation process in order to grab whatever they can for themselves or their constituency. Sometimes it is a matter of gently taking whatever they are able to take. Other times it is more blatant, a game of seizing, appropriating, and plundering. In the mind of the claimer, negotiation is a means of accumulation. It is not about fairness, evenhandedness, or justice. Negotiation is a sport of conquest, domination, and winning. It is distributional: "The more others get, the less I get; and I want to get as much as possible for myself."

Creators engage in the negotiation process as an inventive learning exercise. For them it is a means of forging linkages between parties sharing a linked destiny. By building relationships, creators are able to coordinate efforts, enhance resource expansion, and spur inventiveness. Negotiation becomes an entrepreneurial venture through which the parties discover that by working together, each will have more to share and more to divide. Satisfaction with the process and with their relationship generates rewarding opportunities for future cooperation.

Whether creator or claimer, you negotiate in order to improve your lot: you want to get something. Your willingness to engage and remain in the process depends on your belief that there is something to be gained for the effort.

In Chapter One we discussed the Prisoner's Dilemma and the application of game theory to real-life negotiations. Players exchange *X*'s and *Y*'s over an opaque wall; when combined and calculated these *X*'s and *Y*'s translate into positive or negative benefit for each side. *X* reflects the claimer strategy and *Y* reflects the creator strategy. How do different mixes of strategies determine outcome patterns?

Consider two teams of negotiators: Tom and Tina (Team T) and Bill and Beth (Team B). Their negotiation outcome is reported as the score each achieves in the exchanges.

What if the Team T players are consistent claimers and the Team B players are consistent creators? While Team B is naively building a friendly relationship across the wall, Team T is grabbing points shamelessly. Team T does not care about relationships, and the players on Team B eventually discover that they have been futilely attempting a constructive linkage while losing their negotiation points. Team T reaps abundant spoils from the negotiation, and Team B is left with nothing. When creators negotiate with claimers—and the creators do not change their style—then the creators are most likely to lose in the process.

What if Team T and Team B are both claimers? Then each comes out with negative scores. Each invests tremendous effort in beating the other and they both lose. In the process of claiming, the two expend time, energy, and resources that otherwise could be divided as the spoils of mutual effort. In the real world of a claimer-claimer contest, calculate total assets, including tangibles divided, such as money, space, and property, along with intangibles lost, such as time, opportunities, and satisfaction. Claimers view a negotiation as a win-lose proposition, and they invest ample resources in attempting to ensure their win. When both teams are claimers, their combined investment, when measured against the total resources they could divide, represents their losses. In addition the experience of the negotiation itself is a liability. The resentment and desire for revenge besieging both teams make future accommodation less likely. This is particularly true when those on Team T and Team B are colleagues working in the same organization.

What if Team T and Team B are both creators? They combine their strategies and efforts to achieve a mutually beneficial outcome. The back-and-forth of the negotiation becomes an opportunity for valuable learning, discovery, and trust building. In the real world their new relationship is an added dividend of the process. Negotiators cultivate new settlement options, discern hidden prospects, and devise otherwise unapparent solutions. The mutual satisfaction that results from each negotiation breakthrough spurs them to further resourcefulness. They build a synergy of ideas, solutions, and benefits.

The claimer-creator distinction reveals the negotiation template you bring to the process. It defines your fundamental approach to other people and the elements you are exchanging. Are you a giver, a taker, or a sharer? What values, code of conduct, and principles guide you?

So too, the claimer-creator distinction reveals the template your negotiation counterparts bring to the table. By understanding their negotiation style and strategy, you are able to analyze and even predict their approach and attitude to ideas and proposals. This insight is invaluable, particularly when you must frequently negotiate with the same people.

Negotiation Outcomes

How do these different claimer and creator strategies combine to affect negotiation outcomes: zero-sum, negative-sum, and positive-sum results?

Imagine that Tom and Beth work in the same office. Each is doing a project that requires five marbles. There are only five marbles in the office and it is not possible to bring in additional marbles.

They have a *zero-sum* outcome when they divide the marbles so that if Tom gets four then Beth only gets one, or if Beth gets five then Tom gets zero. They start with five marbles and they end with five marbles. Nothing was gained and nothing was lost in the negotiation, a zero-sum outcome.

They have a *negative-sum* outcome when they decide to split the marbles in half. Each of them gets two and a half marbles. They started with five marbles, but because a divided marble is worthless, they have only four workable marbles at the end. Or worse, if the negotiation is so rancorous that they destroy three marbles as they go back and forth, then they will have started with five marbles and have only two in the end. These are examples of negative-sum negotiation.

They achieve a *positive-sum* outcome when they negotiate what they are each trying to accomplish and what they require to do it. They discover that Tom needs all five marbles and he does his work each morning from nine o'clock until noon. Beth also requires all five marbles for her project but does her work from one in the afternoon until four. They agree that Tom will get the five marbles in the morning and Beth will get them in the afternoon. They have taken five marbles and achieved ten marbles of benefit. This illustrates a positive-sum outcome because taken together they have more in the end than when they started.

The positive-sum outcome resulted from Tom and Beth's willingness to engage as negotiation creators. When they were both claimers, they achieved a negative-sum outcome. And if there was an imbalance in their claimer-creator strategy and impetus, one received more than the other. If, for example, Beth was concerned about Tom's feelings and did not want to upset him, she could have allowed him the majority of the marbles.

In zero-sum negotiation, nothing is gained or lost in the process: the sum of available resources remains the same though the distribution may be unequal. In negative-sum negotiation, the destructive process of bargaining causes a reduction in resources available. In positive-sum negotiation, the constructive process of learning has a multiplier effect on the use of and availability of resources.

Generating Options

Trust is the foundation on which negotiation rests. Relationships are the glue that holds it together as it evolves. And imagination supplies the wings on which it flies.

An inventive imagination is among the most important qualities of the very best negotiators. When people begin a negotiation, the eventual outcome is yet a mystery: they might become frustrated and descend into bickering; they might achieve only a partly effective outcome; they might attain a solution far exceeding their original expectations. Who knows? Their result derives from their combined negotiation frames and their interpersonal skills along with the resonance of their interactions. Without imagination, it is unlikely that they will conjure up much more than the mundane and the self-evident. However, when each brings ingenuity, curiosity, and resourcefulness to the process, they can uncover otherwise unanticipated solutions and opportunities. They can combine intellectual and interpersonal risk taking with pragmatic creativity to envision new solutions. They can understand the possibilities and limits of what might be done and how to make it happen. They are creators in the best sense of the word.

For those with imagination, negotiation itself becomes an opportunity for invention. Problems are puzzles. The thrill of negotiation derives from the parties' esprit de corps as they work at shifting the pieces to find a better fit. Courage inspires the parties to ascend above the common thinking that the puzzle can't be effectively solved. Courage is particularly important for people or groups that are in conflict. It takes imagination to envision rapprochement, and it takes will power to make it happen. When imaginative negotiation clicks, the reward is innovation of the highest order.

In classes, we ask our students to do the arm wrestling exercise. We give them the following instructions: "You know, we've been doing a lot of talking. How about a bit of physical exercise? I'd like you to link up with the person sitting next to you in an arm wrestling position. Your task, in thirty seconds, is to get the back of the hand of the other person down as many times as possible. Count how many times you get it down. Wait until I say, 'Go.' " We pause for five seconds and then shout, "Go!"

A majority of the students begin zealously pushing against one another. The arm muscles flex, the faces contort, and often they become locked and immobilized, unable to budge one another. When we shout, "Stop," they sit back in uncomfortable resignation. They have struggled.

Other students, after the shout of "Go," start rapidly swinging their arms back and forth. They are having a great time. Their pace intensifies over the thirty seconds. When we shout, "Stop," they laugh.

Once the room has calmed down, we ask, "How many people have gotten 5 points or less?" Most of the students raise their hands. Then we go around the room asking the students who raised their hands, "How many did you get?" We hear, "I got 1"; "I got zero"; "I got 3."

Then we ask "How many people have gotten 5 points or more?" With glee, those around the room who engaged in rapid back-and-forth movement shoot their hands into the air. This time when we go around the room, we hear, "We got 50"; "We got 36"; "We got 100!"

What happened? Those who saw the exercise as a contest—the negotiation claimers—heard the phrase "arm wrestling position" and assumed the game to be a win-lose proposition. They positioned themselves to get as many points as possible for themselves and to deny points to their opponent. Their productivity was very low, their arms became sore in the process, and they were unlikely to want to repeat the competition in the future. Of greatest significance, everyone who played the game as a contest reported his or her score as what "I got."

By contrast, those who viewed the game as a *whole image negotiation* viewed the person with whom they were paired with the attitude "you want to get the back of my hand down and I want to get the back of your hand down." They recognized their interdependence in achieving a shared objective. This realization required imagination, because most people who hear "arm wrestling position" ready themselves for a contest between themselves and their paired opponent, rather than a team activity with their paired partner. Those who saw it as a team activity played to obtain mutual benefit: first they waved their arms in one direction so one person got a point and then they quickly waved their arms in the other direction so the other person got a point. Of greatest significance, in achieving a whole image negotiation outcome, they uniformly reported their scores in terms of *we*, not *I*.

It takes a potent imagination to discover this better option. Generating creative negotiation opportunities requires widening the parties' palette of choices for selecting a mutually acceptable settlement or outcome. When incorporated into the negotiation process, imagination sparks the ingenuity of the human spirit. It replaces the fear of losing with the hope of achievement. It is fear that provokes the claimer. It is hope that inspires the creator.

Stuart Schilling has been with Oppidania Medical Center for nearly nine years. A philosopher by training, he translated his interest in applied philosophy and health care into a career in medical bioethics. He divides his time between teaching at the medical school and meeting as needed with staff, patients, and families at the hospital. He has gained the respect of the hospital staff as a good listener and inspired problem solver.

The request for this afternoon's meeting came earlier in the day from Tanya Tarrington, head nurse on Nine West, a general medical floor. The problem, as she had earlier explained to Schilling, is a difference of opinion regarding a do not resuscitate (DNR) order for an elderly gentleman who has been on the floor for more than two weeks. The internist and the cardiologist who have been working with the patient disagree on whether a DNR order is appropriate. Tarrington is concerned about the mixed signals the family is getting, and both physicians have agreed that a bioethics consult is a good idea. Schilling and Tarrington have decided that at this point, it would be best to include themselves, the two physicians, and a social worker who has been working with the family.

Victor Vining is the cardiologist who has been attending the patient, Mr. Ulrich, who was admitted with a myocardial infarction. Wendell White is the internist; he has been following Mr. Ulrich since a previous hospitalization, two years ago, with pneumonia. Ziva Zartman is the social worker who has been seeing the patient and family from the start of the current admission.

The five professionals have gathered in a brightly decorated consultation room usually used for meetings between care teams and the families of patients. Dr. White speaks first. He explains that Mr. Ulrich, a seventy-eight-year-old male, is a patient with nine lives. When he had pneumonia, the staff thought he wouldn't make it and he pulled through marvelously. Since then he has suffered an aneurysm and a severe infection in his foot. After each bout, he has recovered to return to his cherished game of golf. Dr. White concludes that it's simply too early to write this patient off.

Vining waits for his colleague to finish and then presents his opinion on the case. He reports that Mr. Ulrich had been conscious, though very weak, for the first few days of his hospitalization. Vining quotes the patient's remarks: "Doctor, if this can't work, I don't want heroics. This could be it for me." Vining goes on to delineate the patient's medical condition, which, he concludes, is grim. Given the circumstances of the case and the real costs for the hospital, Vining feels it is irresponsible not to recommend that the family sign a DNR order.

Ziva Zartman speaks next. She describes the torment facing the family. She agrees with Dr. White: Mr. Ulrich's previous miraculous recoveries have instilled a sense of hope in them. Yet they also feel that this illness is different. She goes on to explain that they are so distraught and confused that they have pleaded with her just to get a clear recommendation from the medical staff. Mr. Ulrich's daughter has said that the family just can't bear facing an unclear set of choices. Mr. Ulrich, oddly enough, never made a living will, and neither his wife nor the children know what to do.

Tanya Tarrington is the final speaker. She agrees with Dr. White that Mr. Ulrich truly is a miracle patient who has repeatedly defied the odds. She remembers him from two years ago, and how at the time it had seemed unlikely that he would survive. She ordinarily wouldn't be optimistic about a patient as sick as Mr. Ulrich, though there are enough surprises in his medical chart to make her unusually cautious. The problem for the hospital, she explains, is that he is too sick to be discharged to a nursing home. In all honesty, she adds, his continued hospitalization is a financial drain on the hospital. Realistically, they can't ignore the financial consequences of their recommendation.

Schilling first asks for clarification on some points, and then begins his work. Even though the issue of whether to seek a DNR order has been presented as a yes or no decision, he perceives a range of other options for the team to consider.

Schilling scans the table, making eye contact with each of the participants. "Well, it seems to me that this is one of those difficult cases in which we end up making a decision even if we don't. If we can't decide on whether to recommend the DNR, then that is a decision de facto with clear implications, as Tanya has explained. On one hand, we do not want to put the patient and family through unnecessary suffering and the hospital through unnecessary expense. On the other hand, if there is hope for recovery, we don't want to give up prematurely."

As a rule, Schilling doesn't tell people what to do. He sees his role as helping the responsible parties make their own decision.

He turns to Dr. White. "Wendell, as things stand right now, you are reluctant to recommend the DNR. What could happen, or what might you learn, that would change your mind?" The question reframes White's thinking, away from the stance of defending Mr. Ulrich's survival. He shares several clinical indicators, changes over a specific period of time. He adds that if the family members have a change in attitude, if they become willing to give up, that would be an important factor for him: first, because he would want to comply with their wishes and, second, because it would relieve him of any concerns regarding a lawsuit down the road.

Schilling next turns to Vining. He asks, "Victor, what would convince you not to recommend the DNR?" Vining likewise is prompted to reconsider his position in favor. He points to clinical indicators similar to those offered by White. He also wants to be sensitive to the family's wishes and notes that they seem to be reacting more to their grief than to the medical realities facing the patient. He also reminds the group that Mr. Ulrich may have realized that he has reached the end of his road. Tarrington, White, and Zartman each say that until Vining mentioned it, they were unaware of the patient's remark about giving up. Vining is surprised; he thought the patient had shared his sentiments with others at the hospital.

Schilling breaks the silence as each of the people at the table rethinks his or her approach to the case. "It seems that there are three factors here: time, clinical indicators, and the family." He goes through each factor individually. They agree that forty-eight hours is a reasonable waiting period in order to monitor the clinical indicators and determine whether there is improvement or decline. The clinical indicators they will watch for are acceptable to both White and Vining. If there is improvement or status quo, then a DNR order will not be recommended. If there is a decline in the patient's condition, they will recommend that the family sign a DNR order. The group agrees that Zartman will discuss this decision with the family today, explaining to them that the hospital wants to feel certain that the most appropriate and sensitive recommendation is being made. If the family members decide to ask for a DNR order before the waiting period is up, they may do so. If they want to hold out longer, an extension not to exceed three days will be acceptable. Both White and Vining agree that this is a reasonable approach.

"Stuart, thank you for making yourself available on such short notice," Tarrington says. The meeting breaks up and Zartman heads back to Mr. Ulrich's room to meet with the family.

From the monumental to the mundane, the multiparty decisions that you face in health care are by their nature complex. The decision-making models you employ shape the quality of your choices. Collaborative models offer opportunities to build a wealth of constructive options from which you and others can choose. Especially when there is conflict, you can improve outcomes by engaging those involved to generate together a range of settlement options. This creative approach enhances both the processes of your endeavors as well as the outcomes you achieve.

The rapid pace of change in health policy, business, science, technology, and population demographics demands those working in the system to frequently modify and adapt what they are doing. Comfortable work patterns in a health care organization must change in line with these external pressures. At times the long-standing frames used to orchestrate working relationships must be adjusted. How does one lead, negotiate, and reframe these changes so that in both process and substance, they are added value and not a troubling distraction for your health organization?

CHAPTER 6

REFRAMING TO SPUR MOMENTUM

YOU PERFORM many roles as a negotiator. You get, give, teach, learn, guide, motivate, and instigate. And when the negotiation hits a standstill, there is another vital role to play: you and others become champions for a reframing of what all the parties are doing and are trying to accomplish (see Bazerman & Neale, 1992; Stulberg, 1987; Mayer, 2000).

In the previous chapter, we described a classic game theory puzzle, the arm wrestling exercise. Most of the pairs employ an adversarial frame when engaging in this task. They push at one another for the allotted thirty seconds and achieve low scores through their interactions. Other pairs develop a collaborative frame and spend the time furiously swinging back and forth. They achieve a high number of points and uniformly report their score as a joint endeavor.

Yet other pairs begin with an adversarial frame, and then midway through the exercise they reframe their strategy in a collaborative frame. Their explanations for this reframing provide valuable parallels to the problems and processes for encouraging change and adaptation in health organizations.

Some of the individuals in these pairs recognize together and on their own that they are achieving little when they are locked in a stalemate. They look at one another and say, in one form or another, "This makes no sense," and spontaneously start swinging back and forth. This aha moment also occurs in organizations when mutual frustration leads to constructive discussion, providing the impetus for reframing and change. Others among the pairs who started out pushing at one another notice people close by furiously rocking their arms back and forth. As a result they change their strategy too and copy what they observe. This is an example of importing outside ideas and strategies to advance organizational learning.

Perhaps the most poignant story was told by a young, petite nurse in one of our sessions who found herself arm wrestling with an older, burly, prominent surgeon whom she had never before met. She explained after the exercise:

> I looked at this clearly strong and powerful gentleman and realized that there was no way I could out-muscle him and no way I could argue convincingly to have him let me pin his arm as easily as he would pin mine. So, when the exercise began, I went limp and let him get the first point. He looked at me quizzically and we went back to the up position, and again I went limp and let him get a point. This time he seemed even more perplexed, as if he was here for a rough-and-tumble arm wrestle and I would not engage. Realizing that I could not talk him through a change, I looked him straight in the eye, which puzzled him even more. In that moment, he somehow saw me for who I was and released the pressure on my hand. I slowly began directing both our arms back and forth. And then he shouted out on his own, "Oh, I get it," and he started investing the same strength and energy in getting us to move back and forth as he earlier put into trying to beat me. I knew from the outset that he had more muscle power than me and that if this was a mere test of strength, I would have no chance of succeeding. I also knew that for him to change, I had to let him figure it out for himself. That realization couldn't come from me. So I let him have those two points and then I let him figure it out from there. We nurses do that all the time. This is how we get things done in the hospital.

As this young nurse told her story, everyone else in the room was transfixed. It was an example of how less powerful yet knowledgeable people in health organizations wield influence to leverage and reframe the opinions and actions of those who might not otherwise pay attention.

At the break in the seminar the surgeon reflected on his experience. "That was among the most profound moments in my life," he said, in a tone that was both humble and genuine. "I never really appreciated that I do that to people. I see the world as one big contest and I always fight to win no matter what. I was blind to this young woman who sat before me. She was just an obstacle to overcome. Wow."

At times the most persuasive method for encouraging a reframe is to create the conditions under which people—through logical analysis and conclusion—can discover it on their own. As the young nurse explained, there are many who have learned this lesson and who routinely use this strategy.

Why Reframe?

Given the volatile environment in which health care operates, change is ever present. The partner of pressure for change is resistance to change. This is an often told story in health care. The resistance to adoption of electronic health records is just one example of the United States lagging far behind other industrialized countries in advancing technology that can improve quality, increase safety, and lower the costs of care. Numerous obstacles have arisen to impede progress on this topic. Why would reframing be important for this and other challenges that face the health system?

In Chapter One, we presented the dilemma of the cone in the cube, with different people looking at the same object through different peepholes and arriving at very different conclusions about what they see. When their field of vision is narrow—proscribed by the confined hole through which they peer—their decisions and conclusions are likewise narrowly limited. In the high stakes world of health care, with so much at stake—one's career or professional reputation, the budget, legal safeguards, and proficiency—parties often retreat to the comfortable corner of what is known and predictable. Changing one's purview has its risks.

The process of reframing requires people to become curious. Perhaps their view is obscured. Perhaps there is more to be known and understood. Perhaps the options are not as frightening as first feared. Reframing is what encourages parties to accumulate more information, question their assumptions, and consider a wider set of options. They begin to see their problem from a multidimensional rather than unidimensional or two-dimensional viewpoint. Through reframing, the parties transform fundamental elements of their cognitive outlook to seek common ground. They reassess and adjust perceptions and attitudes about the people, problems, history, strategies, outcomes, priorities, and stakes of the negotiation. They seek compatibility.

When parties engage one another with incongruent frames, the negotiation assumes a predictable tone of sluggishness and erosion. For example, progress on other substantive issues is jeopardized when there is basic disagreement about who should be at the table. When irreconcilable suspicion about the true history of the dispute remains, then veiled obstacles deter acceptance of new interpretations. And when the priorities of one party are incompatible with those of another, then the parties are defending divergent purposes at the table. What can be done to overcome these predicaments?

Oscar Ortiz, Artie Ashwood's nurse, had quickly perceived the tension between Artie's mother, Anna, and his girlfriend, Cindy Carrington. Now, hearing loud voices coming from Artie's room, he quickly makes his way to check what is going on.

The shouting suddenly stops when Oscar appears at the door and he notices that all three people are looking expectantly at him. He jumps into the silence. "Is there a problem?" Artie's mother and girlfriend exchange icy glances and then look away.

Artie opens the conversation. "There seems to be a bit of disagreement about where I go tomorrow when I'm discharged. Mom wants me to recover at home, and Cindy wants me at, well, our home. Quite frankly, I'm feeling torn."

"Well, you're already torn up enough, my friend. There's no need to do more damage," Oscar says, hoping his smile will lighten the mood. "Are we talking about where you're living long term, or just for your recuperation?"

"I assume we're talking recuperation," Artie replies. Cindy and Anna are both quiet, allowing this conversation to remain between patient and nurse. Artie turns toward the two women, looking for agreement. They both nod reluctantly.

Oscar continues. "Having hung around this room quite a lot for the past few days, I've gotten the impression that there is not a lot that the two of you think you agree about."

There was a pause, and then Cindy meekly replied, "I guess you could say that."

"Well, in fact, I've found there is one very important thing that you do agree on." Oscar lights up with an ear-to-ear grin and points to Artie. "You both think this fellow here is the most lovable guy in the universe."

The two women sheepishly glance at one another, and unable to restrain themselves, they smile as well. "Now, I do agree he's a nice guy, but I'm not sure I'd go to war over him," Oscar says with an exaggerated wink.

There is suddenly a different feel in the room. The edge is off: there is a sense of relief. Oscar lets the silence linger a few moments so that the harmony can take root.

"Artie's still quite sick. I mean, this guy gets applause for just getting out of bed and taking a hike around the nurses station. It's going to take him a week before he feels well enough to move around on his own. The question here is not where he's going to live for the rest of his life. The question is where can he get the best care for the next few days?"

Artie is tempted to jump in but is afraid that whatever he might say will refuel the fire. Finally Cindy opens up, addressing Oscar. "I guess the problem is that I just started a new job and don't have any time off. If he comes back to our place, he will be alone for most of the day. Artie's mom has a lot of vacation time built up, so she could be with him during the day." Cindy turns toward Anna. "The problem is, I don't want to say good-bye to Artie for the week, but I don't feel comfortable when I'm at your place."

Anna thinks for a moment. Suddenly, a smile opens on her face and her sense of relief is obvious. She places her hand on Cindy's. "I want you to come, and I want you to feel comfortable." She surprises herself just as much as she surprises Cindy.

Oscar has done just enough to turn things around—to reframe the conversation. He gets a thumbs-up from Artie as he leaves the room.

The very exercise of reframing opens a path toward resolution. By devising fresh agreement on elements of their frames, the parties begin movement that nudges them to generate opportunities for settlement. In so doing, they discover that more complementary preferences, information, and hopes yield them better results. They need not agree on each other's perceptions, though they can acknowledge their differences. They need not abandon their objectives, though they might adjust them to enhance compatibility. They are creating a new balance between their distinct concerns.

How do you get the reframing process started? Interrupt the antagonism. Vary the rhythm of the negotiation: say something unexpected; bring in an outside neutral; place new consequences on the table; tell a joke; present a new offer for consideration; invite your enemy out to lunch or for a *walk in the woods*. Unfreeze the cognitive ice jam.

If you are the one who needs to supply the impetus, open with a question, an observation, or a concern. "What do you hope to accomplish?" "I think we're stuck." "Without some progress, we all lose." Trigger curiosity.

Crafting a Fit

Negotiation and conflict resolution is the art of shaping congruity from incongruity.

Incongruity is the condition where the pieces of your puzzle do not fit together or do not fit together well. You want one thing: it can't be had. Expectation diverges from reality. Incongruity is rooted in a mind-set. It impedes reasoning and the ability to imagine new or different options. It is the frustration felt when the world does not seem to make sense. It is the dissonance experienced when good people act in self-serving ways; when good health care is not available for all those who need it; when others in the room don't appreciate the brilliance of what you propose. It is the apprehension that pieces of your life or work are supposed to add up and they do not. It is that discomfort endured when logic disappears. It is the panic suffered when unfairness overwhelms. Incongruity can take you to your instinctual basement.

When experienced in private, incongruity is evidenced by discomfort and confusion. When it comes between people, it manifests as conflict. You naturally resist incongruity in your life, and the people who raise it. The confusion and discord are fantasized away. You want to defeat the opposition.

How do you change your frame of mind? How do you move from fighting incongruity to accepting it when there is no choice? How do you evolve from enduring incongruity to cultivating congruity? A fundamental shift in frame of mind is required.

Reframing in Health Care

The move from framing on the basis of incongruity to reframing in search of congruity produces a pivotal shift in the negotiation process: it changes the premise for the conduct of working relationships. Rather than going to the table with a posture ready to demand and compete—the win-lose strategy—you approach it seeking solutions that further the opportunity to find a gain-gain outcome. Rather than defeating the other side, you hear and respond to their legitimate interests. You reshape the assumptions for engaging one another. You seek connection, relationship, and fit.

Health care work bursts with incongruity. It operates in the realm of highly charged problems and questions that often elude unambiguous solutions. The domain of one specialization overlaps and sometimes conflicts with another: who owns what part of the body? Money is not always allocated in ways that maximize its impact on the population: do we treat disease or prevent it? Patient care decision-making authority is given to people without direct clinical involvement: will the cost of care be covered by the patient's insurance? There is concern for liability, reputation, and professional autonomy. And when the system is embroiled in health policy, business, technological, workforce, and demographic changes, unknowns and incongruities can be overwhelming.

The divisions that emerge from the resulting confusion often manifest as adversarial confrontations that yield winners and losers. This pattern is so ingrained in the operation of health care that some believe it is the best way to operate. Pieces of the system battle to save and promote themselves, making the operation as a whole even more illogical, incongruous, and disjointed.

Devising a more compatible balance is essential to creating a better system. Your capacity to lead and to achieve that balance depends on the methods used to get there: product arises from process. There are essential methods and tools for negotiators to master: changing language to reframe, communicating through listening, communicating through responding and engaging, applying negotiation jujitsu, allowing for negotiation face-saving, understanding negotiation ripeness, using a negotiation map, and engaging humor, which when it works serves as negotiation lubrication. Once engrained in your negotiating personality, these ways of being describe the talents and insights you bring to the process.

Changing Language to Reframe

The substance of a negotiation is framed and reframed by the words you choose, the way you arrange them, the way you deliver them, what filters of the other person they pass through, and how the other person responds. With a simple change of one word for another, you can convey a different meaning and frame to what you say and to how it is understood. The word to change is *but*.

Remove the word *but* from your vocabulary and replace it with the word *and*. This small yet profound change can reframe what you say, think, and do, forming a congruity of thought and conclusion. More important, it will reframe the way others understand and respond to what you are saying as you remove contradiction from your speech.

For example, "I wanted to attend the staff meeting, *but* I could not," is an incongruous statement: first you say *yes* and then you say *no*. There is a subtle yet important difference in meaning when you say, "I wanted to attend the staff meeting, *and* I could not." Rather than expressing two opposing drives, you combine two desires that regrettably had to be balanced. You express two statements that correspond to one another. In place of a defense for your absence, you offer an explanation: "A new patient was admitted and there was no one else to do the workup." If your intention to otherwise attend the meeting is trusted, the *and* that connects your two obligations will prompt a much different reaction from your colleagues than a *but*. Their anger and their disappointment will be allayed. They will more readily accept that you had a difficult set of expectations to balance.

Substituting *and* for *but* is subtle. Try inserting it into your speech pattern: when you say *and*, the reaction to what you say will be transformed. You will build connection between divergent statements. Try it in a negotiation: "I would love to give you additional office space, *and* I just don't have it." Follow the statement with an exploration of the other party's interests: is there a way to satisfy the person's needs within the limitations of the square footage you do have? You reframe the negotiation from territorialism to a quest to satisfy legitimate interests. If the two halves of the sentence were linked by *but*, there would be an implication of lesser worth, disregard, imbalance, and favoritism. The statement "but I just don't have it" has a ring of finality to it; the answer is no.

It works both ways: "I do understand that you can't shift offices now *and* that limits the productivity of our unit." You have acknowledged the limitations facing the other party as you reveal the consequences of those limitations. If there is mutual concern about reduced potential and productivity, then you have opened the door to finding solutions. You have reframed the discussion from a no to a common desire to find a solution for a shared problem. If instead of *and* you used *but*, it would sound as though you were posing a threat: "but that limits the productivity of our unit." The other party might react defensively.

Incorporating the word *and* into your speech reframes your search for congruity. You balance pieces of your puzzle to seek compatibility in place of confrontation. You accept real limitations and creatively explore the field of available innovative options. You recognize that not all interests of all parties can be fully satisfied. You seek solutions that allow all the parties reasonable gains from the negotiation process, and you put more items on the table rather than removing them.

Communicating Through Listening

Negotiation is a form of expression. Through what is said and done, negotiators reveal their objectives. They disclose their concerns. They signal consequences. They divulge information. They suggest alternatives. And they clarify misinterpretations.

There is a wealth of valuable information to be exchanged during a negotiation, but frequently this information is lost. The parties are not listening to each other. They are so taken with their next line, their overriding apprehension, and their compelling emotion, that they don't pay attention. Both their brains and their ears are in the basement. They frustrate others who feel unable to get through to them. The people speaking expect a mindful response to what they are saying, and the other party is preoccupied.

Negotiation is most important as a form of communication. It is a teaching tool. It requires exchange of information. Yet often one side becomes impatient when the other side disregards offers, concerns, and suggestions. The people on the first side feel belittled and disenfranchised, and they don't like it. They become reluctant to continue.

When the parties are not actively listening to one another, they are likely to reach an impasse. What is being said by one is not being heard by the other. It is not integrated into the building of better options. The parties are not creating an exchange of information. Frustration grows. How can you and the others better pay attention? The answer lies in *active listening*.

Active listening is a dynamic process for hearing and responding. It requires some measure of intentional and expressive repeating, reflecting, and reacting to what the other person says. You demonstrate to others that what they are saying is penetrating, that you are working with the information they are sharing. Active listening requires effort. You substantiate your interest in devising a workable solution by engaging with other people around the table.

Active listening means you assimilate and synthesize what you are hearing. Your responses begin with formulations such as, "Let me be certain that I understand what you are saying." From there, you have a range of possible responses, from agreement to acknowledgment to reflection.

The response you give that is most satisfying to others is repetition of their point and then agreement: for example, "Based on what you have found and what you report, I concur that knee surgery is the best and perhaps only real option in this case." Agreement does not mean that you underrate your concerns. You can agree, and then add your *and* to specify what you desire in return. Or you might simply agree, and by gracefully acknowledging what you learned from the other party, recover a measure of relationship and trust for your next negotiation.

If you do not want to signal agreement, demonstrate concern through acknowledgment: "I appreciate that there is a great deal of anxiety in your department regarding the budget crisis." Acknowledgment is an effective way to calm the other parties without conceding your standpoint. You demonstrate your attention to their concerns without admitting culpability. Likewise, you do not obligate yourself to meet their demands.

Finally, if your disagreement runs so deep that you cannot show even acknowledgment, merely reflect what the other person says: "You seem very concerned about the new admitting procedures." Though you have neither agreed with the statement nor acknowledged it as legitimate, you have nonetheless actively responded to what was said. You have sent at least a signal of recognition.

Listening by itself is rarely considered a form of expression. When negotiating, however, the attention, respect, and recognition you show others is an important means for you to build a wider set of options. It is not merely nodding your head. It is demonstrating to others that you are paying attention, a low-cost yet high-impact way to add value at your negotiation table.

Communicating Through Responding and Engaging

Communication involves both *form* and *intent*. Agreement, acknowledgment, and reflection are forms of reacting to others: how you respond. Intent is the substance of a response: what you mean. Are you merely responding to others' overt statements, or are you stretching further to explore their underlying interests? By attending to underlying interests as well as to form, you open new options for resolution. You signal your intent to engage and satisfy some measure of the other side's expectations.

When you respond to overt requests or demands, you mirror what the other party is asking. You clarify, reiterate, and signal your understanding, as in these examples: "You want the weekend off." "You are unhappy in your current position." "The department is not able to raise your salary." You are not agreeing to the request at this point, though with your response, you allay any concerns the person may have about whether in fact you heard and understood what he or she said.

Responding to underlying interests sends a potent signal that you are receptive and sympathetic. You demonstrate your concern for the breadth of what has been expressed, and you show that you are astute enough to figure it out.

You respond to the process preferences, emotional needs, and substantive expectations that motivate the other person—those key elements of interest-based negotiation discussed in Chapter Four. In response to a request for time off, you might add, "You need time to prepare for your son's birthday." To the employee dissatisfied with his or her position, you might say, "You feel overstressed in the job." And to the boss who has turned down your request for a pay raise, you might reflect back what he said as, "You would like to better compensate me, and the budget won't allow it."

Placing underlying interests on the table opens a new, implicit question: is it possible to find a resolution that satisfies the interests of both or all sides? This question is particularly important when it is impossible to completely satisfy a request: "I can't give you the whole weekend off. I could give you a half day off on both Saturday and Sunday by extending the hours of two other people. I know that you have to shop and prepare, and obviously be there for the party. Which half of each of these days would work best for you?" Here, you maintained your staffing levels while you also offered genuine understanding, concern, and choice to the other person. "The stress you now feel on the job wasn't there three months ago. What's changed, and what might we do to get ourselves back on track?" In this instance, you have established your sincere attention and eagerness to uncover your employee's concerns and suggestions. "I understand that the department is short on cash. Would you be willing to explore other ways to adjust my remuneration?" With these words, you open the door to finding a solution while simultaneously addressing the constraints and hopes of both sides. In each case you are engaging and seeking compatibility in order to balance different interests.

Active listening generates the cadence of negotiation. It sets the tempo and builds hope and momentum. It engages the parties by moving them from exchanging information to exploring interests. In so doing, they forge the impetus for an exchange based on mutual interests, thereby increasing the likelihood that they will be able to consummate their deal.

A cautionary note: active listening backfires when it is interpreted as patronizing, paternalistic, or pandering. If the other person perceives your response as rote, trivial, incredulous, or erroneous, your efforts will only generate further suspicion. Negotiation technique, absent the essential ingredients of trust, sincerity, and integrity, is only technique.

Applying Negotiation Jujitsu

Active listening is relatively sensible in practice during a civilized exchange of ideas, information, and requests. Conflict, however, often involves heated emotions and passions. The dialogue coming your way is rife with anger and aggression. You are assaulted with insult, disparagement, hostility, and scorn. Basement behavior by one person pulls others instinctually down in the same direction. People go into survival mode, and what is barked often further aggravates the situation.

Once in the basement, you go into *flight, fight, or freeze* mode. Your instinctual response is to be self-protective. You may want to run away. You may try to crush the offensive by outdoing it: throwing your opponents an even more scathing insult, crafting an even more ghastly threat, or overpowering with an even more outrageous act. Your impulse is to react, to defend and defeat. Or you may be shocked into stupefying and embarrassing silence. Although these reactions might provide some immediate gratification, comfort, or solace to you, they cause the conflict to escalate. What is the option?

Imagine a fist flying at you. You could attempt to stop or crush it, coping as best you can with the resulting shattering collision. Or you could absorb it: grasp it, hold it, and gently slow it down. In so doing, there is no crash or explosion. This is a gentler landing. Borrowing a term from the martial arts, this has been called *negotiation jujitsu* (Fisher, Ury, & Patton, 1991).

Negotiation jujitsu is a technique for diffusing the tensions and emotions that accompany conflict while keeping you in control of your emotional responses. It serves two purposes. First, it calms the other person, giving him or her a chance to release anger and frustration. The other person likely anticipates that you will strike back. Your response, to patiently listen and understand, surprises and calms the other party. You have opened the door to reframing by doing something unexpected. You create a new frame in which there is regard and respect.

Second, negotiation jujitsu offers you a handy brace. It helps you maintain control of your own emotions and instincts when someone is shouting at you. It helps to get you out of your basement. Negotiation jujitsu keeps you focused and preserves your patience as the other person vents his or her feelings. Imagine using your left hand to absorb the verbal blows directed at you. You may have to do this several times, repeating it as the person cools down. Finally, when the other party has witnessed your willingness to hear and respond, there is more openness to reframing.

After reducing the anxiety and hostility coming from the other side, you are able to offer an alternative frame; imagine this as lifting your right hand, palm up and giving. You have signaled that you are amenable to considering the other person's interests as well as your own. You demonstrate the legitimacy of his concerns as you implicitly ask him to do the same: "I hear you, and I hope you hear me." You have diffused the situation by finding a balance that looks for a mutually beneficial solution. Negotiation jujitsu does not validate that the other side is right or wrong. It merely states that you have clearly heard the other party and you recognize his concerns. And then it allows you to state what is in your power to effect.

Negotiation jujitsu is a form of active listening. It is useful in health care situations where emotions are often deeply passionate. It calms a hysterical parent reacting to a child's illness, dissatisfied employees angry about their assignments, a disgruntled patient frustrated by the cold chicken soup. Instructing the parent to knock it off, telling the employees to get a job elsewhere, and informing the patient that you couldn't care less about the meal: these responses only escalate the situation. You hope to cool passions by remaining cool yourself. An early measure of empathy and attention goes a long way toward preventing what could later become an onerous dispute.

Katherine Knight, the nurse manager of the intensive care unit, senses there is a problem as soon as she enters Janice Johnson's office. Janice, the vice president of nursing, looks pensive and distracted as Katherine takes a seat across the desk from her boss.

Johnson looks down at her desk as if she is reading reports as she speaks. "Katherine, I've been reviewing the budget figures for each of the departments. Your increase from last year on the salary line is 10 percent above other departments. Your overtime is way up from last year, and in reviewing your own time sheets, you personally seem to be spending much less time at the hospital." With that, she looks up and glares at Knight.

Knight is astounded. First, this is not Janice's usual style. Something is terribly wrong. Second, Janice had to know that the staffing issue in the ICU is not an isolated problem, and that it is being addressed with the transfer of Heather

Harriford to the general medical floor. Finally, Janice knows that Katherine's mother had been ill this year and that Katherine had needed time off to take care of her. Janice had approved the leave time. So Johnson's attack hits Knight as unjust micromanagement of a nursing unit. It is wrong.

Knight guesses that something else might be going on: Janice seems to be in the basement. Knight wants to figure out what is really going on. Whatever it is, she does not want to escalate the situation by opening with a challenge to Janice's allegations. Knight descends to the basement herself, takes a deep breath, and counts to herself slowly: "one, two, three." Then, with her wits about her, she takes another deep breath and responds as calmly as she can.

"Janice, I know that our salary figures were up this year. This has been disappointing to me as well, especially given the financial crunch facing the hospital." Having shared a common concern for the problem, she next wants to gain a better understanding of what's going on. Is it possible that there's something of which she is unaware? She continues, "Tell me, were there any particular surprises in the monthly reports that just came out?"

Johnson's tone softens. "No, there were no surprises. It was just that, relatively speaking, your department sticks out like a sore thumb on these accounting sheets."

"That is not good," Knight agrees. "Do you think that with the transfer of Heather Harriford to the medical floor, our salary and fringe benefits line will improve?" She raises the matter gently. She is being careful not to embarrass Janice if the problem is that Janice has overlooked a major staff shift that has not yet shown up on the accounting report.

"Oh, yes, Harriford. That obviously isn't reflected in this report as the transfer is just taking place now. Well, that could bring you more in line."

Knight is relieved that Johnson seems to be reacting to the stresses of the hospital's financial situation rather than trying to micromanage the unit. With that in mind, Knight decides to share some of her activities in order to assure Janice that the financial issues are being handled. "Janice, I am also concerned about the overtime issue. I met yesterday with Charlotte Chung, the triage nurse on the night shift in the emergency department. She is working with Dr. Lumberg and the other physicians in emergency to reassess their protocols for ICU admissions. If we can safely reduce the work load on the night shift, we will be much less dependent on overtime." She continues to fight the urge to tell Johnson to leave the details to her.

Johnson sits back in her chair with a look of retreat. "That's good," she responds, though now even more distracted.

Knight continues. "You remember that my mother has been ill for the past few months. Obviously, it has been an enormous strain for me and my family, and it had to affect the department to some extent as well. People have been great, very supportive. Anyway, she's back home now, and my father is pretty much able to take care of her. I should be back on my regular schedule next week."

"Oh, yes, I'm sorry. I forgot about your mother. Is she feeling better?"

"Miraculously, yes. She needed a total hip replacement and she was quite depressed. She's doing better now, thanks."

Johnson changes her tone, becoming more reflective. "I don't know what we are going to do, Katherine. I have to find someplace to cut our costs; I mean significantly. I am searching for some easy problems to fix. The department simply does not have much room to give. After our last round of cuts, we are pretty much down to bare bones."

"You have to know that your unit heads are behind you," Knight replies. "This is tough for all of us. You can use us. If we each in our own little way can contribute something, the combination could be significant for the hospital as a whole."

The meeting ends on an upbeat note. Knight has reframed the discussion. She has taken it from confrontation to collaboration. And in the process, the two leaders have gained much more with which to work.

Allowing Negotiation Face-Saving

One of the parties in a negotiation declares an ultimatum and draws a line in the sand. Preposterous conditions are demanded for any change in position: conditions known to be untenable. The individual is tenacious, persistent, and unrelenting. There is seemingly no room for change. This intransigent attitude leads to declarations such as, "This hospital will never accept another Medicaid patient!" "From now on, absolutely no more evening hours!" and, "We are going to find a different hospital in which to practice. Good-bye and good riddance!"

This type of angry declaration both burns and creates a standoff. Any progress toward a mutually satisfying solution ends. The conflict resembles a showdown at high noon: a macho duel. Negotiation turns into confrontation. The question becomes who is going to conquer whom?

This is obviously a dangerous situation. The level of combat often escalates disproportionately to the original issue. Information, events, and perceptions are distorted to justify the alleged menace. Such misrepresentations only cloud the real issues. The destruction resulting from the confrontation will likely injure innocent bystanders, people who are neither party to the original issue nor able to contribute to its resolution. Patients and staff members are common casualties of the vengeful feuds of hospital leaders.

What can be done to reframe this sort of stubbornness? The individual who made the statement is trapped in a box, with little room for escape. He or she has taken a rigid stance that is unlikely to be conceded or end well. Demands are framed as win-lose choices. Whether you are one of the parties involved, a mediator, or even the perpetrator, there is a maneuver that can be helpful: we call it the art of *negotiation face-saving*.

Take the original statement and think of placing it in a box, a cognitive frame of reference: this is box 1. Define the specific context, and explain the statement so that it makes logical sense within that frame or given what was known at the time. For example, "When you said that the hospital would never accept another Medicaid patient, you were under a great deal of pressure." Or, "... you understood there were some financial improprieties, which turned out to be mistaken." Or, "... you thought the head of cardiology was lobbying to have you fired by the board." Or, "... you were reacting to news of another malpractice suit being brought against one of the staff." Or, "... you were unaware of how the community would react."

Looked at from this sort of perspective, it is likely that the original, inflated declaration has a coherent and valid frame of reference. The statement is reasonable in its original context: box 1 made sense at that time. Now, create a new box, with different considerations: "Given your frustration at that time, you made a decision. Now there is new information that you did not have when you made that first decision." What you have done with this comment is to legitimize a new context and therefore a modified statement. You have given the stubborn party a pragmatic justification to support a reframing. You have offered a graceful exit from a difficult trap. You have maintained the individual's dignity without compromising that of others. The new box, box 2, is a sensible place to move into, now that the situation has been placed in a new light. It is a pragmatic way to help someone to retroactively climb up and out of the basement.

At the point when the parties are firing combative and destructive declarations (and, one hopes, the arrows are only spoken words), most are aware that dire consequences lie ahead for someone. They are caught in the spiral of their own escalation, outwardly confident though inwardly fearful of the consequences and humiliation of defeat. Reframing the dispute to allow a dignified return to the table is the purpose of negotiation face-saving. It is a magnificent maneuver, opening interest-based negotiation when most assume it is near impossible. You allow the parties to shift from box 1 to box 2. You might even find at times that you can use the maneuver for yourself, when you realize you have said something that on further consideration you regret. Negotiation face-saving is a potential way to repair the damage without losing your dignity.

With the current pressures for change, one hears in the vocabulary of health care frequent military metaphors: we are going to *attack* the market, *overcome* the hospital across town, *quash* the competition, and *undermine* the other department. These statements become the battle cries that encourage positional lines to be drawn. Given the necessity for coordination and connection of services among health care providers, this sort of mind-set only obstructs good health service. Reframing these ultimatums provides a step toward enhancing both the premises and the purpose of the system.

Understanding Negotiation Ripeness

Negotiation works on a timeline. It has a tempo: sometimes measured in hours, sometimes in days, weeks, years, or decades. As with the punch line of a good joke, everything depends on timing.

Reaching agreement requires time to vent, think, consider, stew, consult, and ready oneself to settle. When you are ready, you are *ripe* for resolution. You want to reap the benefits of settlement. You want the pressure of the issue off your back. You want to move on to other business. Whatever it is, you want to get it over with.

Ripeness is a point in time. On one side of ripeness lies *too soon* and on the other side *too late.*

When it is too soon, one or both parties simply are not ready to settle. They may need more time to mull their emotions. If they are angry, they want to burn off steam before they encounter the other side. If they are perplexed, they want to gather more information to formulate a judicious choice. If there were parallel discussions elsewhere, they want to learn how these were settled, as a point of leverage. There could be advantage in holding off a settlement discussion. They are annoyed and perhaps adamant if someone forces the issue before they are ready.

When it is too late, one or both parties are bitter about the costs and consequences of not settling earlier. They are past ripeness and to the point of bitterness. They know what they had hoped for. Those opportunities are over and gone. The dollars are gone. Negotiation and settlement at this point are foregone. They are angry and disappointed about the original matters awaiting discussion, as well as about the fact that these have yet to be discussed. Each side's distrust of the other side is reinforced: people can't even get themselves to the table, to say nothing for getting themselves to settlement.

Ripeness is a problem when everyone is not ready at the same time, when what is too soon for one person is too late for another. The *when* of settlement becomes a new bone of contention.

Consider a simple example: a couple falls into the ripeness trap when they have a disagreement. He wants to get the matter out and over with right away in order to return to a more pleasant rapport. She prefers to sit on it for a while, vent her anger and frustration, and only then get it over with. The husband, ripe for resolution, pushes the matter, further aggravating his wife. Getting nowhere, he gives up in frustration. By the time she is ready to settle, he is steaming about having wasted the day. His unwillingness to finally wrap the matter up further exacerbates the problem.

The couple finally resolve to negotiate ripeness. They determine that after a disagreement, they will settle immediately on a time to talk: nothing more: "Let's talk this over during lunch." This assures the wife that she will have time to vent. It also assures the husband that the day will not be lost. When they finally do talk, both will be ready. Finding resolution on that original disagreement will be greatly eased. They have negotiated ripeness.

The same principle applies to your professional work.

Of course, compared to the complexity of a health care organization, the husband and wife have a simple problem to solve. The time is theirs as are the consequences. In health care, time itself teems with significance, value, and opportunity, either lost or grasped. That significance affects the cost and impact of time on your negotiations.

Income, fees, and quality in health care are calculated and perceived in measures of time: length of patient stay in the hospital, time spent in the surgical suite, number of patients seen per hour, and from the patient's perspective, "amount of time the doctor [or nurse] spent with me." Whether it be delay, indecision, or hustle, time translates into dollars and cents. Health professionals sell their time. If employed by someone else, their time is not all their own. If self-employed, their time is their money.

Time is also a variable in health service outcomes. The timing of when patients are seen may affect their health status, especially if their condition is serious. If the condition is not life threatening and they wait, the delay adds to their stress. Treatment and convalescence are measured in units of time: hours, days, months. Health care already works in a realm of stress and pressure. When time is not appropriately respected, that stress expands.

With time so valuable, lack of consensus about negotiation timing seriously complicates the process of negotiation. When it causes what is perceived as an unnecessary delay in progress, resentment builds. Timing becomes a point of leverage when it is more important to one side than the other: "I'll discuss the matter now if you would be willing to . . ." Or, "I won't negotiate with you now unless you will . . ."

Attending to ripeness requires a balance of patience and perseverance. This is particularly important when negotiators are coping with different external pressures and staff priorities. Because substantive progress is more likely when there is agreement on ripeness, it is wise for the parties to frame and agree upon a timeline early in their negotiations.

Using a Negotiation Map

Patterns of clinical interaction set the tone for health care negotiation, because the topic of clinical care—even in the far reaches of Washington policymaking—evokes emotions about life and death, the quality of life, and one's sense of social and financial well-being. In the clinic, high-volume, brief, and intense meetings of great consequence typify the culture of health care negotiation. In the course of a day, a clinician typically encounters numerous people, each different. Discussions ordinarily are for short periods of time. Decisions are quick. For the patient, what is discussed is of great significance. The professional must move efficiently from one conversation to the next, cognizant of the unique medical and personal circumstances of each.

If you are a medical professional or administrator, you keep the pace by using shortcuts: cues that help you achieve a rapid understanding of the problem and the person. Like a detective, you quickly case the joint, you collect information, and you draw a cognitive map to organize what you have learned (Figure 6.1). You assess the facts and the people, placing them in categories and adjusting your decisions and interactions accordingly. If you do not correctly systematize all the information available to you—including the vast store of research upon which evidence-based clinical and management decisions are to be reached—the choices you make and actions you take will be far below optimal.

There are many factors weighed as you organize and frame all this information. There is the data side, including evidence, laboratory results, and costs. And there is the social and negotiation side, which includes the organizational positions of the people involved and their personal characteristics. Your observations intermingle, leaving you with impressions that affect what you do: the information you exchange, the decisions you make, and the actions you take. Thanks to your quick assessments, you conduct your business without taking a detailed history of each situation and each individual involved.

You hope that your diagnoses are accurate and your conclusions about the information and the people are valid. A quick journey through uncharted territory

FIGURE 6.1 Negotiation Map

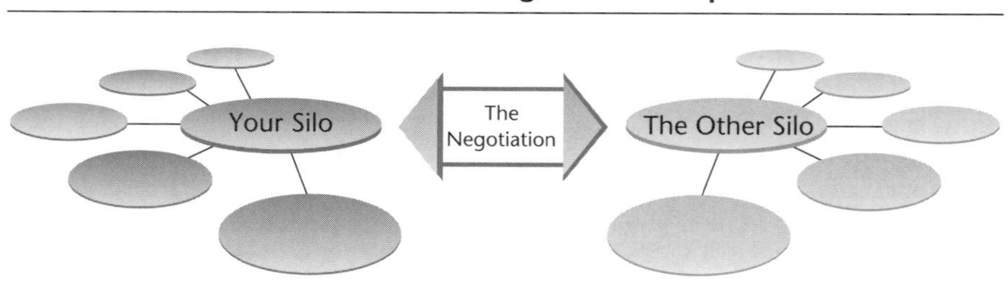

is helped by a good map. If the map is flawed, you encounter significant obstacles to negotiation progress. You misinterpret cues, neglect important information, and react inappropriately. Similarly, if other negotiators inaccurately appraise you, what you say and do is then misinterpreted, and your offers of conciliation are then unheard, your concerns are ignored, and your efforts to settle are futile: you are in conflict. Such misunderstandings distract from the work to be done. To get back on track when mired in conflict, all parties must reframe their expectations and their patterns of exchange.

The *negotiation map* is not merely a cerebral version of the organization chart. That chart only partially describes the division of power and influence in the organization, because leverage is derived from more than just one's place in the hierarchy of the institution. What you know, whom you know, the value of what you have to offer, and your relationships with others contribute to your formal power and also to your informal influence. For example, how do different people in the organization view your authority and sway within the system? More than just "organizational politics," the negotiation map captures the range of changing opinion, which is affected by and affects the what, who, and why of bargaining both within the system and well beyond. The map shifts and changes ever so slightly with each negotiation.

Your understanding of the negotiation map is essential to your framing and reframing of the solutions feasible across distinct organizational, clinical, or system circumstances. Can you devise a policy for the medical staff that cardiology, surgery, and psychiatry can all accept? Can you assist the patient's family, the medical staff, and the hospital's general counsel in reaching agreement on a DNR (do not resuscitate) order? Finding a balance between multiple constituencies with their different home teams is fundamental to accomplishing consensus in a large complex institution. It is more than organizational politics because some of these people are not on the chart of organizational decision-making authority.

There are two dimensions to a negotiation map. Representational negotiation describes its organizational aspects. Symbolic negotiation explains the personal and interpersonal aspects.

Representational Negotiation. Imagine you are negotiating the purchase of a car from an individual who owns it privately. You have no spouse, colleague, or friend to whom you must report. No one will say, "You spent $15,000 for that junk heap!?" Likewise, the person negotiating the sale of the car has no one to whom he or she must answer. No one will say, "You sold the car for just $15,000!?" There are just two people involved in the exchange. These two own all the decisions and they bear all the consequences. No one else is involved. This is called *simple negotiation.*

Minutes after the news breaks online, Arlan Abbington, chairman of Oppidania Medical Center's board of trustees, calls Iris Inkwater and instructs her to arrange an immediate, emergency meeting of the executive committee of the board. It is quickly set for midday.

Every member of the committee is present when Abbington opens the session at noon in the OMC's large conference room. The lunch buffet has hardly been touched. "First, thank you all for coming on such short notice. I am sure that by now you have all heard the news." Early that morning news broke that Community Health Plan (CHP) had signed an exclusive contract with Urbania Medical Center. The contract includes a feeder arrangement with two of the smaller community hospitals on the west side of the city. Beginning in just sixty days, all CHP-covered patients will be directed to use Urbania.

As soon as Abbington finishes his summary of the situation, Dr. Benjamin Bennington, a retired physician who has been on the board for two years, asks urgently, "What about CHP patients who are being seen by physicians here at Oppidania?"

"This is an exclusive contract between CHP and Urbania," Inkwater responds. "In exchange for lower rates of reimbursement, they get all the CHP patients. If those patients want their hospitalization covered, they must go there. If their physician doesn't have privileges there, and most of our staff don't, then the patients have to change physicians or change plans."

"But that's devastating for the medical staff," Bennington blurts at Inkwater, as if she had devised the new rules.

"Dr. Bennington, it's not only devastating for the physicians on our staff and their patients, it's also devastating for the hospital. We stand to lose more than $57 million from our budgeted revenue with this shift. We knew that CHP was contemplating some changes, and we were attempting to show them a good-faith effort to bring costs down. They never made a counteroffer to us. Furthermore, the link between the two community hospitals and Urbania is a surprise. We had been talking to one of those sites, Perpetual Memorial. We've also had discussions with two of the east side hospitals, and with this news, those talks are going into high gear."

"Well, Iris, talks are one thing. What are we going to do about this immediately?" Catherine Cartwright injected. Cartwright is a major figure in the community and has been on the board longer than anyone else. "You know this is going to mean a lot of bake sales for the volunteers," she says ruefully.

Inkwater smiles. "Yes, I know, Catherine, though I think we're talking about some very expensive cakes." Iris had learned firsthand how combative Cartwright can be, and she is happy that they are on the same side. She is counting on Cartwright to rally the board.

Abbington turns the conversation. "Iris, what is the picture as you see it?"

Inkwater stands up and walks slowly around the table. "There are several factors to consider. First, there is no question that Oppidania retains a far better reputation than Urbania. I've made some calls and the word on the street is that CHP is already catching hell from corporate benefits officers and from its members. You should read the online comments that have been posted to this morning's story in the *Oppidania Journal*; and it's only been a few hours." She goes on to explain that people don't like to be made to switch doctors or switch hospitals. Furthermore, she expects that the community hospital doctors who have smooth-working relationships with OMC staff members will be outraged at having to change their referral patterns. "My inbox is already overflowing with e-mail messages. My PDA hasn't stopped buzzing. Everyone has an opinion and it's gotten very hot," she continues. "CHP took a calculated risk. We could lose. They could lose. With open enrollment time coming up, they may find that a lot of people in town want to switch to another health plan—or at least that's our hope."

"If they have the option to switch," says Bennington. "I keep reading that employers are tightening up choices and concentrating their business with fewer insurers to get better rates."

Abbington listens intently and then asks, "Does it make any sense, though, to just sit and wait for things to happen? What if the allure of lower rates is compelling to our patients or their employers?"

"We're not waiting," Inkwater retorts. "We have already made a preliminary outreach to one of CHP's main competitors, Arena Health Insurance. I sit on the board of the ballet with their CEO so we have a relationship. They are interested in a possible exclusive relationship with us; though I am sure we will have to bargain hard to get a livable rate of reimbursement. The sense I'm getting is that they were thrilled with the CHP move. They believe that they can draw patients away from CHP with only a marginally higher cost. Their premise is that patients' primary loyalty is to their physicians and to their hospital and not to their insurer."

"But where does that leave our physicians?" Bennington asks.

"Most of our medical staff accept both CHP and AHI, and most employers in town also offer a choice, though AHI is slightly more expensive. If we are left only with AHI, it will be a different flow of patients, and there *will* be patients. The people at AHI think that CHP's strategic mistake is that its leadership believes the market will move based on cost alone. AHI knows the reputation of our medical staff and the high quality of their work, and they believe our good reputation will rub off on their own public image. They are talking about a marketing blitz that emphasizes what's best for your family's health and future. If you're an optimist, you could conjure up a picture in which our covered lives actually go up with this move. Right now though, we just don't know."

"Iris, I think it is safe to say that the board is behind you in pursuing negotiations with AHI," Abbington says. He looks at the other members, and they each nod. "It seems you are taking the high ground on this matter and that is smart. We have quality and reputation on our side, and there is no use risking that for a bitter contest that will get us nowhere."

"Thanks, Arlan. I appreciate that," Inkwater replies. "It is comforting to know that our situation is not quite as dire as the media would have us believe. We do have some tough times ahead, and AHI is going to want a tight budget to maintain its competitiveness. We can pull through this one, and I think we can do it without adding another bake sale, Catherine."

"Well, Iris, if you have that sale, you know I'll bring my famous brownies," Cartwright says reassuringly. "From what I've heard, I don't think that CHP has acted very fairly. I think that we go out and kick some butt." There are chuckles around the table at the coarse language from the refined senior member of the board. The meeting is adjourned with a sense of cautious hope.

Simple negotiation is rare in health care, where decisions and actions typically spread out to a vast, integrally intertwined network of others with a stake in the outcome. In a highly interconnected system, what one person does inevitably affects others. This becomes problematic when one person acts on the assumption that a negotiation falls into the simple category and others assume otherwise because they are affected by it. You experience this problem when your staff, supervisor, or patient—or for that matter your significant other—says, "You agreed to what!?" They are reacting to the effect your action has upon them. In your dealings, you represent them and they bear the consequences of both your accomplishments and your shortcomings.

Representational negotiation typifies the system-based interactions of health care. Because of the integral connections among departments, functions, and people, the deeds of one person impose upon or enhance those of others. When you speak to a patient about benefits and procedures, you represent the policies of the hospital, and implicitly, the policies of the patient's insurer. When you agree in a meeting to new obligations for your staff, you represent their work and interests. When the board of directors assigns you to negotiate a consolidation agreement with another institution, you represent your hospital's objectives and concerns. Information, reactions, and implications flow through the organization via everyday exchanges and negotiations. Recognizing and working with these formal and informal connections is the essence of systems thinking.

Your negotiation map (Figure 6.1) assists you in charting who influences you and whom you influence. It helps you assess the nature, power, and significance of that influence. You know that if you are at a task force meeting about to agree on a change in staff policy, you must first know what range of changes will be acceptable for your department, your supervisors, and your staff. In the course of representing them, it is wise to check to ensure that what you agree to on their behalf is acceptable to them. Furthermore, you recognize the range of acceptable conditions for other people at the table. Each person at the table speaks for constituencies that are best consulted before a final decision is reached.

These constituencies, the people for whom you speak, are your *home teams*. If you work in a complex health center, you are likely to have many home teams. A male nurse for example has many different home teams. He has allegiances to the nursing department as a whole; to the other nurses and the profession; to the physicians, technicians, and assistants on the wing where he works; to the overall medical center; and to the group of male nurses who share his unique vantage point. A female obstetrician likewise has social allegiances to the OB department, to the medical staff as a whole, to her office staff, to the medical center, and to female physicians who likewise share her distinct experiences. You have an interdependent relationship with each of your home teams: you need them for support and encouragement, and they depend upon you for the same.

Therefore, when you negotiate, you attend to the effect of your actions and decisions on your constituencies. If you agree to an arrangement that is unacceptable to your staff, you will likely have a rebellion on your hands. They will decry your disloyalty and wonder about your real allegiances: they may suspect that you are responding to a mandate from your own supervisor or pursuing personal gain at their expense. They may not appreciate the onerous struggles and choices you faced during a meeting at which none of them were present.

Likewise, you want to understand the representational considerations brought to the table by others. Might they be anxious about the reaction of their home team to the agreement being crafted? "I could reluctantly go along with reducing the staff-to-patient ratio, though I have real concerns that both our staff and our patients would walk out in protest." Is this a real concern or simply a ploy?

Finally, you want to ensure that your agreements do not disintegrate when they are presented to others' home teams. "I had wanted to join in the new project. The problem was that when I described it to my department, they were firmly against it." The wise negotiator is concerned not only about his or her own home team. Similar concern is shown for those of others. If the deal falls apart once it gets back to someone else's home team, then you are stuck. Put the question on the table. "How is your department—or your boss—going to react to this proposal?" "What has been your experience in bringing similar agreements back to your institution?" Reading between the lines of their answers, you will learn both about strands of authority within their home team as well as their influence with that team. You can then craft an agreement that you believe will sell on their turf as well as your own.

Symbolic Negotiation. At times when you interact with someone else, you get the impression that they are not reacting to you for who you are and what you value. Rather, they are responding to what you *symbolize* for them. It could be a variation of, for example, white, male, Midwesterner, Anglo-Saxon, bearded, physician. Each of those qualifiers may come with preconceptions, either positive or negative, based on the other person's own characteristics, experience, and expectations. The possible variations and affinities within and across categories of people are endless.

In health care work, the quick interactions, negotiations, and decision making require the use of shorthand methods to comprehend and efficiently classify situations and the people involved. In the abstract there is nothing right or wrong about this phenomenon: we all do it all the time. The problem arises when the quick assessment does not in fact fit the person. When "white male" invariably equates to "insensitive, domineering, and narrow-minded," then effective interpersonal interaction is hindered. Personal characteristics, race, employer, profession, gender, and culture can likewise produce rigid assessments damaging to meaningful negotiation.

Frequently individuals are playing out larger, unresolved, societal tensions as they interact in everyday negotiations. Both men and women struggle with readjustments of gender relations in their day-to-day interactions. Employees of different organizations shoulder the tensions between their institutions as they discuss the transfer of a patient. Similarly, patients vent general frustrations with "the doggone health care system" when they arrive at a clinic.

Given the nature of the work, symbolic negotiation takes on particularly complex overtones in health care. For the terminal patient, the physician might eerily come to symbolize death. For worried and distressed parents, the pediatric ward and everyone who works therein may signify hope for them and their child. And for a laid-off employee, the supervisor symbolizes rejection and calamity. What a health care employee or institution does can have extraordinary meaning for others. And perceptions of that action, whether good or bad, can be ascribed to all related individuals or institutions. One of the authors (Lenny Marcus), when speaking with a politician, identified himself as working at one of the large teaching hospitals in town. When the politician found out where Lenny worked, he beamed. "You guys did a great job taking care of me when I was sick. I'd do anything for you." The fact that Lenny was not a clinician was irrelevant to the discussion. Similarly, Lenny was once introduced at a meeting as a faculty member of a large university. Someone at the meeting who had had a bad experience with that institution began criticizing him, treating him as a symbol of the school even though he had nothing to do with the source of her complaint.

The question is not only what you symbolize for others. The flip side is what they symbolize for you. Does that symbolic meaning you attach to them limit your negotiation effectiveness? Are you overeager to agree with others simply because they are physically attractive? Are you reluctant to reach a mutually beneficial agreement with others when you're distracted by their poor taste in wardrobe? And most important, are there certain types of people, quirks, or characteristics that send you ballistic: for example, people who in your view are pushy, arrogant, timid, jerky, or underqualified?

If certain characteristics send you to the basement, this response has the potential to compromise your effectiveness. You may find, for example, that certain characteristics unleash a fusillade of frustration inside you. The person with these characteristics has taken you to the basement by pressing one of your toxic "buttons"—by the power of association he or she has ignited your fight, flight, or freeze response. Unless you understand and check your reactions when dealing with people with characteristics irksome to you, your toxic buttons will be pushed at the discretion of others. What you do and what you say will be out of your grasp. When you do not control your buttons, you will likely be impelled to do something counter to your own interests: make a comment you later regret, threaten in a way that escalates the conflict, or do something else that damages you as much as it does others. Know your buttons. Someone else could purposely aggravate you in order to impel you to say something that will later be used against you. Even very smart people can be pushed to say or do some very dumb things. When your button has been pushed, call a time out or do what is necessary to regain your composure and get out of the basement.

What happens when your shorthand symbolic assessments do not fit the people with whom you are dealing? Then it is time to reframe. Get to know others for who they are and what they hope to achieve. Likewise, reveal yourself to them for who you are: let them know your own values and concerns. Reframe from stereotypes and symbols to real individuals and genuine relationships.

Using Humor: Negotiation Lubrication

A chapter on negotiation reframing would be incomplete without some mention of humor. When it works, a well-placed joke, clever observation, or quick-witted comment is the most potent way to invigorate a dormant negotiation. It offers perspective, a release of tension, and sense of togetherness. What is the relationship between humor and negotiation?

Laughter is one reaction to incongruity. Jokes are funny when there is a paradoxical situation that is resolved in a zany manner. Punch lines evoke a release of tension because they are unexpected, timely, and clever.

Conflict resolution likewise reconciles incongruity. Two parties in a tense face-off confront one another with seemingly incompatible demands. It appears that nothing can bring them together. If found, compatibility will be applauded because it is unexpected, timely, and clever.

A cautionary note on humor: not all humor is helpful in calming negotiation tensions. Certainly humor that is demeaning of others, that is insensitive to the situation at hand, or that is otherwise out of place can torpedo a meaningful discussion. Wisdom and balance in the use of humor is critical, especially in negotiations that involve sensitive, interpersonal circumstances. That which is humorous to one person may fall flat with another. Be sensitive to cultural differences and other considerations that may lead your joke to be misconstrued no matter how benevolent your intentions.

When it succeeds, humor confers a human quality to the negotiation process. And bottom line, good negotiation and good reframing are about elevating our best human qualities.

Renegotiating Health Care

The work of health care involves achieving a tentative balance between what is believed to be true on one hand and the actual facts on the table on the other hand. In a field of endeavor so rooted in scientific inquiry, it might seem incongruous that belief and fact do not routinely coincide. It is telling that just a few years ago, *evidence-based medicine* rang as a new cause and movement in clinical judgment. Wouldn't one have thought evidence to be the basis of decision making all along?

In an ideal world, belief and fact concur. The two are in synchrony when what you actually do equates with what you aspire to accomplish. That fit bestows a genuine satisfaction and quality upon your work. What you achieve in your professional life fulfills fundamental values about people, relationships, rewards, and results. Your work is a principled means of fulfilling your personal mission.

When belief and reality do not mesh, what you do contends with what you believe. The pieces of your professional life are in contradiction: they do not fit. Your work is riddled with seeming myth. You proclaim quality care when what you do is ration care. You affirm your commitment to patients even though your focus is a fixation on profit. Your actions are a cover for your intentions. You laud the wardrobe of the naked emperor.

The question is whether the community of people who populate the health system can achieve a new balance: new beliefs that mesh with new realities and worthwhile outcomes.

What we have in this country is often referred to as a *health care system*. In fact, what has been built is a *disease eradication system*. This system does a remarkable job in, for example, saving the life of a one-pound, premature infant: in that case the technological capabilities and willingness to spend are nearly limitless. Yet there is reluctance to invest a concomitant effort in maintaining the health of a square mile of infants in an inner city. Medical and nursing students are trained to treat disease, with far less emphasis on promoting health. Reimbursement covers medical procedures delivered, yet there is no compensation for procedures avoided. The myth is reinforced that machines, buildings, and treatments equate to good health care.

Many of those facts of the past are changing. There is fresh energy for health care reform, even if the visions for that reform cover a wide range of possibilities. Patients are changing: there is an emerging consensus that people want to be healthy, they want health insurance at an affordable cost, and they want it for everybody. The workforce is changing: the student profile is evolving, and with it there are new curricula, remodeled reimbursement systems, and funding streams that signal a different set of assumptions and incentives. And new technologies are able to learn and accomplish extraordinary tasks at a pace that far outshines their human counterparts. These new themes and trends demand a renegotiation of health care: reframing what is being done and the very purposes for doing it. These changes are manifest in the groundbreaking policies, procedures, and regulations that are increasingly governing interactions among the many stakeholders in the system. In your practice and your negotiation map, you negotiate and renegotiate this balance every day.

Because some of these changes threaten those who benefited before, advancing through the obstacles of reframing is often an uncomfortable expedition: working through the anger and frustration of the resistance is a loathsome though necessary step in the process. If you can progress from venting to learning, option building, resolution, and agreement, the effort will have been worthwhile.

There are numerous impediments along the way. Such barriers are to be expected, as they often are the typical phenomena of conflict itself. Those caught in conflict must find a common path to reach the bounty of settlement. It is a matter of adjusting and readjusting until the riddles are unraveled and the resolution revealed.

Staying on board throughout this evolution requires reframing: shifting what you think, changing what you do, and modifying the methods by which you do it.

After the last of the other board members have said their good-byes, Arlan Abbington follows Iris Inkwater into her office. Inkwater is still feeling a bit overwhelmed by the flood of messages that erupted with the news of the CHP decision.

Abbington has never felt more acutely taken with the "fiduciary responsibility" he assumed when he was handed the chairmanship of the board than he does right now. His many years in banking have provided him with abundant business sense and experience. His physician son has schooled him in what it means to practice medicine these days. His wife, a retired nurse, has many friends in the field who keep him abreast of trends in health care. And his long-time fascination with the health system has kept him a voracious reader of periodicals designed for trustees and hospital managers. He knows that if he had it to do again, he would likely have worked in health care. It's too late now to give up his banking career, though taking the helm of the Oppidania Medical Center board is, he feels, the next best thing to being in the thick of the action.

Although he is not happy about the turn of events, this is the kind of puzzle and challenge Abbington loves. Rather than being demoralized by the news he is energized. He knows that this may actually be an opportunity. The community could rally around Oppidania. CHP and Urbania could turn out to be the bad guys if their sudden alliance is perceived as a scheme of convenience rather than a plan for better health care. It may also prompt some necessary changes within OMC. As he always tells his colleagues at the bank, "never waste a good crisis."

Although he is excited, Abbington is also sensitive to the strain that this is putting on Iris Inkwater as CEO. Despite her bravado in the boardroom, he now reads nervousness and maybe a hint of panic in her face and body language. She twitches with every vibration of her phone.

"Is that your fourth cup of coffee? Or your fifth?" he asks. "Sit down and take a deep breath."

Inkwater falls back on the leather couch in her office and sighs; "Arlan, what are we going to do?"

Abbington sits across from her and leans toward her. "What are we going to do?" he replies. "We're going to make the most of this."

"What do you mean? We're watching a big chunk of our business just fly out the door. I tried to put on a good face in there, but frankly, I don't really have a plan. I was prepared for a negotiation but this really blindsided me."

Though they have very different roles within the hospital, Abbington and Inkwater have crafted a comfortable and constructive working relationship. Abbington has also taken on a mentoring role with the CEO. "Iris, you have shared with me for some time now that you need to shake this place up. With health reform playing out and the economy being what it is, there have been a lot of changes to the marketplace. You have lamented that your staff want to operate as if the good old days are here to stay. You haven't really been able to move them beyond incremental changes in the way you do business, right?"

"Look, Arlan, change doesn't come in one day. Well, a lot of change came today. But we didn't evolve from monkeys to humans overnight. Change takes time. We're making progress."

"Are you really happy with the progress you've been making, Iris?" He taps his finger firmly on the coffee table as he speaks. "Are you ahead of the curve, behind the curve, or are you not quite sure where the curve is?"

"Well, that's a fair question. Today, to be quite honest, I'm not sure where exactly the curve is. I learned a long time ago that if you are in a leadership position and you're totally surprised like this, you should take it as a wake-up call. I knew there were rumblings going on, but I wasn't aware that we would be hit like this. As much as I've complained about others, I have to admit that I'm not fully comfortable either with the pace of change and the aggressiveness that we're seeing in health care these days. Maybe you're more used to this in the world of banking and finance. For me, this is a shocker."

"And if that's how you're feeling," Abbington replies, "imagine how others on the management committee, your department heads, medical leadership, and staff are feeling. This hospital is in the basement. All these people are looking to you for leadership. Get into gear. Turn this into an opportunity to redefine the change curve in this hospital and in this community, Iris. This is no time to mourn what was. The only option is to actively work to define what will be."

Abbington's words hang in the silence as Inkwater ponders just what acting on them would mean. She looks up at the Edward Hopper print hanging on the far wall. It shows Highland Light on Cape Cod in a scene of summer serenity, with the lighthouse standing tall and strong. Yet the lighthouse is not alone: it is part of a complex, a support system. Inkwater has always kept this print in her office and uses it to help center and ground herself in times of turbulence. As she gazes on its simple, solid buildings and placid sky, she realizes that first she has to climb out of the basement. Then she has to get her senior leadership and the clinical staff out of the basement. And then together, she thinks, we have to move forward in a new and different way. We have to lead the market not lag behind.

"OK, Arlan. I'm getting convinced." She moves forward in her seat and looks him in the eye. "I really value your wisdom at times like this. Do you have any suggestions on how to get started?"

"Yes, I've been through some ups and downs at the bank over the years. You need to bring this hospital together one step at a time. I suggest you pull all your senior people together for a retreat. Signal your urgency by scheduling it for next weekend. It should be an opportunity for you and others to put your concerns and ideas for moving forward constructively on the table. You, Iris, need to be an active participant in this process so I suggest you bring in an outside facilitator.

We once had a pretty significant market bump at the bank, and I did something just like this and it worked.''

''That makes sense to me. So you've done this before. Do you have some recommendations for our retreat?''

''Recently I met two guys at a trustee conference who talked about the Walk in the Woods. It's a method for problem solving. One is a doc and the other is a PhD. They know health care and they could be a help. They also have a good sense of humor together, and we certainly could use some humor and perspective here.''

Inkwater gives a gentle laugh. ''Yes, I could use a reason to smile. This sounds like the beginning of a plan.''

By late afternoon, Inkwater has Benny Bourne and Larry Larkin on the phone. They both are on faculty at a university out west, and both, fortunately, were available to take the call. Bourne's background is as a surgeon and Larkin's is social science.

Inkwater presents the predicament facing Oppidania, starting with the CHP shocker and then describing some of the other internal issues facing the hospital. In concluding, she asks, ''So, what do you guys think? Is this a terminal condition?''

Bourne speaks first. ''Well, Iris, there is good news and bad news. The good news is that you are not the only hospital facing this sort of a scenario. We are working with hospitals across the country, and there is a ripple effect spreading out like an earthquake from Washington. The fact is that people in D.C. might know how to craft and pass legislation and Wall Street might know how to trade stocks, but neither knows how to run a health system or a hospital. The market is changing faster than anyone imagined possible, and oftentimes it's hard to predict an outcome because we haven't seen exactly these sorts of pressures before. Medicare and Medicaid are morphing and so is the private market. So you're not alone. The bad news is the same as the good news. You're not the only hospital facing this scenario. So everyone is learning how to scramble fast. From our perch, we think that there are places that will emerge as better institutions from this phase and some that will collapse. That is the choice point and there is not a lot of room for error.''

Larkin jumps in after Bourne. ''Benny is right. This is a time to be strategic in what you do and how you go about doing it.'' He goes on to describe some of significant differences in how hospitals are responding: those that are able to bring their departments and staff together into a comprehensive plan and operation are doing better than those caught up in old internal rivalries. He explains that these rivalries get worse because, when people are feeling panicked and believe they are struggling to survive, ''they start to engage in what looks like civil war, and as people inside the organization attack one another, they thereby weaken the organization in its outside market. Conversely, the 'together' systems come out of their change process stronger, leaner, more flexible, and more responsive to the market. When you can achieve a comprehensive plan and operation, you create a competitive edge that appeals to your customers: insurers, benefits officers, and even government regulators. When you're a together institution, your quality marks go up, and given that those numbers are now easily available to everyone, the patients, potential patients, consumers—whatever you want to call them—are paying attention. That translates into volume, and as you know, volume these days translates into viability."

It all makes sense to Inkwater. "OK, now for the tough question: are you available to come out here next weekend?" Larkin and Bourne check their calendars. They are both free. The three of them review the basic terms of an agreement and then discuss the need to quickly arrange a series of phone interviews with key stakeholders: Larkin and Bourne must become familiar with the people, the system, and the issues before arriving for the retreat. The Walk in the Woods it will be.

Renegotiation based on common interests is a fitting manner for charting both the new challenges and the new opportunities.

And what is the destination? A health system that keeps people healthy, thanks to an infrastructure and a wealth of collaborative professional expertise that facilitate the process.

CHAPTER 7

THE WALK IN THE WOODS

AFTER YEARS of research, teaching, and guiding the complex steps required to move from an impasse, through problem solving, and to agreement, we developed a model of interest-based negotiation that we call the Walk in the Woods. The Walk is a step-by-step method for steering negotiators, mediators, facilitators, and participants through the negotiation process. It is designed to assist those at the table to identify legitimate interests among the stakeholders; to reframe the understanding of those different viewpoints; to trigger imaginative solution building; and to clarify the give-and-get exchanges in pursuit of a mutually beneficial outcome.

Our motive for developing the model was in large part pedagogical. How could we teach health care professionals—very smart people expert in the clinical and management aspects of their enterprises—to learn how to better interact and negotiate with one another? We were impressed with the high stakes, the smarts, and the high level of emotion involved in health care negotiations. These have a distinct intensity and essence that makes them different from business dealings or day-to-day interpersonal exchanges. Life or death outcomes, professional failure or success, ego, status, and large sums of money are often at stake or in the periphery. Just as caregivers learn a specific order for conducting a physical exam—which directs them to carefully detect and thereby not overlook critical clinical factors—negotiators too can learn and adopt an order that guides them to work through essential components of interest-based negotiation.

The Walk in the Woods is named for the classic 1982 problem-solving saga of two Cold War nuclear arms reduction negotiators. Delegations from the United States and the Soviet Union were meeting at a pastoral retreat center located outside Geneva, Switzerland. Paul Nitze led the U.S. delegation and Yuli Kvitsinsky led the Soviet delegation (Blessing, 1988).

Facing a desperate impasse in their talks, the two sides called for a break. As the story is told, during this pause in the formal meetings, Nitze and Kvitsinsky bumped into one another and together agreed to take—in this bucolic retreat center—a walk in the woods. The conversation opened with discussion of the impasse and its complexities. It continued on to stories about their backgrounds, careers, and families. It eventually reached the topic of their mutual desire to break the impasse. As the walk progressed, the two came upon both shared and divergent concerns, interests, and objectives. They eventually achieved a genuine understanding for what their two countries faced in the escalating arms race and what they might accomplish if they were to reconfigure operating premises. With that, they explored how they might realize significant mutual force reduction, a particularly noteworthy ambition given Nitze's reputation as a hardliner on relations with the Soviets. As the walk concluded, they settled on a set of options and solutions designed to break the impasse. Although their agreement was subsequently rejected by both Moscow and Washington, the saga of their meeting was immortalized in a Broadway play and came in the literature to exemplify the advantages of informal interpersonal bargaining and interest-based negotiation (Kremenyuk, 2002).

The Walk in the Woods as presented here is a structured negotiation and conflict resolution exercise that focuses attention on the interests, motives, and objectives of those participating (Watkins, 2002). The method is designed to enhance the transparency, the efficiency, and ultimately the satisfaction of an exchange by expanding systematically the range of interests and objectives incorporated in that exchange (Ury, Brett, & Goldberg, 1988). When adversarial interaction finds parties in conflict, this structured, four-part progression for renegotiating working relationships can assist negotiators in constructively integrating the ideas, ambitions, and concerns of the many parties who have a stake in both the process and its outcome. This method and its premises can be used to facilitate complex multiparty negotiation, to mediate conflict, or as a personal discipline, to privately guide an individual through the steps and thinking of interest-based negotiation.

The Steps of the Walk in the Woods

The Walk is a step-by-step method of assisting stakeholders in finding a resolution for complex problems. In practice, the Walk serves as a detour from the normal course of discussion (Figure 7.1). Why do we describe it as a detour?

In typical problem solving, parties to a negotiation proceed straight to solutions, debating the relative merits of one solution over the other. This is often done without a consensus on the definition of the problem or an understanding of how it might be distinctly perceived or experienced by different constituencies

FIGURE 7.1 The Steps of the Walk in the Woods

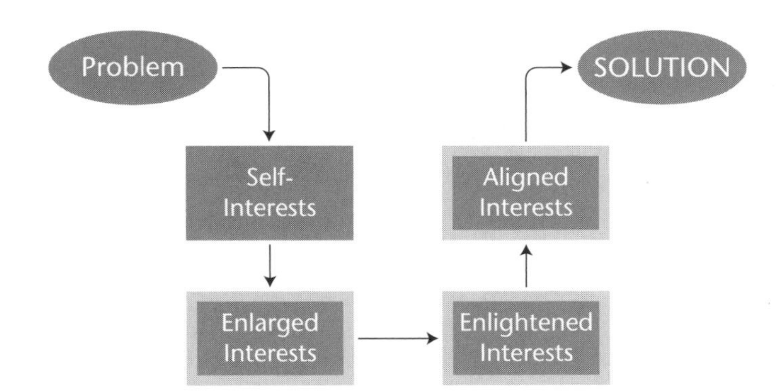

and how it might therefore specifically affect these stakeholders. In extolling the merits of one solution over others, parties typically advocate for opportunities that benefit their own interests and disparage solutions that advance the interests of others. The contest is waged by wielding their relative power or control of necessary resources or by taking the moral high ground, as in "my solution is better than yours because it is more ethically correct."

The Walk circumvents this entanglement by providing a transparent process to, first, understand the problem from multiple perspectives and then—based on the resultant reframing that occurs—to build responsive solutions through a joint enterprise (Susskind & Cruikshank, 1987). By first gaining a fresh perspective on just what the problem is, the parties are less likely to debate solutions that ultimately solve just a portion of their shared conundrum. Participants become less defensive and more willing to engage in the dialogue and creative enterprise of solution building because offensive solutions that ignore fundamental interests are unlikely to gain traction (Jones, 2005; Slaikeu & Hasson, 1998).

There are four steps to the Walk in the Woods. Each step entails a specific negotiation activity. That activity generates an outcome that prepares negotiators for the action required in the next step (Heifetz, 1994). The steps are designed and ordered to allow participants to explore and exchange the hoped-for outcomes that motivate them through the process. After explicating all their motives and working to transform them, parties are more likely to join together to develop solutions based on their combined motivations. The following brief description of the four steps will give you an overview of this process.

The first of the four steps is *self-interests*. Each party states his or her interests: what he or she hopes to gain or achieve in the negotiation. Implicit in this discussion is revelation of what individually motivates each party to the process.

In the process, all parties are encouraged to actively listen to one another in a nonadversarial manner. Often parties will remark at the end of this step that this was the first time they felt that individual participants were genuinely paying attention to what others had to say.

In the second step, the *enlarged interests*, the parties—having heard the interests around the table during step 1—are asked to list what they view as points of agreement among these interests. This comes as something of a surprise, as people tend to focus the bulk of their attention on points of disagreement. Following that, the parties are asked to create a second list, this one noting the points of disagreement. Typically, even in highly contentious conflicts, the parties discover that their points of agreement far outnumber their disagreements. Why does this happen? Often the parties share a common set of values, a similar recognition of the downsides of a continuing conflict, and a common understanding of the possible advantages of a mutually beneficial solution. From this discussion, they discover their overlapping motivations, an extension of what was learned in step 1. Often, parties will remark at the end of this step that if they agree on so much, there must be some way to resolve their points of disagreement. This realization is the initial source of the reframing that occurs during step 2.

In the third step, the *enlightened interests*, the parties together craft new ideas and possibilities that, prior to this discussion, they would otherwise have been unlikely even to contemplate. The reframing that has occurred in step 2 encourages a fresh look at their sources of disagreement. It generates the possibility that inventive opportunities for agreement may be discoverable. The participants are asked—through explorative and creative brainstorming—to list innovative options that could contribute to resolving the issues that divide them. These new options newly motivate the parties. This third step introduces the *no commitment zone*. When this zone is in force, participants can explore fresh and unorthodox ideas and options without being concerned that new and unrealistic expectations will be raised as a result.

The fourth and final step, the *aligned interests*, is the bargaining, give-and-get phase, when the parties finalize arrangements of the deal they have been negotiating. If they are truly motivated toward an interest-based solution, then the participants on each side are working toward their own advancement by enhancing the accomplishments of their partners at the table. In concrete terms, each party articulates what it hopes to *get* in the negotiation and what it is willing to *give* in order to consummate the deal. The solution accomplished reflects the shared interests and motivations of the parties to the process, thereby generating buy-in for the outcome that they have negotiated.

In the next sections the steps of the Walk in the Woods will be more fully explored, with guidelines for putting the method into practice.

Arlan Abbington, the chairman of the Oppidania Medical Center (OMC) board, is a member of the Oppidania Tennis and Racket Club, and he arranges to use a conference room at the club for OMC's retreat. There is no question that everyone needs to get away from the hospital, and the high ceilings, comfortable chairs, beautiful woodwork, noncafeteria cuisine, and inspiring art at the club provide a more conducive atmosphere for discussion. The usually formal group of OMC leaders is instantly more collegial in their "retreat wear" of polo shirts, jeans, and running shoes.

The medical center CEO, Iris Inkwater, opens the meeting, welcoming everyone to the club, thanking Arlan for opening the club to them, and expressing her hope that the retreat will signal a new beginning for OMC. Around the table are the hospital's twenty-eight leading thinkers, movers, and shakers: the executive committee of the board, the hospital's vice presidents and department directors, and the leaders of the medical staff. She thanks them for rearranging their schedules on short notice and then introduces Benny Bourne and Larry Larkin.

"Everyone needs to be an active participant in this process—including me," she says. "That's why we've brought in outside facilitators. These two gentlemen come highly recommended by Arlan. So let's get started."

Bourne and Larkin have requested that tables and chairs be set up to form a single U-shaped table. They walk to their stools on the open side of the U; easels with markers lined up on either side. The group sizes them up: some with excitement and others with nervousness and skepticism.

Bourne, with a smile, opens the retreat process. "Thank you, Iris, and thanks to each of you for joining this conversation today. Larry and I have had the opportunity to work with a number of hospitals and systems experiencing the shock of rapid change that we understand you are now experiencing here at Oppidania." Bourne goes on to discuss the strategic advantages of developing a strong consensus within the institution in order to be more responsive to new competitive forces in the marketplace. He outlines the goal for the day: to come up with a set of strategic priorities linked to operational imperatives that everyone in the room agrees are critical to Oppidania's short- and long-term survival.

Larkin picks up the introduction from there. He and Bourne have done this together many times before, and the pace and tempo of their exchange is both engaging and promising. Their comfort with one another and their confidence at the front of the room engender a sense of fresh hope.

"So today we're going to go on a Walk in the Woods," Larkin continues with a gesture to the clump of fresh pines that can be seen just outside. "We're not going to be doing it out there though, as nice a day as it is. We're going to be doing it here around the table." He then gives the group the background on the Walk process and its purpose, how it works, and what it intends to accomplish.

He concludes: "The point of this retreat and the point of the Walk itself are the same: if solutions are going to emerge that work for Oppidania, they have to derive from the leadership in this room. You have to invest in making them work, and as leaders, you have to bring along everyone else who is not today in this room. If you can build consensus here, the strength that emerges from that cohesion will be an important organizational asset you have for moving forward."

Larkin then turns to his colleague and, with a mock bow, announces, "Benny is going to start us through the first step of the Walk, learning about everyone's self-interests."

Step 1: Self-Interests

Concept: Uncovering the Interests. The purpose of the first step of the Walk is to give each party the opportunity to express his or her self-interests as well as to hear and appreciate the self-interests of others. Negotiations reach an impasse when each stakeholder pursues his or her own agenda with little regard for the objectives or concerns of others (Bryson, 2004). Those different agendas, when they promote escalating degrees of selfishness, limit attention to a narrow set of objectives—"it's all about me."

Interest-based negotiation intends to address and to some extent satisfy the interests—mutual or different—that stakeholders bring to the table. Interests include the goals, objectives, ideas, concerns, and hopes that these stakeholders aim to address and satisfy through the negotiation (Ury, 1991). For people working together, interest-based negotiation implicitly reduces the effort invested in battling one another and increases efforts directed toward achieving mutual gain. To encourage the expression of interests, a *safe zone* of mutual respect and recognition must be an explicit feature of the process. *Positional negotiation*, by contrast, intends to establish winners and losers. The premise of positional bargaining is that one's objectives are best met by attaining victory, control, or dominance. This is the difference between a safe zone, in which one could achieve a mutually beneficial solution, and a dangerous environment, in which one could be handed a serious defeat.

This first step of the Walk in the Woods intends to set an appropriate tone. The opening may include a statement such as this: "We are here to achieve an interest-based solution to our problem. It will require us to fairly state what we hope to achieve in these negotiations. Even more important, it will require us to fairly and respectfully hear what others have to say. Because of the nature of our interdependence, finding a solution that is mutually satisfying demands that we first understand what each stakeholder brings to the table."

Method: Engaging the Parties. When preparing for a Walk, the first question is, Who will be at the table? Arriving at the answer is not as easy as it may appear. It requires identifying the key stakeholders. These stakeholders include those people who believe they have a say in the matter as well as those people who will be significantly affected by the outcome. Because this definition could comprise an unwieldy number of participants, it is common for large constituencies to be represented at the table rather than participating en mass. Where one draws the line between inclusion and exclusion is critical. Omitting someone whose buy-in is essential or including someone perceived as an enemy could engender resistance to the negotiated solution, no matter how well it reflects everyone's interests or desires. Similarly, creating an uneven balance at the table—whereby some constituencies or viewpoints are more generously represented than others—could threaten the ultimate acceptance and legitimacy of the outcome (Kritek, 1994). And certainly, including each and every person with a stake in the outcome could create an enormous group and require an impossibly large venue.

In general, smaller is better. With fewer people, there is more direct dialogue and less likelihood of grandstanding. Nevertheless it is important to ensure that all key stakeholders, ideas, and viewpoints are represented. Often the best litmus test is the anticipated outcome of the Walk. If a particular constituency were excluded, would its members be motivated or able to undermine the result of the process? If the answer is yes, this group should be represented. Does a particular stakeholder reflect a point of view that would otherwise be missing at the table? If so, then he or she should be there. These questions offer guidelines, recognizing that who is and who is not at the table is often a matter of sensitive negotiation in and of itself.

Once the participants have been selected and the table is set, it is time to begin the Walk. In practice, during the opening self-interests step, each party or a representative of each constituency will make a statement about their perception of the problem or issues being negotiated, their particular interests in relation to that problem or issue, and what they hope to achieve through this process. If a facilitator or mediator is guiding the process, it is common for him or her to call on people around the table, to elicit their statements, and then to summarize the key points. If it is a meeting or negotiation without a facilitator, then each party in turn is given the chance to state his or her mind regarding the issues on the table. And if it is an interpersonal discussion in which just one person is familiar with the Walk, the method becomes a personal guide that prompts and encourages expression and eliciting of legitimate interests rather than contentious positions (Mayer, 2000).

The purpose of the Walk in the Woods is to help parties build or restore confidence and ultimately trust in one another. The process helps them recognize that those on the other side of the table are not necessarily the opposition and thus to be defeated. It begins to identify the advantages and the results that could derive from truly working together: simultaneously, uncovering both motive and incentive for those participating.

Parties often come to the table in a positional frame of mind. They do not trust the other side. They are convinced that the other side has deceitful and perhaps selfish intentions. They come in a protective mode, seeking at least to hold their ground and at best to conquer their opponents.

What is required for people who implicitly do not have a trusting relationship to begin talking and even listening to one another? Expecting people to abruptly establish trust is to ask for the near impossible. Even the word *trust* is often too charged and too personal.

There is an alternative. In place of trust, it is best to focus attention on *confidence*, and to ask, for example, "What would it take for you to have the confidence that the other side will in fact do what they have agreed to do?" And, "What could you do to give the other side confidence that you will carry out what you have agreed to do?" These questions place the emphasis on the present and the immediate future rather than on the past. Whereas *trust* refers to deep-seated matters of relationships and beliefs, confidence building refers to specific actions and behaviors. It could take years to repair the suspicions arising from the past, though nothing could do more to speed the process of interest-based negotiation than some successes and confidence building in the present and into the future (Cloke & Goldsmith, 2000).

Having established what it would take to build confidence, one can then ask each of the parties to discuss their self-interests. "What do you hope to accomplish?" "What resources do you need in order to meet those objectives?" "What obstacles do you face?" "What resources can you bring to the table?" "How do you view others at the table?"

Parties are encouraged to answer these questions in a straightforward, nonadversarial way. They are also encouraged to respect the *no zinger rule*, a prohibition on words, gestures, actions, or derisive remarks that could derail the constructive and safe expression of interests. The purpose of step 1 of the Walk is to educate others at the table in a way that makes it as easy as possible to listen, hear, and understand. Obviously, if these comments are interspersed with jabs, the discussion will soon deteriorate into name-calling and accusations.

The most important ingredient of the process is the listening. Participants are encouraged to listen *actively*. This requires hearing and understanding of what is being said. Instructions for active listening might include, "Make it clear to others that you are paying attention, that you care about what they are saying, and that you are trying to understand." It is remarkable how often listening is lacking at a negotiation table. The most important information out of which the most resourceful solutions could emerge is obscured because negotiators are not paying attention.

Listening actively is not costly nor does it require extra time. And yet it can generate a wealth of new value and confidence. Most important, nothing is lost in the attempt. Done well, it allows all participants to gain a new appreciation for the hopes, objectives, problems, and constraints facing each person at the table (Tannen, 1990).

Transitioning to the Next Step. The first step of the Walk has reached its conclusion when those at the table have come to appreciate the legitimate differences among themselves and to recognize that those distinctions need not necessarily be fodder for belligerency. Even though the parties may not agree with one another, they are able to see the logic behind diverging points of view. There is often a fresh respect among participants, an encouraging sense of relief that differences are on the table, and an engaging fascination that a process has been initiated to better understand and work with issues of importance. By the end of this first step, the parties have a much broader definition of their shared problem, they see how it is viewed differently by different players, and they accept the ultimate necessity to balance these different perspectives if a solution is to be achieved. The cone in the cube analogy discussed earlier is an appropriate image for the observations and insights that derive from this first step of the Walk in the Woods—people now understand that the problems they face are multidimensional.

Once the parties really begin to hear, understand, and engage with one another, they are ready to explore multiple opportunities to reframe their differences and potentially even find ways to *expand the pie*, create a set of options that they have not yet considered or perhaps even discovered. Hence the next step of the Walk is designed to get the parties to enlarge their interests.

"Remember that what you say here is important and what you hear is even more important," Benny Bourne tells the OMC leaders as their session gets under way. "Each of you needs to be frank in stating your self-interests—that is the only way that everyone will know what they are."

He explains that the goal is to synthesize the best thinking from around the table and make the most of the opportunities that arise. "You benefit in this room from many different perspectives on the same set of problems," he says as he surveys the group. "You have trustees, managers, clinicians. You have people with many years of experience in health care and some with much less. And you have people who are being squeezed by the current pressures facing Oppidania along with some of the people who are doing the squeezing." Bourne makes a motion with his hands like crushing an orange and elicits smiles around the table. "It's no fun being squeezed, and it may come as a surprise to those under pressure that the squeezers probably aren't enjoying the process too much either." One step at a time, Bourne is intentionally broadening their focus of attention away from "good guys" and "bad guys." He wants to engender an image of people all facing a shared set of constraints and potentially shared solutions. He is by design setting the stage: here is a puzzle and we are here to figure it out, together reconfiguring the pieces and then constructively and productively piecing them together.

Larry Larkin steps forward as Bourne returns to his stool. They have a practiced rhythm that subtly models teamwork for the group. "Our first question is about priorities. If the Oppidania Medical Center is going to make the most of the transitions going on in health care today, including the fairly dramatic news you recently received, what are your priorities? I would like you now to take a few minutes to privately write them down. What are the top three strategic priorities for Oppidania along with what are the operational imperatives for each?" He gives an example: if one of the strategic priorities is reducing costs, how can OMC put that into place operationally? He suggests talking about improvements in information technology platforms to enhance efficiency and reduce workforce expenses. Another strategic priority might be expanding the "book of business" to grow patient volume. Operationally this could mean expanding niche markets such as sports medicine, launching an aggressive marketing campaign to brand new services, and recasting the image of the hospital as a great place to get care.

"It is perfectly acceptable to talk about sticking with what you consider a current top priority. Remember though, you only get *three*," he admonishes.

There are chuckles around the table, and someone comments, "There are going to be some people in this room who are going to have a hard time controlling themselves. I mean, only three!" The lighthearted tone about what is an onerous topic relieves some of the tension around the table.

"The whole point of the exercise," Larkin interjects, "is to get you focused. Of course, you each could come up with a bazillion priorities. So as you are coming up with your three top ones, focus on your domain and not 'this place would be really efficient if *everybody else* got their act together.' You will have five minutes, so spend it focused on priorities in your sphere of work or in relation to a topic with which you are familiar.''

''What Larry is saying is that it is not your individual comments alone that are important,'' Bourne says. ''The value of the exercise is what you will come up with together. Themes will emerge as we go around the room. New ideas will surface and there will be synergy in putting your ideas together. So don't worry if your three priorities don't fix every problem that the hospital faces. Just make sure that you have identified the priorities in your scope of work or expertise. No one knows that work or set of responsibilities better than you, and so it's better if you help in figuring them out.'' And then with a playful smile crossing his face, he concludes, ''Otherwise, someone else will have to do it for you, and we all know that is no fun.''

There is a point to the way Larkin and Bourne are structuring the early work of the group. They are familiar with the proclivity of organizational leaders to divert attention onto the problems and solutions of someone else. The ''fix *them* and leave *me* alone'' syndrome is an easy trap to fall into, consuming a lot of the talking and reaping little in the way of substantive improvements. Larkin and Bourne's goal is to direct the attention of people in this room toward responsibility for the decisions, actions, and results that they can reap through the retreat, and with that, set the stage for ultimate implementation of these solutions. One advantage of the Walk process is that it elicits this motivation.

For the next five minutes, the room is silent. People write. A few rise to refill their coffee cups. Some look up and glance about the room. Others ponder reflectively. As simple as the question is, it presents everyone with a perplexing challenge.

With a look at his watch, Bourne claps his hands to bring the group back together, ''OK, everybody ready? As we go around the room, Larry and I will write down your top three priorities and the operational imperatives.''

Larkin jokes, ''Remember that I'm an academic and he's a doctor so if what we write is illegible, let us know. And remember, even more important than what you say, pay attention. Listen. There will be many gems that come up around this table. Their value though is ultimately in what you are able to do with them, how you will be able to put them together.''

What ensues is a ninety-minute series of short and rich presentations. People listen. There are surprises—someone saying something that implies a sacrifice that wasn't expected. There are puzzles—a suggestion that seems out of sync with everything that is going on. And most important there are themes. Although many strategic imperatives match one another, the operational implications spark a range of new and even exciting ideas. By the time the group gets to the morning coffee break, Bourne and Larkin have assembled a colorful collection of easel paper that now covers the wall on the side of the room without windows.

As people get up to recaffeinate, Iris Inkwater scans the rich collection of thinking adorning the wall. She feels both excited and a bit intimidated. There is so much here to absorb. Obviously and fortunately, this is a really smart group of people, able to develop a dynamic collection of ideas. She has a new appreciation for the folk assembled here, and most important, she is feeling a new sense of hope and confidence.

Step 2: Enlarged Interests

Concept: Discovering Shared Interests. The purpose of this second step of the Walk is to help parties reframe their understanding of what they are negotiating. This shift in thinking moves them from a natural state of unidimensional and two-dimensional thinking to a multidimensional problem-solving perspective. What is implied in these different dimensions of negotiation perspective?

The dimensions of a negotiation may consist of, among other things, the amount of tangible and intangible gains that each party independently hopes to achieve, the relative power and influence of each of the stakeholders, and the varied histories and experiences that affect what occurs at the present table (Bazerman, 1998). Each negotiation carries its own unique set of dimensions. Therefore one facet of the analytical process is identifying just what the relevant dimensions of a particular negotiation are and then working to account for them through the negotiation process. Failing to do so is tantamount to negotiating blind (LeBaron, 2002).

The unidimensional perspective considers a problem simply as a matter of satisfying "my own" wants and desires, ignoring other dimensions as if they do not exist or do not merit consideration. A unidimensional negotiator expects self-satisfaction, irrespective and sometimes even to the detriment of others. In the mind of the unidimensional negotiator, successful negotiation is about satisfying his or her objectives, with little or no consideration for the needs or concerns of others. Negotiation success is measured exclusively in terms of outcome, with scant consideration for process or the substantive impact upon and opinion of others.

The unidimensional perspective on negotiation often sparks resistance from others at the negotiation table who see it as selfish and are loath to accommodate such expectations. This resistance manifests as a positional response, instigating a tendency toward two-dimensional problem solving, which typically means a fight.

The two-dimensional perspective sees the problem as *us versus them* (Bacharach & Lawler, 1981). The negotiators confront one another as opponents with rigid demands. Others at the table are seen as obstacles to be circumvented. Any gain or credit for the *other* side is seen as a loss for *us*, so the parties become as concerned with constraining others as they are in winning gains for themselves. Two-dimensional problem solvers are singularly focused upon attaining victory and avoiding defeat. They use positional and confrontational strategies and tactics to get their way. Two-dimensional problem solving is typified as classic, win-lose adversarial behavior.

Uni- and two-dimensional negotiators show little concern about the interests of others. Rather, these other parties are seen as obstacles and opponents to be overcome. The purpose for knowing and understanding others is to better beat them: learn their vulnerabilities, develop a strategy to exploit them, and then head for victory (Cloke & Goldsmith, 2000). In their minds, the process of gaining information has a very circumscribed and selfish purpose.

By contrast multidimensional problem solving attends to the differences in perspectives, ambitions, and desires of the many parties whose combined efforts ultimately will determine the success or failure of the process and its outcome. Multidimensional problem solvers see a broad array of factors that must be considered if a deal is to be reached. For starters, they look at their own situation with an ordered perspective: they are able to distinguish that which they *must* get from that which they would *like* to get. In other words they prioritize their interests, recognizing that they are more likely to gain what is important to them if they are willing to give on elements that are less important. Beyond that, they are actively curious about and aware of the ways others at the table order their interests. They view others, and opportunities to assist one another, as productive means toward shared ends. Multidimensional problem solvers recognize that their best chance to achieve their own interests is by working with others to satisfy theirs.

In this step, then, participants' interests are enlarged through transforming their uni- and two-dimensional perspectives on the problem into a multidimensional perspective. This is what is meant by *reframing*.

It is common as one approaches a negotiation to have a *frame*, a mental model, for what the problem is and what is to be achieved (Senge, 1994). The data used to assemble that frame are self-generated and serve a combination of legitimate self-interests and downright selfish interests. However, once parties have been exposed to the interests of others around the table, this newly acquired information can reshape their understanding of both the process and possible outcome of the negotiation. To encourage them in turning this analytical perspective into a new frame, it is useful to systematically assemble that new data in a way that fosters its constructive reinterpretation (Argyris & Schön, 1996). How can this be accomplished?

In the typical me-against-you frame of mind, it is common to focus on points of disagreement and how they might be advantageously resolved. In the enlarged interests phase of the Walk, a new focus is placed upon the often invisible points of agreement.

Method: Reframing the Negotiation. In practice a facilitator or one of the parties will simply pose the question, "What is it that everyone around the table agrees on?" Typically, two easels are used (Isenhart & Spangle, 2000), one headlined "Agreement" and the other headlined "Disagreement" (a useful image even if it does not fit the circumstances of every negotiation).

It is important to list points of agreement first. This list will often include principles and values shared by the parties, an expression of a common desire to resolve the issues or reach consensus, the often surprising mutual acknowledgment of the downside of not reaching agreement, and a vision for what might be achieved if the problem could be amicably settled. With a bit of grounded imagination, this list can be quite long and very revealing. There is frequently an aha moment that emerges as the parties realize that on the most important issues, they actually do agree. They recognize that many of their interests and their motivations are overlapping, and with that, they see the possibility of developing an agreement that can advance those shared motives, values, and interests. That realization is what prompts the new understanding of what they are negotiating about, the reframing that opens the possibility that the Walk will take them to unforeseen conversations.

Next, on the second sheet of easel paper, the disagreements are listed. It is rare to find that the number of points of disagreement exceeds the number of points of agreement. Those points of disagreement look quite different to the participants when seen in light of the newly minted and enlarged points of agreement. They often seem less important and more resolvable alongside the sometimes profound points of agreement. The reframing process is complete when the parties discover a fresh perspective on the shared problem and a renewed energy and hope for finding a resolution.

In combative two-dimensional problem solving, it is common for the sides to focus far more attention on what divides them than on what might unite them. The exercise in this step of exploring points of agreement and disagreement may reveal the merits of seeing the other side as a possible ally to be recruited rather than merely an enemy to be defeated. If this reframing can be achieved, it allows all sides to choosing to invest their energies in exploring shared solutions over simply scheming to defeat one another. It is a discovery process because, in most cases, the parties did not previously recognize the mutuality of their concerns, obstacles, and objectives.

In the course of this less confrontational dialogue—as they actively listen to one another—the parties often find that there might be innovative solutions to their shared problems. These solutions were formerly obscured by their preoccupation with what divided them over what could in fact unite them. As this phase of the negotiation concludes, it is not uncommon for someone to say, "If we agree on so much, we have to find a way to resolve those points of disagreement."

Transitioning to the Next Step. The constructive dialogue that is at the center of this phase of the Walk in the Woods encourages the parties to see their own situation, and the circumstances that they share, from a new and different angle. They not only better understand their side of the problem. They also appreciate the problem from the perspective of others—thus seeing its many dimensions. It is this broadened view that is at the center of multidimensional problem solving.

The parties recognize in this process that their shared problems are not a simple matter of good guys and bad guys. Such a simplistic view is replaced by a real appreciation for the issues that all sides are grappling with—what they each need in order to meet legitimate objectives. There is also fresh awareness that together they might even be able to help solve each other's problems. They might build options that neither could have considered if working alone.

What is the outcome of this phase of the process? Each side has generated a bigger picture of the work to be done. Each has reframed the problem. They all see themselves as part of something larger: an interdependent system of people whose successes and failures directly affect the fate of others in their surroundings (Marcus, 2003). It puts what they do—the problems they confront and the potential they face—into a whole new perspective.

It is the change in the mood of the negotiation and the new possibilities that are opened that propels the parties into step 3 of their Walk in the Woods. This next step translates the previous *aha* moments, the discoveries of enlarged interests, into enlightened interests—new ideas, creative options, and innovative solutions. It builds upon the widened perspectives and new confidence that the parties are establishing together.

It is a particularly lively and friendly coffee break. People who don't regularly interact are engaged in discussing what was said during the first step of the Walk in the Woods. Physicians approach trustees. Finance people talk with clinicians. Old-timers are animatedly discussing ideas with more recent recruits. A sense of wonder and optimism is overtaking the room, along with a realization of how hard, different, and potentially even exciting the future could be.

Bourne calls them all back to their seats for the next step of the Walk, working toward enlarged interests. At the front of the room, the two easel boards are headlined respectively "Agreement" and "Disagreement." Larkin poses a question, "Did you notice anything as we went around the room during the self-interests step of the Walk?"

David Dickenson, the vice president of human resources, raises his hand. "Yes, it was fascinating how common themes came up around the table. There was a lot of talk about the workforce and how we might be able to get the same amount of work done with fewer people. There was also a lot between the lines about our values. We are a value-driven institution and a value-driven group of people here. I think it showed. There are certain things we are not going to sacrifice, chief among them the commitment to high standards of quality of care."

Janice Johnson, nursing vice president, raises her hand as well and Bourne gestures toward her. "Actually, I heard it a bit differently. We are a labor-intensive operation. The work we do is hands-on, and there is no way around that. I heard a lot about productivity. How do we help our people to become more productive without placing new burdens on them that ultimately frustrate them, making them less productive? My concern is that in solving one problem we may end up creating new and even more dangerous problems. We are caught in the cross fire. The policy wonks want us to cut costs and at the same time they mandate nurse-to-patient numbers that are expensive. I mean, when we talk quality we have to remember it's not simply a nice slogan; it takes people to make it work."

Rajeev Rao, chief financial officer for OMC, dives into the debate: "Actually, I heard an interesting combination of perspectives as we went around the room. Janice, I think you're right about nurse-patient ratios. They are a central tenet of quality of care, and for sure they are a metric that has gotten a lot of deserved attention. That said, I think everyone is looking at what we can do to make the life and the work of our nurses less burdensome so they can be more productive and, with that, find ways to do good and to do it in a more streamlined way. I was hearing options as we went around the room."

Larkin jumps back in. "Now you see the point of the enlarged interests step of the Walk. Benny and I had the same observations. There were some very important themes of agreement that we heard as you went around the room, though you will be better able to identify the specifics because you live here and interact together on a regular basis. So first, let's list what you saw as points of agreement. After that, we'll move on to points of disagreement."

Everyone is suddenly quiet as they stare at the wall with the array of strategic priorities and operational imperatives that were delineated in the first step of the Walk. Some jot notes. Others stand up to get a better look. Everyone is thinking.

Finally, Fred Fisher, OMC's medical director, breaks the silence, "Well, I think we can all agree that this is not fun." There is an uncomfortable titter in the room. Stand-up comics in nightclubs get hecklers; facilitators know that it is uncomfortable tackling tough issues and it sometimes evokes its own form of resentment. Larkin and Bourne glance at one another; they know what to do next.

Bourne, as a fellow doctor, turns to Fisher, "Fred, I could not agree with you more." By concurring with Fisher he demonstrates that this is a legitimate sentiment, which the leadership of the hospital will have to recognize and acknowledge. At the same time, he also wants to keep Fisher engaged in the process, as he is an important figure in the institution. "When I walked out of medical school," Bourne continues, "I was given a diploma and what I thought was a golden ticket to professional fulfillment and autonomy. Sure, practicing medicine was going to be tough but everything surrounding the clinical work would be easy: there would be generous reimbursements, a hospital to cater to me, and patients who would bestow upon me their abundant gratitude. What could be bad?" Bourne shrugged his shoulders. "And then someone changed the rules and didn't pass out the new rule book to us. Doctors no longer received a free lunch at the hospital, administrators began to push us about utilization rates, and Internet-savvy patients started questioning all aspects of their care. Suddenly we were strangers in a strange land."

"We could sit here and lament it. At the end of the day though, it is what it is. We are in a different world now. Fred, believe me, I know this is a tough transition. And we doctors need to be engaged in this process more now than ever before. It is up to us to ensure that we maintain a doctor-friendly environment, because if we don't, the road is only going to get rougher. There is a lot that medicine must uphold as the system transforms, and you're right, it's not fun, though it is critically important."

The other participants looked back and forth at each other, wondering how Fred would respond. He sighs heavily. "You're right, Benny, but as I told you during the break, this isn't easy for a guy who has been around this block too many times before. I have to admit though, it's even less fun if someone else is calling the shots for me. OK, so you want to know what we all agree on? Here's my real answer. I think we agree that we have to distinguish ourselves as an institution. That means we have to provide extraordinary clinical services and be aggressive drivers of quality of care. It is our strategic advantage compared to our competitors, and if we keep that singular focus, other things will line up for us."

Larry Lumberg, medical director of the emergency department, decides this is a good time for him to enter the dialogue. He has been included in the retreat not because of the seniority of his position but because he is respected by his peers as thoughtful and direct. "I think if you look at the list, quality and the advantage it creates for us pop up repeatedly, though I think they are part of a much larger balance." He explains the importance of looking at everything through the lens of the market because market forces drive many of the challenges they face. "For example, I see that people talked not so much about reducing costs but rather about improving efficiencies," he says. "This is a subtle yet important difference." He continues his analysis, turning to quality. "I see specific services and activities where we can focus attention and get a lot of bang for our buck. With that, we create market advantage: better care at a better price. I think, by contrast, our competitors will cut quality in their zeal to cut costs, which might work in the short run and it will catch up with them over time." Focusing on Fred Fisher across the table, he concludes, "And I think we're smart enough to figure out how to do it. There is a lot of good thinking here."

Larkin walks over to the easel titled "Agreement," notes what has just been said, and then announces, "OK. That was a good start. What else?"

For the next sixty minutes, the group pulls out themes of agreement from the many comments and ideas collected during the self-interests step of the Walk. Iris Inkwater notes to herself that there have been a number of eye-openers. The expected divides between administrative and clinical people have not appeared: in fact, there is broad accord on what needs to be done about both costs and quality. New ideas are gaining broader support than she would have imagined, and even Fred Fisher is making contributions.

Dickenson raises his hand again. "If I may, it seems that we've reached a consensus: the hospital must find better ways to keep the humans doing what only humans can do, and to let machines and computers do what they can do at lower expense."

When the list of key themes is exhausted, Bourne changes the topic: "OK, now that we have this impressive list of agreements, what is it that you disagree about?"

Arlan Abbington, the board chair, is perplexed. "We seem to agree on so much. What is there to disagree on?"

In fact, there were a number of points of disagreement. Clinicians called for trimming down what they perceived as top-heavy management. Managers believed clinicians could be far more precise in their patient care judgments in order to avoid wasting time and money. Some in the room were in favor of consolidating operations with other health systems, whereas others believed that would dilute the OMC brand. One person commented, "We're at the top of our game. Why would we want to align with someone downstream?" and another disagreed, saying, "This is about market share. If we leverage our reputation to expand volume, we are in a much stronger position in the market."

As the retreat approaches the lunch break, Larkin moves to the center of the room: "Now that we concluded the first two steps of the Walk in the Woods, what are your observations about where OMC is and where you might go from here?"

Perry Pudolski, OMC chief operations officer, takes a stab at it. "On the one hand the points of disagreement we identified are significant and, for the most part, aren't really new. I mean, we have to admit that we've been over much of that terrain countless times. On the other hand the points of agreement are really interesting. There are some really exciting ideas and opportunities there. And from my perspective, if we can agree on so much from the get-go, I am sure we can find ways to resolve those points of disagreement."

To everyone's surprise—and to the delight of many—Fred Fisher follows on: "I agree with Perry. I can tell you from my Navy days that I would rather be on a ship that's going somewhere than sitting in port waiting for orders. This place has a lot going for it, and I think we could actually turn the corner with some of these points here. The question, of course, is how we can put them into action. If we can somehow reduce the pain of the transition then good things could come out of this."

With that Bourne concludes the morning session and the group heads toward the bountiful buffet in the adjoining room.

Step 3: Enlightened Interests

Concept: Explore New Thinking. Top-notch negotiators share a common characteristic: the capacity to imagine. They are able to comprehend problems and develop solutions that others who do not share the same visionary aptitude are simply unable to see. Why is imagination so important?

Negotiation at its best is a process for finding and taking advantage of opportunities: a chance to explore options and discover an outcome that does not already exist. The most creative negotiators smartly hunt for possible advantages and devise ways to make them happen. For example, in a complex organization with interdependent components, it is impossible to fully achieve one's objectives without working resourcefully in concert with many others. Therefore seeking gain at the expense of one's cohorts is imprudent. Conversely, advantage generated in concert with them can be synergistic. And it often takes a dose of grounded imagination to find these healthier options.

Engaging imaginative thinking is both difficult and important. Why? Young people are encouraged to imagine: early education curricula are designed to cultivate radiant creativity. With time and the process of personal and professional socialization, that gift and propensity for creativity fades, replaced by reliance upon familiar patterns, comfortable solutions, and the securities of the known and tested. People accumulate a mound of "baggage" as their lives and careers progress: biases, sour experiences, resistance to change, and downright stubbornness. Time constraints and pressure may compel the path of least resistance and acceptance of interim or less desirable solutions. This mind-set gets in the way of imaginative problem solving and obscures what could be achieved through the negotiation process. Uncovering an innovative solution requires abandoning one's accustomed blinders for at least long enough to become inventive.

The purpose of the enlightened interests step of the Walk is to systematically generate the fresh and innovative ideas that can spark such a synergy of action and interaction. This step comes at the point—just after the substance of the negotiation has been reframed—when negotiating parties recognize the potentially untapped and valuable benefits that could accrue from a working partnership, a mutually beneficial solution, or a peaceful settlement of their conflict. This recognition engenders newfound confidence and motivation that is a far cry from the reticence and resistance with which they likely initiated the process.

An infusion of genuinely creative and inspired thinking at this step of the Walk engenders fresh ideas, though it is especially difficult to activate if the parties are in a highly polarized conflict. What can mitigate the dangers? There is one rule that can help you avoid a destructive pitfall that would increase polarization during this step of the Walk. The discussion of enlightened interests occurs in a *no commitment zone* of safety. Ideas can be proposed, explored, or pondered without fear that someone will slyly slide a contract under one's nose just as the creativity has reached its peak. This rule frees participants from the fears and constraints of an obligation cast too early in the process.

Just as listing points of agreement and disagreement was a useful exercise during the enlarged interests step, an exercise to encourage creative problem solving and to practice mini-deal making is at the heart of the enlightened interests. How is this accomplished?

Method: Generating New Opportunities. Once again, go to your real—or at least "virtual"—easel board. Instruct the parties to brainstorm (Fisher & Ury, 1981). During brainstorming, have them generate as many creative ideas as possible. There should be no commentary, no editing, and no disagreement with what is being said as it is recorded on the board. Allow new and inventive ideas to flow so they can stimulate even more fertile possibilities. For example, go around the table and have each party offer an innovative idea in the form of a sentence starting with the word *imagine*: "Imagine if we could . . ." In addition to encouraging positive and productive ideas, urge participants to consider what could happen if the problem or conflict is not resolved. Spur them on with evocative questions: "What *out-of-the-box* options can you think of that might move us toward a solution of this problem?" Try open-ended questions, such as asking them what might happen if they tried a specific provocative idea. Encourage them to think about both the short-term and long-term implications: "If the problem is solved, what are the benefits? And if not, what are the costs?" Remember: genius in the form of innovative and exciting possibilities often arises by merging seemingly outrageous and unconventional ideas. Record each of the comments, observations, and ideas resulting from these questions so they can be part of the subsequent analytical process.

For the sake of illustration, assume that forty new ideas and possibilities have been listed on your easel board. Each of these points has a different potential meaning or set of implications for each of the participants. Negotiators felt safe in putting these ideas on the board because at this point they are nothing more than playful and exploratory thoughts considered on the pathway toward a workable solution. Among them are options that are promising, impossible, funny, frightening, and exciting. The question now is what to do with them.

Just as one warms up before engaging in serious exercise, parties to a negotiation can use an opportunity to warm up in advance of the real deal making that will occur during the final step of the Walk. The second phase of the enlightened interests step offers this opportunity. How is this done?

After the brainstorming list is complete, every point is individually discussed and assigned a number: 1, 2, or 3. The criteria used to categorize each point depends on the nature of the issues being negotiated. For example, ideas could be categorized by level of agreement. If everyone agrees on a point, it gets a 1. If there is clear disagreement, it gets a 3. And if there is ambiguity about agreement or disagreement, the idea is assigned a 2. Similarly, the categorization could be by feasibility, time frame (what could be done in the next week, month, or year), or sell-ability (likelihood of being acceptable to represented constituencies, such as a board of directors, staff, or a labor union). After going through each point, do one last review of the ideas that received a 2—a maybe—asking whether what was learned through the exercise could modify and thereby nudge any point up into the 1 grouping or down to the 3 category. Or perhaps, a proposed solution that received a 2 could be modified or traded for something else in order to turn it into a 1. Points assigned a 1 are the *deal makers* and those given a 3 are the *deal breakers*. It is just as important to know what is impossible as it is important to forge the newly possible.

Next, start a fresh list of only the points that garnered a 1. It is this set of ideas that will be carried into the next step of the Walk as the substantive bargaining gets under way.

When they are leading a Walk in the Woods retreat, Bourne and Larkin rarely enjoy a leisurely lunch. They use the time to get a deeper read on the room. Larkin checks in with Iris Inkwater, Arlan Abbington, and Perry Pudolski to glean their sense for how things are going. Inkwater and Abbington are very upbeat, and Puldolski expresses concern about whether a concrete outcome will emerge from all this talk. Bourne speaks with Fisher and Lumberg. Fisher is surprised at how much ground they have covered so quickly. Lumberg is warily cautious, warning Bourne to be careful of a setup: "Don't be surprised if people stop singing 'Kumbaya' once we get to some hard decisions."

As he finishes talking with Lumberg, Bourne notices Janice Johnson eating by herself. She is clearly unhappy. Bourne pulls a chair up next to hers. "What's on your mind, Janice?"

"I know where this is going by the end of the day," she says. "When things get tough, the first thing they do around here is try to solve the problem on the backs of nursing. I've been through this before and I can feel the wave coming. And it's not going to be good for my nurses."

"Keep with us, Janice," Bourne urges. "Your perspective is important." As the lunch hour is drawing to a close, Bourne then excuses himself to go to compare notes with Larkin.

It is close to one o'clock, and Bourne encourages the participants to fill their coffee cups and get ready to move on to the enlightened interests step of the Walk.

"You accomplished a great deal this morning in steps 1 and 2 of the Walk," Bourne says to the reassembled group. "We call self- and enlarged interests the *learning steps* because you have gotten a good and detailed picture of all the different perspectives that you have at the hospital. Now it's time to build the options that you can take into charting OMC's strategic direction and operational imperatives."

Larkin then describes step 3, the enlightened interests segment of the Walk. He emphasizes that this step features a no commitment zone in which offers can be made, actions suggested, and even wild new ideas floated without fear that they will be considered firm obligations. The purpose is to explore new possibilities, new ways of doing business, and new opportunities, without concern for the implicit commitments.

Perry Pudolski challenges Larkin. "If we are making suggestions without committing to follow through, then what's the point? I mean, all we're going to get is a lot of hot air."

Bourne takes up the challenge: "That's a valid point, Perry. This step of the Walk precedes the last step, where we will establish aligned interests and where we will get concrete, tangible commitments. Before we get there, we want to take a moment to encourage some productive creativity so that we don't just circulate and then argue all the same old ideas in that final phase. What we have also found is that there are a lot of both real and hidden constraints to really inspired thinking. People are afraid of change. They are concerned about increased burdens. And quite frankly, many of the best ideas are often lost because people are afraid of looking silly. Therefore, just before we get concrete, we erect this little inventive zone to encourage barrier-free thinking. We know it's a bit of a leap. Would you be willing to make the jump with us?" Pudolski signals his acceptance but Bourne is not convinced: "Perry, how about this. Can we check in with you a bit later on this question?"

Pudolski nods more enthusiastically. "You've got a deal."

Larkin walks to the center of the U formed by the tables to provide instructions for the process of developing enlightened interests. "Now we'll have another few moments of silence. I want you to write the word *imagine* at the top of your piece of paper." Larkin pauses. Knowing that this is an unusual instruction for this sort of a group, he waits until he sees people actually writing it down. "Good, now you've taken the first step in this process. Consider this. Let's say it's the year 1900 and I have asked you to imagine what health care would be like in the year 2000. That would be an extraordinarily tall order. Hard to imagine: CAT scans, MRIs, joint replacements—I could go on and on. People who observe the evolution of science and technology estimate that we will create more knowledge this year than in the previous 1,000 years combined. It's hard to imagine, right?" Bourne and Larkin glance around the room and people are transfixed.

Bourne continues the introduction, "As OMC leaders, you need to be looking at a five-year horizon at least. That's what it takes to plan and act strategically. Once you have the horizon in sight, then you ask yourselves what we need to do today, tomorrow, and over the next five years to get there. A lot is going to change in health care over the next five years. And Oppidania is either going to be leading that change here in town or following behind it. With that pace of innovation and adaptation, there won't be much room for followers. So with that background, under your word *imagine*, I want you to describe what innovative things you could all be doing to lead the curve, to move beyond your current set of dilemmas, and to turn Oppidania Medical Center into the leading organization that it aspires to be. Imagine the outcome and imagine what it will take to get there. You have ten minutes. Keep in mind what we discussed this morning. Are there any more questions?" There were none, and people settled into quiet, intent work.

Ten minutes later, Bourne and Larkin are at the front of the room by the easel boards ready to record what will follow. Over the next hour, they go around the table and everyone has the chance to share his or her *imagine* notes. The thoughts range from the brilliant to the mundane. Yet even the mundane ideas have kernels of opportunity embedded in them. Once the overlapping new ideas are lumped together, the exercise yields forty distinct proposals that the group did not have that morning.

Lumberg's idea reflects the sort of progressive thinking that has pervaded the room. ''Imagine,'' he reads, ''that when a patient arrives at our emergency room, we are able to assess, diagnose, and move them through our system to expeditiously reach a decision on their disposition with accuracy and at a pace that exceeds the expectations of patients and the clinical staff.'' He explains that the electronic medical record (EMR) currently being used has cumbersome features that significantly slow the process. It takes a long time to get lab results back, to engage everyone who needs to be part of the decision, and to fend off other distractions. He shares what he has been reading about new EMR platforms that have been shown to cut that time by half or even more. ''If we could see that kind of improved efficiency in the emergency department, it would trickle throughout the hospital like a welcome infection. We could greatly reduce the cost of getting a patient in, through, and out of our system. And furthermore, it would be a great marketing angle: a better emergency room experience would be an attractive draw for patients.''

Rajeev Rao, OMC's CFO counters, ''I don't want to squelch creative thinking; however, I have to insert a dose of reality here. We have already invested a lot into our EMR system and it is not something that you can easily replace. I mean we have to be looking at ways to save money, not spend more.''

Lumberg wants his tone to be friendly, so he responds carefully to Rao: ''I think you're right about saving money. That said, money is squandered every day on each patient who comes through our ER. All that I am suggesting is that we do a cost-benefit analysis on an upgraded system. Based on what I am hearing from colleagues at other hospitals, the numbers look really good. And I think that is the point of this exercise. Yes, we can't go off spending money carelessly. I think we can, however, be more analytical in what we are doing and, with that, find all sorts of ways to improve efficiencies and the patient care experience.''

Rao tips his pen toward Lumberg in a friendly salute, ''I can sign on to that. As long as we are intentional and analytical about what we are doing, we may find short-term investments that generate great long-term returns. Yeah, I'm willing to have that discussion.''

Bourne walks into the U. ''What you have just seen is the essence of the enlightened interests step. What we do next, and thank you Larry and Rajeev for that demonstration, is to go through each idea and assign it a number.'' Bourne explains that when there is agreement that the idea is worth pursuing, the idea gets a 1. When there is disagreement, it gets a 3. And when people are uncertain about whether it is worth following up, it gets a 2.

Bourne says, "Everything that is a number 1—a *deal maker*—will be brought along into the next step, where we focus on the aligned interests and come up with strategic and operational steps for going forward—the commitments Larry was looking for. Every idea that gets a 2 merits a discussion, just as we saw here about the emergency department and the EMR. That discussion could elevate the idea into another deal maker, and it will then go into the 1 column. Or if it really is unacceptable to a constituency around the table, it goes into the *deal breaker* column, number 3. In other words, advocating that proposal in its unchanged form would significantly alienate one or more of the stakeholders here to the point that it does not deserve further attention."

Larkin continues, "OK, this is a pretty easy process. I will read each of the forty options. If you think it is a 1, something you would sign onto in its proposed form, raise one finger. If not, raise three. Or if you could sign on with some modifications, put up two fingers. Be clear—my eyesight is not what it used to be. If I get all 1's on a proposal, it's a 1. All 3's, and it's a 3. Any proposal for which there is a mix becomes a 2. Here we go."

It takes the group ten minutes to make it through the forty ideas. About half of the ideas make it into group 1. A few are relegated to group 3—imaginative though not realistic. And the rest await in group 2. The subsequent mini-discussions about these 2's elicit a range of objection, advocacy, and questioning. In the course of this, many of these ideas evolve and look different by the time the discussion ends—the result of a bit of compromise, a lot of clarification, and a dose of good communication.

And by the time they arrive at the afternoon coffee break at the conclusion of the enlightened interests step, the participants have twenty-five new, energizing ideas and proposals that they did not have when they started the day. Just before adjourning the discussion, Bourne walks over to Perry Pudolski and asks out loud, "OK, Perry, how are we doing?" Both Bourne and Larkin had noticed Pudolski's enthusiasm during the exercise. "This is great," Perry replies. "We're making good progress."

With that, tired though resolute smiles break out around the room as everyone stands up for a well-deserved breather.

Transitioning to the Next Step. In addition to providing substantive points for later negotiation, in what way has this sorting exercise been a warm-up for the bargaining that occurs during the aligned interests step of the Walk?

Assuming that the enlightened interests generated those forty new items, the negotiators have just had forty opportunities to engage in mini-deal making.

The low-stakes and no commitment discussion about each item gave them a chance to get to know one another, to experience how they perceive the issues and outcomes differently, and to practice arriving at an agreement about the number each item was assigned. Every point that achieved a 1 or a 3 represents an agreement. Every item that received a 2 is a matter of disagreement and perhaps further negotiation.

Note the behavior that is often present during this step of the Walk. The sometimes zany discussion evokes laughter, storytelling, and a fluid discussion among the participants. Typically, it is a fun, funny, and stress-relieving experience. Whereas participants might have started the Walk in a contentious frame of mind, by the time they are well into and engaged in the enlightened interests step, they begin to see the shared problem or conflict as being on one side of the table and themselves as being on the other side, striving to resolve it together.

It is common for this brainstorming exercise to establish a reservoir of new ideas and even a measure of goodwill. The imaginative dialogue that occurs during the enlightened interests step is reflective, responsive, and invigorating. The creative exchange catalyzes hope and new confidence that workable solutions can be found. Just as it opens doors to new opportunities, the low-stakes discussion allows participants to discover doors they never knew existed. Intuitive, inventive insight takes its place with the pragmatism of linear thinking. The necessary risk taking, flexibility, and openness to innovative ideas is buttressed by the new confidence found in the first two steps of the Walk in the Woods. The familiarity and practice experienced through the exercise has created a set of resourceful ideas and productive motivations that will take participants into the next step.

In the course of the enlightened interests discussion, the parties generate new dimensions to complement the multidimensional understanding achieved during the prior step of the Walk. As they transition toward the aligned interests step, they will employ those new dimensions to build a multidimensional solution to their shared problem.

Step 4: Aligned Interests

Concept: Redefining Success. The first three steps of the Walk serve as prelude to the bargaining—the actual *getting* and *giving*—that occurs during the step of achieving aligned interests. The purpose of this step, as implied in its name, is to guide the parties toward an aligned outcome—decisions, exchanges, and relationships—that link and balance what they each hope to achieve. This is the destination point, where—depending on the nature of the Walk—the deal is struck, the conflict is settled, or the partnership is endorsed.

When the parties to a negotiation begin their Walk, they each likely have a definition for what they would see as a "successful" outcome. Success of course has a number of important connotations, speaking to more than just the actual booty acquired at the table. It also encompasses—among many other ingredients—the achieved status, image, relationships, and implications for future negotiations. Success, as opposed to winning, accounts for the complexities and interactions of the negotiation above and beyond the tangible take.

Success at the outset of a Walk is most often defined in relatively narrow, unidimensional terms: the parties each seek victory. That frame of reference defines how their acquisitions could enhance their well-being or advance their cause. The purpose of their Walk is to expand that horizon, in other words to redefine success so that it integrates considerations beyond the unidimensional (Schelling, 1960; Thompson, 2001). The process has transported them from a uni- and two-dimensional understanding of their positions to an integrated multidimensional perspective on their problem; they have gone beyond a cone in the cube approach. By the time they reach this final stage of the Walk, they are ready to transform their multidimensional problem into a multidimensional solution. The impetus toward and discovery of that otherwise unattainable solution is the essence of their mutual triumph.

If the parties at this point have in fact achieved this redefinition of success, then the discussion during the concluding step of the Walk will be significantly different from what otherwise would have occurred. This difference is the added value of the process. It reframes what the parties are negotiating toward; it changes the criteria used to assess whether the goal was attained and rewrites the story the parties will tell about both the outcome and the process of their negotiation (Slaikeu, 1996).

Method: Prioritizing and Expanding Interests. In real life individuals do not get everything they desire. Each individual sets priorities and then allocates time, assets, and effort to achieve that which is deemed most important. In negotiation this process is made explicit, not simply in the confines of each stakeholder's personal thinking and behavior. It is at the core of the interchange between two or more stakeholders who must align their priorities to best satisfy their different interests.

To align priorities, the gives and gets are described, defined, and ranked. Each party to the negotiation has his or her order and hierarchy of interests. In practice, during the bargaining phase of this concluding step, the participants articulate what they *must*, *want to*, and *would like to* get in order to consummate the deal. It is almost always the case that lists differ around the table. In similar fashion, the parties articulate what they are *eager*, *willing*, and *unwilling* to give in order to achieve an agreement. Over the course of this discussion, it is likely that some of the items topping people's lists will drop into a secondary position as parties recognize the value of flexibility on the road to crafting a deal. The discussion during this step creates conditions that encourage the parties to adapt their lists as long as the dividend—an agreement—satisfies a desirable combination of interests.

It is not uncommon for this discussion to begin with the momentary feel of horse trading: the horse seller exaggerates the beauty of the animal while the buyer points emphatically to its scruffiness. With a bit of refocusing, the stakeholders are reminded of what brought them to the table and what has been learned through the Walk: their shared interest in consummating this trade at a fair price and in a manner that encourages continued trade into the future.

Once the priorities of the give-and-get have been articulated, the discussion moves toward fleshing out the actual exchanges necessary to achieve consensus. It is common to hear, "I would be willing to ... in exchange for ..." At this point the parties discuss the matters to which they are willing and not willing to commit; the strategy, logistics, pragmatics, and timeline for accomplishing their objectives; and the implications of the deal for future collaboration and negotiation (Bacharach & Lawler, 1981). In other words, they are in effect saying, "I would be willing to satisfy some of your top priorities if you would be willing to satisfy some of mine." The mesh of gears—the alignment—is reached as the parties recognize how their different yet overlapping interests allow them to satisfy another person or group as a means to satisfy themselves.

Ultimately, if the negotiation is going to end in a deal, each party must achieve some recognizable gain: each must *get* something. The things they get certainly need not be the same and need not even be of equal monetary value.

The value of what each stakeholder gains in the process—whether it is tangible, such as money, or intangible, such as recognition—is gauged by the importance it has for him or her. A deal is reached if the parties are able to think imaginatively about what they value and what they are gaining by having come to a deal—the very frame of mind that the Walk hopes to inspire. There is certainly value in the cache they take from the table. There is also value—if they are negotiating a conflict—to the ceasefire: the savings realized by not having to wage battle and the goodwill engendered by the deal. If it is a business arrangement, there is value not only in the current dollars on the table. There are also future deals and opportunities opened by the agreement. And if it is a matter of negotiating a working relationship, there is value in the exchange of knowledge, synergy of ideas, and boosted morale that come with developing a satisfying partnership. By attributing a clear value to these multiple dimensions of the deal being achieved—many of which are intangible and therefore defy monetary significance—negotiators discover that there is much more available for exchange than they had previously thought and therefore much more to be gained through a creative and interest-based approach to crafting an agreement. In this way the parties truly expand the pie: each gets more because there is more to be gotten.

Transitioning Toward the Conclusion. The reformulated definition of success reached during this aligning of interests is this: "If I succeed, you succeed; and if you succeed, I succeed. Therefore let's work toward achieving mutual success."

What occurs in this final step of the Walk is the *so what* of the process: the commitment, the transaction, or the conflict resolution. At the outset of the Walk, the parties articulated the problem, process, and purpose for their coming together. The Walk has provided them with a structured, directed, and deliberate platform for working toward an alignment of their interests. It is at this point that they can assess their progress in achieving a working relationship that has spawned a viable agreement.

The arrangement must meet several tests if it is to be upheld over the long run. It must be acceptable to each of the constituents. It must make conspicuously clear what each stakeholder has to gain and what each stakeholder has put on the table. As each side evaluates the deal, it must meet—in its balance—the test of fairness (Bazerman & Neal, 1995). If it does, it will likely fulfill its long-term challenge: the test of time.

The intent has been to find common ground. The time when the bargain is being finalized is not the moment to inflate desires or to exaggerate needs. Rather, this is the time to seek a just balance, pledge to work together, and begin to anticipate the rewards of the resolution. Each party gets more because the parties together have conceived more. Each party is just as concerned about the others' satisfaction as about his or her own and that of his or her constituents. The deal the parties are accepting is based on a synergy of intent and outcome. If it achieves its potential, it will spawn its own additional successes. The parties create the *whole* that is at the heart of whole image negotiation (see Chapter Five).

The process is punctuated in a form appropriate to the nature of the specific negotiation. Whatever that form might be—a memorandum of understanding, a letter, or a contract—it is useful to write down the agreement, being careful that the language, spirit, and depiction of the process and outcome are acceptable both to those who participated and to those who did not—all of those who will ultimately judge what occurred. It is likely that what has been accomplished is worthy of the time and effort invested: it should be duly documented and celebrated. Reaching agreement is not to be taken lightly. It is hard work, requiring a wealth of patience, perspective, and flexibility. What has been achieved is significant not only for what it clarifies about the past but also, and even more important, the agreement is significant for what it opens for the future.

Bourne and Larkin use most of the break to ready themselves for the home stretch of the retreat. Much has been accomplished to this point. The self-interests step engaged everyone in the group and cleared up a number of the reservations people had brought into the room, though not all of them. Robust reframing occurred during the enlarged interests step. And a bevy of new ideas emerged out of the enlightened interests step. All of that process would have to come together in this final step of the Walk in the Woods, in which they would work to establish aligned interests.

"OK, Larry, this is where the rubber meets the road—and not the sky. We have to keep them grounded," Bourne says. He looks out at the group now energetically engaged in conversation around the coffee urn.

Bourne corrals everyone back around the table, and Larkin opens the final session. "You have generated twenty-five new and creative ideas for charting a fresh course for OMC. Not every idea is the same in scope. Several of them propose significant strategic changes: for example, idea 17 on our list is 'imagine reconstructing the hospital as a patient-centric organization that builds around care quality and patient satisfaction.' Others of them are more tactical: for example, idea 3 on the list, which imagines a new building to expand the number of community doctors with offices adjacent to the hospital. And some, such as the EMR upgrade that we discussed before, are more logistical."

Bourne steps forward. "Any change you adopt will have to combine strategy, tactics, and logistics. If you have one and not the others, you won't effectively progress. For example, if you develop your strategy without pragmatic ways to put it into practice, then you will simply have a collection of flowery words. Or if you have a lot of logistical steps that don't combine into a cohesive plan of action to reach a clear goal, what you do with one hand won't leverage and encourage what you are doing with the other. You will end up with a lot of activity but not necessarily significant productivity, and that's not good. Hospitals can lean too much in one direction or the other. What you, as leaders of this institution, must find right now is the sweet spot: just the right combination and balance of strategy, tactics, and logistics."

"So scan the list of ideas on these easel boards," Larkin instructs. "Let's start with those that are strategic. What are they?" Three strategic themes emerge. (1) Build OMC into a patient-centric hospital focused on care quality and patient satisfaction. (A note is appended to this strategy to say that this does not imply that OMC is not focused on these things today; this is a new theme.) (2) Expand the community focus of the hospital and support for the hospital to the community of neighborhood-based caregivers, who together can see OMC as a resource for their health and health care needs. (3) Bolster the research and scientific profile of OMC so that it is even more recognized for the excellence of its patient care and academic credentials.

It is Iris Inkwater who voices what many in the room seem to be feeling: "All of these ideas are great. Who wouldn't want to be working in a hospital that did all three of these at once? My problem in looking at the list is that what it implies is that we are doing everything all the time. It is a bit overwhelming."

Larkin nods and smiles at her, "You're absolutely right, Iris. Accomplishing just one of these strategic objectives is a monumental task when you think about what each individually demands. Here though is your advantage in linking these different pieces together into a cohesive framework such that one activity leverages and supports the others. You have the advantage—as leaders working together intentionally—to influence and accomplish a lot and, with that, to achieve broader impact. Let me give you a very pragmatic example. How many of you when you are driving to work are doing more than simply driving?"

"What do you mean?" Pudolski asks.

"I mean," says Larkin, "that you structure the time to multitask so that you accomplish far more than just getting to work."

Janice Johnson jumps in with a chuckle. "Oh, I get a lot more done during my commute. I'm on the phone. I'm listening to the radio to get the news. And I'll admit that I text, though I promise, only when I'm stopped at a red light."

"Exactly," Bourne comments, "and I'll bet, Janice, that when you get in the car, you know where everything is that you'll need so you can make the most of your time on the road."

"You better believe I have everything I need in easy reach. Otherwise I'd waste time or be unsafe on the road."

Larkin picks up on her comment. "That is exactly what we are saying. If you have a cohesive plan, you can put the pieces together to envision and accomplish far more than if all these possibilities," he says with a gesture to the easel boards, "were separate activities. Think connectivity of thinking and activity as you put together your strategy and the logistical and tactical moves that will drive you to implementation." They silently contemplate what that will mean.

Bourne lets the quiet hang for some moments before he takes up the activity. "Now let's move to the next layer of this discussion. How do you view the tactical ideas that were put forth? A tactic is a plan or action taken to achieve a desired outcome. Your strategies define your outcomes. Now, what will you do to get to each outcome? For example, making more space available for physician offices is a tactic that would help you achieve a more community-based presence as well as build the patient-centric focus you have identified. As you look through the list, identify tactical moves and actions you could take, and identify the ways each advances your strategic advantages."

The next forty-five minutes bubble with robust and lively conversation that draws lines connecting strategic objectives with the ways to achieve them. There is enthusiastic give-and-get across the room. One person offers to jump-start a patient education initiative, and someone else offers assistance in the way of information, advice, and even personnel support.

Finally, Larkin announces, "We have arrived at the logistics. Logistics encompass the details of daily work that either facilitate or obstruct getting the job done. Because logistics can make such a difference in the efficiency and effectiveness of work in health care organizations, people often raise logistical matters to strategic importance. That creates a lot of confusion. Be clear on what your strategy is and what your tactics for that strategy are, and then drive to create a logistical framework that aggressively supports them. You will better meet your objectives and you will be less likely to be distracted."

Larry Lumberg crosses his arms and leans back in this chair. "I'm not sure I understand. Are you saying that logistics aren't important?"

"Not at all," Larkin replies, "they are critically important. They just can't be conflated with strategy."

"But if our EMR is not working well, that's not a good strategy," Lumberg replies.

"If your goal is patient-centric care, then you want quick, accurate, and effective communication," explains Larkin. "And the better you do that, the more patient-centric you will be. The question of one EMR over another is a logistical matter, and the better your choice, the more likely you are to achieve your strategy. There are many logistical aspects to your strategic objectives, and the cost analysis you discussed earlier helps you to systematically and fairly assess those options."

Bourne walks up to Lumberg. "I understand what you are saying and your concerns. We physicians live and work in the world of logistics. When logistics work well, life is great. We get our jobs done and we are happy. When logistics don't work well, then as we know, life is hell. OMC has to be careful to be sure that its logistics are as robust as its strategy. This is where physicians and health care managers often fail to understand one another. Managers think physicians are caught up in the details and don't see the bigger picture of running a complex institution. Doctors complain that managers can't make the trains run on time. And you know," Bourne pauses before producing the punch line, "that's why we actually have so few real trains running in this country. The old-time train barons thought it was all about the trains and didn't realize that it's all about transportation. So trains lost out here as a mode of transportation, although that didn't happen in other parts of the world. What we are talking about here, for OMC, is high-quality, cost-efficient, top-notch health and health care. Figure out how to do that—and a fabulous EMR is part of making that work—and you all do well here. It's not an impossible puzzle to figure out."

"OK, I see; I get it." Lumberg seems satisfied.

As the discussion of logistics progresses, the power of linking strategic objectives to logistical activities both clarifies and simplifies the conversation. Those around the table, including Lumberg, are clear on what they need to get in order to make the system work better. And they are equally clear on what they are willing to do—to give—in order to make it happen. There is a lively and inspired exchange of ideas, proposals, and concessions.

As the retreat draws to a close—with agreement around the room on the strategic objectives and under each objective the list of tactical drivers and logistical arrangements needed to make each happen—Rajeev Rao comments, "It feels like we are drawing straight lines between what we are trying to do, the frameworks to drive it forward, and then the details to actually make it happen. They fit together like nice logical lines drawn to link strategy, tactics, and logistics together and then all the strategies, all the tactics, and all the logistics have a synergy too. This is looking like a kind of matrix design to move ahead. As you might guess with my being the CFO, my left brain is dominant and this makes great sense to me."

Larkin smiles. "That's why we call this last step of the Walk in the Woods aligned interests. This is really what you have accomplished through this exercise. You not only have learned a great deal, as Benny pointed out earlier about the first two steps, you have also found a way to align yourselves as leaders with steps for moving OMC to a new vision, with a way to get there. You are all to be commended."

Bourne follows with his concluding comments. "Before you get too self-congratulatory however, you as the leadership group of OMC still have a lot of work to do. This is just the beginning. Have you noticed that what students consider *graduation* we academics call *commencement*? You have graduated from self-interests to aligned interests. And you still have to take this rudimentary framework of alignment and turn it into an actionable plan. If you didn't have this though, you probably would be mired in defensive moves in responding to your new situation. When we first met you and interviewed you, we both observed that you seemed to be in a state of collective panic. You don't have to panic. Yes, you are facing some tough decisions and some rough seas ahead. What impressed us through this day is that you have a lot of assets that you can all draw upon. You have a great and deserved reputation. You are well respected in this community and far beyond. And what we have seen today is that you have a leadership body that 'gets it.' You are willing to roll up your sleeves and draft a new direction for OMC. For that, I also commend you."

At that point, with the Walk in the Woods concluded, Inkwater steps to the front of the room. "First, I want to thank Benny and Larry. That was a tremendous job." The room erupts into enthusiastic applause and the two humbly bow. "Now, as our friends here have said, we have a lot of work to do. We covered more ground today than I ever imagined we could, and everyone in this room deserves abundant kudos for making that happen. So I offer my heartfelt thanks to each and every one of you. And here is my pledge. We have a number of meetings coming up. Many of those meetings are part of our routine schedule. What we came up with here today will headline each meeting—the board meeting, senior executive meeting, and department heads meeting. Before too much time passes, we have to start talking about this with our broader constituencies so everyone at OMC can get on board, knowing what it is we want to get done. I will take responsibility for starting the ball rolling and building up the momentum. And I need each of you to do the same with your corner of this organization." Inkwater looks around the room making eye contact with the people she needs to move the message forward. She is encouraged by the nods she sees in return, in particular from the thought leaders like Fisher, Abbington, and Johnson. "There is every reason to pull this place together and to make great things happen, and after this day, I have every confidence that we will succeed."

And with that, the Walk, the retreat, and an era for OMC end. And a new era begins.

The Walk in the Woods in Practice

Picture someone pounding a nail into a piece of wood. The right hand lifts the hammer into the air ready to bring it down with force on to the carefully positioned nail. Instead, the hammer misses its mark and inflicts a crushing blow on the left hand. Ouch!

Might the left hand in retribution grab a knife to cut off the right hand? Obviously not. It is unthinkable. Our anatomy acts as a connected whole. The left and right hands are interdependent.

The same could well be true for people working in the same organization, leaders endeavoring to put together a merger of two organizations, or professionals seeking to reconfigure their shared practice. If the stakeholders negotiate on the premise of a *whole image negotiation,* the parts engage on the premise of imagining and finding a reshaped whole that provides them *mutual and shared benefit.* That is the value added by the Walk, the premise one builds in leading others through the process, and the objective of generating buy-in the agreements that are created.

Understanding the Value Added by the Walk

Negotiation is a perplexing process. There are a multitude of factors at play. Some of these factors are knowable and others are not. Important data are available to some at the table and not to others. And even for what is known, it is often difficult to pay attention to and account for everything that must or could be considered.

This reality creates its own pitfalls and dangers. Overwhelmed and bewildered, parties may opt to heed a limited set of variables, to the exclusion of those that may be critical to finding a solution. They may be distracted by variables that seem to demand the most attention. Or they may retreat to their own comfort zones, caring only for what they want to achieve and ignoring the legitimate interests of others. This proclivity to isolate and focus on certain variables and exclude others is a danger in the negotiation process that can yield skewed or otherwise less than optimal results. It can generate new and otherwise avoidable obstacles that themselves impede forward progress. It is an important factor in negotiation failure.

By design, the Walk in the Woods intends to address the problem of collecting, exchanging, and analyzing data critical to negotiation decision making. Though not a perfect or fail-safe process, the Walk explicitly encourages stakeholders to place information on the table, pay attention to what others have added, and then use this fuller picture to drive the direction and objectives of the negotiation. It is an organizing method for the task facing the negotiators (Deutsch & Coleman, 2000). The first two steps, addressing self-interests and enlarged interests, are as we mentioned earlier the learning steps, providing the opportunity to gain the information necessary to construct a deal. The final two steps, addressing enlightened interests and aligned interests, are the action steps, during which options are constructed, prioritized, and put into an order that allows the deal to move forward. Through this process, options, choices, and consequences are made explicit. By deepening the stakeholders' understanding of the multiple dimensions of the problem or conflict that has brought them to the table, the Walk helps stakeholders to distinguish what is more important from what is less important. It is in putting the pieces of that puzzle together that the parties discover a solution that best meets their shared and mutual interests.

This method also helps participants better understand one another and the dynamics that affect the course of their negotiation. And in a more subtle way, the Walk helps parties to better understand themselves. With its focus on interests, it allows each party to explore what it is critical for him or her to achieve in the negotiation, to distinguish real priorities, and to apply these new insights to the emerging solutions and choices being considered. It is common for individuals to start with a measure of unacknowledged or even unrecognized confusion about what is really being negotiated and what is really at stake. At its best, along with the wider range of options from which they can make better informed choices, the Walk offers participants an added measure of clarity and self-confidence (Goleman, 1998).

Enhanced self-confidence is an important ingredient for encouraging parties to have greater confidence in one another. As they better recognize what they individually hope to gain from the process and as they discover opportunities to generate mutual gain in collaboration with others, they are better able to identify points of agreement and generate new ideas. By the time they arrive at the final step of the Walk, they have already achieved important new realizations: about themselves and their own interests, about the overlap between their interests and the interests of others, and about the potential to create change by injecting new ideas and opportunities. These *aha* moments set the stage for success, increasing the odds that the parties will negotiate a solution, settlement, or agreement that might otherwise have been elusive (Shell, 1999). Getting them to this point is a matter of carefully guiding them through the process.

Leading a Walk in the Woods

As indicated earlier, there are any number of ways to use and apply the concepts and methods of the Walk. The three most commonly used approaches are (1) a guided Walk in which an expert leads others not familiar with the process, as in facilitation or mediation; (2) a collaborative Walk in which two or more people familiar with the process use it as a framework for their own discussion or negotiation; and (3) a Walk that a negotiator uses as a personal discipline to informally guide discussion with others not familiar with the process (Kurtzberg & Medvec, 1999). For the purpose of illustration, this discussion will focus on using the Walk to formally facilitate negotiation or resolve conflict.

The first consideration in setting out on a Walk in the Woods is determining who is to be at the table. This must be done in consultation with the potential parties, being careful not to be overly inclusive or overly exclusive.

Once the parties have been determined and are gathered together, the facilitator sets the stage for negotiation. The introduction includes descriptions of the problem that triggered the meeting; of the outcome desired, stated in general terms; and briefly, of the process. This opening should include a concise synopsis of the method: the premise, steps, and transitions for achieving an outcome that incorporates the core interests of those around the table. It is often useful to include the story of the diplomats' Walk in the Woods at Geneva. Participants should be given an opportunity to ask questions about the process, and then move directly to step 1.

As described in the previous sections, each step has its own objectives, methods, and intended outcomes. Each step is designed to lay the groundwork for what comes next. It is useful to begin each step with a brief review of what is to be discussed, why it needs to be talked about, and what the step hopes to achieve. It is useful to conclude each phase with a synopsis of what has been discussed and resolved and the ways in which it leads to what happens next.

As one moves through the Walk, it is important to be flexible. Though the process has been described here as a neat, linear, step-by-step method, in real life it does not always progress in a straight line. At times, for example, in the midst of the enlightened interests conversation someone will want to discuss a self-interest that he or she was reluctant to reveal before now. It is wise, as appropriate to the tone of the discussion at the moment, to go back, hear what the party has to say, and let others comment or further contribute to this new piece of information. In other words, in practice, it is important to go with the flow, show flexibility as a facilitator, and most important, to use the Walk as a vehicle to encourage constructive conversation and discovery of information. The method should not be so rigid that it gets in the way of fluid and valuable discourse.

How long does a Walk usually take? It depends of course on the nature of the problem, the number of people involved, and the complexity of the issues. The approach could be used constructively to organize a two-hour meeting of a group of staff working to proactively resolve an organizational problem. However, when people are taking a complex, high-stakes conflict through the Walk, it can take them a day or even two to frame, reframe, and progress through the steps. And the Walk can likewise be used to guide a short fifteen-minute interpersonal negotiation, helping the parties to listen to one another, understand one another, generate some creative options, and then reach a resolution.

Generating Buy-In

In the course of their Walk, stakeholders discover an array of choices available to them and the resulting consequences linked to each. Often they end up choosing an option that at the outset looked far less than perfect. They do so because in the course of the process, they have come to accept that their goal of a unidimensional, perfect solution is likely an unattainable fantasy. They come to realize that the fantasy outcome could be secured only at an unpalatable cost to others and that in the long run it would not serve their purposes. This is an important shift in thinking, and one that has taken both time and attention to achieve.

As a consequence of this shift, the parties buy into a solution that they might not otherwise have accomplished. They recognize that the outcome reached is likely as good as it can get, given real constraints. A second consequence is that the parties are generally enthusiastic about the outcome they have achieved. They are also encouraged by the support of the other parties at the table, because these others have also accepted an outcome less than what was originally seen as perfect. This measure of buy-in is perhaps the most important dividend of the Walk and the best insurance that what was decided will be implemented in good faith. In other words, all the participants will want the solution to succeed because they created it together, because it strikes a reasonable balance among the array of interests, and because it is serving the priority interests of those about the table.

This important realization would likely not have been derived from an adversarial process. It more likely, and certainly more convincingly, can emerge from the lessons learned during interest-based negotiation. By reducing the hyperbole and posturing in the negotiation process and replacing it with candor mixed with flexibility, parties are encouraged to acknowledge the possible pain that current constraints are placing on everyone at table. And they are likewise encouraged, at that point, to redirect their collective energies toward generating gains that would otherwise elude them. It's a simple formula: more gain equals less pain.

Conclusion

Multidimensional problem solving and the Walk in the Woods serve as guides to decision making among people who share a common purpose and a shared fate. The name of the process itself is a metaphor with intentionally rich and vivid imagery. It evokes the importance of getting away from the conflict or controversy, injecting perspective into the negotiation, meaningfully engaging the stakeholders, and with that, producing something that would not otherwise have emerged. In the end it is the ownership of process and product that is most critical to the success of the experience, for both the stakeholders who will benefit and the facilitator who has led them through the paces.

PART THREE

CONTEST, RESOLUTION, AND CONNECTIVITY

CHAPTER 8

POSITIONAL BARGAINING

WHOLE-IMAGE negotiation—interest-based interaction, collaborative problem solving, and the Walk in the Woods—is our preferred mode for reaching decisions and taking action. These strategies adapt best to the close, interpersonal work that typifies health care. By enhancing constructive exchange, whole-image negotiation synthesizes common purpose and generates opportunities for inventive solutions.

Nevertheless there are situations when aboveboard, interest-based negotiation is not your best strategy. In those circumstances, you will be better off resorting to *positional*, or *distributional, negotiation.* The intent of this chapter is to help you identify those circumstances: What are the cues that alert you to the need for positional tactics? Once you have made the choice to use positional negotiation, what methods and maneuvers can improve your chances for success and reduce the risks of retribution? And how can you incorporate the wisdom of becoming a negotiation chameleon, crafting a balance of interest-based and positional techniques to maximize your objectives?

Before you read further, we would like to post a cautionary note. When we are conducting a training session and we reach the section on positional bargaining, the mood of the room turns. There are some who rub the palms of their hands back and forth and mutter comments such as, "OK, now to the good stuff—this is how to *really* win." For others the topic evokes negative associations; it reminds them of times when positional tactics were used against them, and they really *lost*. Yet others shy away, afraid of engaging in potentially contentious negotiation and concerned that their inadequacies in this area render them "negotiationally challenged."

Conflict and its negotiation involves, in effect, a synthesis of heart, head, and gut, that is, a combination of emotion, intellect, and instinct.

Emotions and passions run high as people are compelled to confront difficult choices and consequences; it is the reality of these choices—often a set of less than optimal or even bad choices—that sweeps them into the negotiation process or that drives them away from its commitments. As we have discussed, the fears sparked by these choices and their consequences send people to the basement. Some freeze, some run away—flight—and others gird for the fight. When the emotions of conflict take you to the basement, will you descend further or will you have the self-discipline and power to rise through your emotions to take a more reasoned approach?

The intellect, when engaged, can encourage the parties to conduct the transaction in a reasonable and civil manner, or it can constrain them to distort the problems and pigeonhole them into meaningless categories. Understanding can easily slip into intellectualizing. From the basement you must rise to engage your mind with balanced and reasoned deliberation.

Instinct can evoke primitive survival impulses that ignite contentious, win-lose conflict. Sometimes it is defensiveness that drives the parties to self-protection. At other times an affinity or sense compels them toward compassion. Each has the potential to degrade or elevate the tone and destination of the negotiation. The parties describe a gut sense for what is right or wrong.

What combination of impulses guides your negotiations?

Adversarial methods derive from your instinctual drive for self-protection. Deep in the basement and fearing your demise, you attempt to guarantee survival through overpowering your enemies, both real and imagined. Control becomes a matter of defense. In a physically violent situation you may pull your arms in tight to protect your body. In a professionally dangerous circumstance you may copy your allies or superiors on an e-mail in an attempt to guard your career. And in a personal predicament, you preserve your self-respect. Fearing brutality and defeat, whether physical, professional, or personal, you alleviate your anxiety by outdoing the destructiveness of the other side. Civility may be abandoned in the quest for victory.

When parties to a negotiation believe their survival is at risk—however loosely defined—they are likely to behave positionally. At times there is an inclination to view even small matters as a gauge of survivability: "If we give on this issue, who knows what will hit us next!" That temperament is a reflection of professional insecurity. That sense of jeopardy has been exacerbated in recent years by the increasingly competitive health care environment. To be sure, the battles for patients and dollars have spawned professional as well as organizational winners and losers. In such a scenario the question of how they can win assumes a vital importance for people who want to ensure their professional futures. Paradoxically, the true winners in the marketplace are learning that the best way to ensure their survival is by finding new ways to work together. Joint ventures, interoperable technologies, consolidations, and mergers—even though difficult to galvanize—provide a protective position of strength in the face of rapid and volatile change. *Collaborate to prevail* is a clever and strategic method of building muscle in a highly competitive environment.

Unraveling Positional Bargaining

Humans invest great energy in cloaking animal instincts in higher-order activities. People eat as do dogs; though dogs don't adorn the activity with silverware, napkins, and classical music. Dogs romping in the park—pushing, biting, and chasing other dogs—can resemble the interaction in many health care organizations, though the dogs do not glamorize their activity as a struggle for professional dignity, "serving the patients," or departmental integrity.

To bring positional negotiation into its appropriate balance with other methods, you must see it for what it is. Defensive and offensive urges are many times real and warranted. To misjudge them, however, could be fatal to your desired outcome. If you persist with interest-based negotiation when others irretrievably seek your professional ruin, you will indeed be defeated. Likewise, when the other side holds out a hand and you perceive a fist, you not only erase his or her good intentions, you become self-destructive in the process. It is a matter of knowing yourself, understanding others, and then cleverly choosing from a set of viable options. The better your understanding and the wider your options, the greater are your chances of achieving satisfying outcomes from your negotiations, especially the tough ones.

When you are negotiating with reason and compassion and the other side is negotiating for conquest and control, you have two choices. First, you can try to move the other party toward your frame: appeal to her head and heart by reframing the problem into an interest-based negotiation. Emphasize your overlapping objectives, common purpose, and mutual desire to avoid negative consequences. By hearing as well as responding to her innate fears, you begin her move beyond those apprehensions. However, when you are genuinely convinced that appealing to her reason and compassion cannot work, then you must put your own guard into gear. Be clear about your objectives, the tactics likely to succeed, and the methods you will use to maintain self-control throughout the process.

As you read this chapter, the tone and tactics of contentious bargaining may ring familiar. So too should the costs and consequences. This chapter is not an endorsement of positional bargaining. Rather, it is a dose of reality. When adversarial negotiation defines the culture of your workplace, then that workplace may feel more akin to the wilds of an untamed jungle than to a setting for attaining the higher purposes of health care. You must learn to play the game judiciously before you can change it.

Public opinion has a funny way of turning complex issues into simple dichotomies. That is the nightmare for the Community Health Plan (CHP). When news spreads of CHP's withdrawal from the Oppidania Medical Center in favor of Urbania Medical Center, a well-intentioned effort to trim health costs and save money for plan subscribers turns sour. Rather than being heralded for bold leadership in curbing health inflation, CHP is now being castigated for threatening the viability of a venerable institution and, in the process, short-changing its customers with bargain-basement health care. Newspaper editorials give the issue reasoned though critical consideration. Radio talk show hosts are not as generous. And public opinion, being what it is, now greatly disfavors CHP and all groups associated with it, especially Urbania Medical Center. One particularly outraged and vocal CHP subscriber has launched a social media campaign based on the theme "our health comes first" and has attracted more than one thousand followers in just a few days.

Urbania, caught in the cross fire, is cast, somewhat unfairly, as the cheaper and clearly inferior alternative to the Oppidania Medical Center. Though Urbania has never shared Oppidania's stellar reputation, no one has ever before gone to the trouble of suggesting that its care is mediocre. Now it seems that everyone in town has his or her favorite Urbania slur story—on topics that range from major gaffes to everyday inefficiencies—and is happy to share it. And even though Oppidania may have its own shortcomings, in the polarized, bad-guys-versus-good-guys mood that has arisen in the city, people seem to have only good things to say about Oppidania (except, of course, the people at CHP). The antagonism reaches a new level of vindictiveness a few days into the dispute when CHP releases Oppidania's price list, detailing what are described as exorbitant costs for everything from an aspirin to a triple-bypass procedure.

The question at Oppidania is how to handle both the public relations response and the strategic countermoves. The general consensus among the organization's leaders is that there is no need to enter the fray directly: everyone else in town is doing it for them. Oppidania can take the high ground, emphasizing its historical and continuing commitment to high-quality patient care and community service. Public perception seems to be that although Oppidania may be slightly more expensive, its life-giving accomplishments make its costs worthwhile. Amid the controversy, another sentiment common to health care debates is being heard: people are willing and should be able to make this health care choice for themselves and their families. Oppidania, in response to media inquiries, outlines the aggressive measures it has taken to reduce costs whenever possible, though never to the detriment of quality patient care.

While Oppidania is keeping a low profile in the fracas, Arena Health Insurance (AHI), CHP's major competitor, is not. Much to the chagrin of the Oppidania leadership, AHI has launched an aggressive marketing campaign featuring full-page newspaper ads touting its continued commitment to high-quality care and patient choice. With upcoming open enrollment periods for a number of major employers, the insurer wants to implant the impression that people who do not choose AHI are risking their health and cheating their families. The leaders at Oppidania, hoping to keep their options open, are afraid that the AHI strategy could backfire on them, just as the CHP strategy has inadvertently damaged Urbania.

After much discussion, Oppidania's executive leaders agree that the best strategy is not to make calls about the matter to any of the key players. They consider contacting Urbania to diminish the possibility of rifts between the two hospitals. They decide that little good can emerge from such a conversation and that it might be interpreted as an apology when none is warranted. They likewise reject the idea of asking AHI to moderate its aggressive ad campaign. As long as there are no overt inaccuracies, it is not up to Oppidania to instruct a major client on how to manage its marketing. And finally, they decide not to call CHP, as they feel that they already have the upper hand in any potential negotiations. It was CHP that had walked away, and it would have to be up to CHP to walk back. The senior staff recognize this as a risky strategy, as it offers only precarious control and limited maneuverability. Nevertheless it keeps their options open, even though the options themselves are not all that attractive. The decision is to wait, anxiously, and see.

For the next few days, neither CHP nor Urbania calls, and the story remains a top one in the local media. The reports run from facts and figures to sappy human interest stories. Finally, a newspaper editorial questions why the health care community is allowing this mess to get so out of hand. This point is picked up by the local public radio affiliate and two of the local television news programs. Pressure builds for the city government to get involved. The city's health department commissioner, Manuel Mendez, however, says that it is up to these private companies to settle the matter on their own. On the advice of the mayor's office he has decided not to get involved, concluding that to do so at this point could lead them all into a political maelstrom with little potential benefit.

The call from CHP finally comes. Nathaniel Norquist, CHP's chief financial officer, asks for a meeting with Iris Inkwater, and it is arranged for the following day. Inkwater spends the afternoon with her senior staff, developing a strategy for the session. They conclude that it is in the best interests of the hospital to resume the relationship with CHP and that if the Oppidania people play it cool, they will probably end up with a favorable financial arrangement.

Given the media attention, Norquist and Inkwater meet for lunch at a quiet restaurant on the outskirts of the city. It is just the two of them, as usual, on neutral turf. They ask for a booth at the back. The opening niceties are brief, tense, and cold: they both know "what's new." Inkwater makes a lame joke about feeling like a secret agent and making sure they weren't followed. She waits for Norquist to make the first substantive move.

"Iris, what can I tell you? We're taking a beating over this deal with Urbania. The exclusive with Urbania might have been a bit rash. We want to reconsider an arrangement with you."

Inkwater sips her iced tea and then tries to sound as noncommittal as possible: "In the spirit of cooperation, I'll refrain from saying anything about looking before leaping. We are willing to consider what you have to offer."

"Iris, what we have to offer is very simple," Norquist says with a shrug of his shoulders. "We'll bring you back on at the same rates we gave Urbania."

She smiles ruefully. "We looked at those figures after our last round. They are fantasy numbers, Nathaniel. We can't see how Urbania is going to survive with those rates. It has to be cutting staff to dangerous levels. We're not willing to have our candy stripers perform nursing functions." Inkwater knows what she is doing. On one hand Norquist needs her now more than she needs him. On the other hand she cannot afford to lose this contract.

"Well, Iris, *that* is a fantasy. Urbania is not using candy stripers in the surgical suites. They did, however, cut where it is appropriate to cut. You know yourself that they are getting a bad rap in the papers. Don't let yourself get caught up in the propaganda." Norquist is trying to divert discussion of this topic as a cost-equals-quality issue by demeaning Inkwater's remarks. It does not work.

"I find that offensive, Nathaniel. We are talking dollars and cents here, and I have a commitment to keep Oppidania viable as a high-quality institution. I am not willing to compromise on that quality." Inkwater wants to paint Norquist into a corner, but Norquist has more maneuvering to do.

"So what will you get for it, Iris? An expensive funeral? Oppidania has simply been unwilling to go through the belt-tightening that every other institution has accepted. That is the reason for this mess. We have our responsibilities as well, Iris."

The discussion is descending to finger-pointing. "Nathaniel, you will get nowhere by personalizing this issue. You have created your own mess, and now you want me to bail you out. We are not willing to do that for you." Inkwater catches herself. What is she saying? The strategy is to play *hard to get* now and only later, with a better offer on the table, to play ball with CHP, because the hospital really does need the contract. She has allowed the conversation to turn into a divisive confrontation.

They both retreat to their salads, eating silently, with the echoes of their last interchange still hanging in the air. Norquist fidgets with his napkin; he is beginning to panic. He has strict instructions to bring back a verbal agreement to continue discussions leading toward reinstating the contract. It has to be done quickly, before the upcoming open enrollment period when enrollees will have the option to switch plans. He can't jeopardize the company's financial viability.

Norquist breaks first. "Well, Iris, if you can't meet the Urbania numbers, what numbers are you talking about?" Norquist knows he may be creating an impossible situation for himself. Urbania would protest being pressed financially if Oppidania gets a better deal. This controversy has been too much in the open to hide anything. And because CHP has already negotiated several contracts with large employers based on the assumptions of the new financial arrangements with Urbania, any increase in costs will hit the plan hard. He has little if any room to maneuver.

Inkwater comes back slowly. She knows that if she says 10 percent more, Norquist will balk. In reality she needs 5 percent. She decides to play the numbers a bit high to leave herself room to come down. "Seven and a half percent, Nathaniel. My numbers people said that the difference between your figures and what is scarcely livable for us is seven point five. If you want us, that is what you will have to pay."

Norquist is worried. "Iris, I will tell you point blank. That number will kill us." Actually, Norquist has some room to move. Before giving in, he wants to see if he can rattle Inkwater and get her to go lower.

Watching his body language and confident in her numbers, Inkwater senses that he is calling her bluff. She is not going to be tricked. "Nathaniel, the numbers are not going to kill you. You've done it to yourself. You are making impossible promises. You've squeezed yourself in two directions. You got carried away with your own assumed ability to control this market. It's not that simple, Nathaniel. No one did this to CHP but CHP."

Norquist is here for a negotiation, not a scolding. He resents Inkwater's lecturing, and he is momentarily overcome with a sudden urge to leave the table. He catches himself. He speaks deliberately. "Iris, you need us as much as we need you. If you are left with AHI alone in this town, they will squeeze you dead, and there will be no one left to bail you out."

"Squeeze us the way you are squeezing, Nathaniel? We are getting nowhere, my friend. I suggest you go back to your shop and think hard about what you are proposing to us. Begin to sound reasonable, and we will be willing to talk."

The meeting ends abruptly. They split the check. Neither Inkwater nor Norquist walks home with what she or he had hoped to achieve.

The banner headline in the next day's morning newspaper summarizes the predicament: "OMC and CHP suspend talks." It is not news that plays well at Oppidania. Nor is it well received at CHP.

Adopting a Positional Approach

There are three sides to the choice for positional negotiation: what you want, what the other party wants, and your appraisal of the exchange. The key for you is attaining your objectives. As you assess the other side, tactics are the gauge. And the back-and-forth between you and the other party defines the relationship and the exchange.

It is a particularly quiet Sunday evening on Six West. There are several empty beds on the floor and no new admissions. Heather Harriford realizes that days like this probably do not help the hospital's financial crunch, though it does make an evening shift easier to get through.

There are several patients who have been on the floor for over a week now, and Harriford is the primary nurse for one of them, Mrs. Helen Hayward. Just a few months ago, Mrs. Hayward was a robust seventy-eight-year-old lady with a discernibly dignified demeanor—definitely "Mrs. Hayward," not "Helen," to the staff. She is now suffering from colon cancer and in steady decline. Harriford can tell that Mrs. Hayward has been a true matriarch, with a strong personality, and the lifeblood of her family. That family is now taking her deterioration badly, and she can sense that they are floundering without her steady direction. Harriford has a warm rapport with Mrs. Hayward and her children, and she finds it rewarding to work with them.

Harriford is at the far end of the nurses' station, making notations in Mrs. Hayward's chart when Dr. Cummings nudges up beside her. At the age of twenty-nine, Chuck Cummings is in the last year of his residency and has an air of supercilious confidence about him. He has that "I just popped out of a fashion magazine" look in the way he dresses and carries himself. Though he has caught the eye of many of the nurses on the floor, Harriford has never found him to be her type. In fact she rather dislikes his macho arrogance and how he struts about for both the staff and the patients.

Chuck Cummings loves a challenge. He also needs to know that every woman he meets adores him. Heather Harriford, for some reason, has shown no susceptibility to his charms, something he finds particularly troublesome because he thinks her to be the most attractive of the nurses on the shift. He has embarked on a mission to overwhelm her coldness and fix this problem. He doesn't believe there is any woman in the hospital who can't be warmed up.

Cummings sidles up against Harriford, as if he were reading the patient record she's working on. He whispers in a deep voice, "Well, well. Aren't you loved by the Hayward family, Heather. They can't stop talking about you." Cummings's face is very close to her ear, and Harriford can feel his breath as he speaks. She pulls away and focuses on the computer screen, continuing to type as she slides the keyboard out of Cummings's range. She no longer feels him touching her.

This Cummings doesn't like. "Are there any of those chocolate chip cookies left?" he asks, trying to get her to engage.

"No," she replies simply and without moving her eyes from the screen.

Cummings likes to be in charge when it comes to women. He decides to change the topic to one that Harriford can't ignore. Maybe this will win her over.

"You know, Mrs. Hayward is in a lot of pain. I want to double her morphine drip. Heather, I want you to take care of it, now." He lowers his head, mockingly trying to get her attention. "Please," he says, like a little boy begging for candy.

Harriford turns around and then steps back to create a more comfortable distance. She keeps her composure and, one word at a time, speaks in measured tones to Cummings. "We tried upping her morphine last night, and she became nauseated and very ill. I don't think it would be a good idea to try that again."

Cummings is exasperated. He is just about to launch into a nurse-doctor lecture when he realizes that there is a far better way to handle this little tiff. He extends both arms and places them on Harriford's shoulders. "Heather," he says, in a tone of clear condescension, "you have to remember who's the doctor here and who is the nurse. Now, there is no reason to play hard to get." At this point his hands are firmly massaging her, and she can feel his fingers gently playing with her bra straps. "I want Mrs. Hayward to get the morphine, and you are her primary nurse. Now, would you do that for me, sweets?" Cummings's hands pulled her toward him, as if he wanted to hug and make up. He was feeling a wonderful sense of victory.

Harriford is burning up inside. One moment suddenly turns into her entire career. Everything she knows and believes flashes in front of her eyes as she stares at Cummings. And she knows that whatever she does next could affect her entire career as well. On the one hand she may have no chance standing up to this macho icon. The whole medical staff would stand behind him. On the other hand this is going on in public, and maybe she just has to take a stand right now.

She feels Cummings's hands caressing her arms. She sees him glance down longingly at her breasts and back to her eyes with an ever-so-slight smile of approval. This is it, she thinks. She tells herself to be calm. "First, I want you to take your hands off me." She is firm. Cummings pulls back, slowly. He looks shocked. The color drains from his face, and he seems momentarily speechless. Harriford has a sense that this is an unusual event for this animal. "I want you to know that you are not to touch me, or for that matter, anyone else here who does not want to be touched. Do you understand?"

"I wasn't touching you. I was just being friendly, that's all." Cummings looks like someone has just knocked the wind out of him. He is trying to keep his composure and it isn't working.

"Second, Mrs. Hayward will have a violent reaction if you load her up with morphine. I think it is medically inadvisable. I refuse to administer the drug because I know it would be harmful. I watched it happen last night when you weren't here."

Cummings takes note of her change of topic. He is relieved that she is turning what could have been a somewhat uncomfortable matter into something easier for him to handle. "Look, *Nurse* Harriford. Whoever you might think you are outside of this hospital, here I am the doctor and you are the nurse.

Patients change their condition every day, and what happened yesterday will not necessarily happen again today. My orders are for you to administer morphine, and I expect that to be done right now."

"Well, *Doctor* Cummings, you might as well know now that I am filing two complaints against you: first, for sexual harassment and, second, for prescribing an inappropriate medication. If you had only spent more time looking at Mrs. Hayward's record and less time playing games with me, maybe you wouldn't have gotten yourself into this mess. It's right here in black and white." Though Harriford is fuming, she is careful to keep the volume of her voice down so no one else can hear what is going on.

"Well, Ms. Harriford. You can do whatever you want. I just want to remind you of one cold, hard fact." He is whispering forcefully. "I am the doctor. And you are the nurse. And in the long run, my years of medical training are far more valuable to this floor and to these patients and to this hospital than all your petty little nursing efforts combined. It's not even a contest. So the only one you're hurting with this little outburst is you, Heather." He wants her intimidated. Maybe a bit of reality will shut her up.

With that, Harriford turns around and walks straight for the sanctuary of the nurses' lounge. Fortunately, it is empty and quiet when she gets there. She is trembling with fright. She is shocked at what Cummings has said. And she is even more shocked by what she has said. She falls on the couch in the corner, sobbing.

Plan your strategy to best accomplish your objectives. When the parties are part of a shared *whole*, then a strategy that offers *gain-gain* potential can work best. When the parties are unalterable adversaries, the only outcome is win or lose. You want to expand your chances for a win that is clean: one that optimizes your short-term objectives as it softens any long-term harm to your own standing. What cues help you make your choice?

Recognizing Positional Relationships

One of our colleagues aspires to an epitaph that reads, "He left the world a better place." He is not a rocket scientist, brain surgeon, or philosopher; by his own description he is just an ordinary person. Making the world a better place is something he works on every day: when he talks with a ticket agent at an airport, when he sees a patient in his clinic, and when he interacts with professional colleagues. *Relationships* for him are not just the long-standing personal connections he has with people he knows well. Even if it exists for just a moment, a relationship is that link with others for which he continually strives.

He is ready to admit a selfish motive: "I figure that one day I'll help someone, they'll help someone else, and finally, maybe weeks later, it will come back to me."

In health service organizations, these sort of short yet intimate encounters are the norm. Patients enter a clinic sick and vulnerable, expose their symptoms and their bodies, and everyone hopes, feel better on the other side of their visits. For patients, the relationships that matter are the interactions that give them confidence that they are being treated as individuals and respected throughout the process.

There are times when a relationship is not important for you. Perhaps the circumstances are urgent and allow little time to attend to others. Perhaps you are distracted or involved with something more important than social capital. Perhaps the value of the tangible transaction—money, space, or status—supersedes the importance of your association: what others think of you is less important than what you tangibly receive from the exchange. You assume there to be little or no utility to the relationship and you bargain accordingly.

Likewise, people on the other side in a negotiation may signal to you that a relationship with you is unimportant to them. This message is conveyed by what is said—and not said—the dirty tricks they play, and their ostensible obsession with winning. They are little concerned with your regard for them. Intimidation, coercion, and impudence characterize their attitude. Negotiation becomes a game of domination. According to the rules of their game of conquest, the victor is entitled to harass the loser. The preferences of the loser are immaterial. After all, if you are truly defeated and no longer around, what you think is irrelevant. The tenor of these sorts of battles is more akin to that of children in a sandbox fighting over who gets the shovel than it is to that of professionals engaged in responsible debate.

Negotiation is a two-way street, and the mode of interaction, implicitly and explicitly, is determined by both sides. You can bring the other parties to the water you are offering, but if they do not want it, you can't make them drink. If they don't care about a relationship, your offering one won't change them. And if they are determinedly antagonistic, you might decide to carefully adopt parallel tactics; you do not want to prep for a civilized debate only to find your opponent armed and ready for a shoot-out.

Employing Positional Tactics

How do you know whether the people on the other side are leaning toward positional or interest-based negotiation? The tactics they use offer the most revealing clues. Paying attention to their moves helps you plan your own. At some point, the time arrives to invoke the reciprocal rule of negotiation: if you play dirty with me, then I'll play a bit dirty with you.

The inventory of positional tactics is of course endless. The following categories are commonly seen in health care settings.

Misinformation

The most common ploy of positional bargaining is to spread bad information. In the work of health care nothing is more harmful than misinformation: falsehood, deception, fabrication, fraud, deceit, pretext, exaggeration, and unfounded rumor—and let us not forget omission. Why?

Information is the currency of decision making. Whether it is a matter of finances, administration, personnel, or patient care, the scientific proclivity of health care craves logical conclusions. Distortions foster a precarious atmosphere for clinical and managerial work. Misinformation detracts from both process and product: like a virus, bad information takes on a life of its own. Those trapped in the cycle of misinformation justify their misjudgments by defending their information. Soon fantasy turns into fact as organizational myth is born and cultivated.

When you are convinced that rumors and innuendo about you are intentional and not the result of miscommunication or mistake, you are faced with a situation that warrants decisive action. By tolerating deception, you implicitly concede to it. This is your cue to adopt a more positional strategy.

Why would someone propagate misinformation? This behavior usually arises from a combination of character and purpose. For some, such deceit is an acceptable tactic because they believe "all's fair in love and war"—and in negotiation. Perhaps it was used on them by parents, supervisors, or colleagues, and by virtue of this experience it has become acceptable for them to use it on others. It is a customary practice to them.

How else might a person justify duplicity? For some, commitment to a higher purpose sanctions conduct that by itself is disdained: that is, the end justifies the means. Misdeeds are cloaked in the sanctity of the cause, and the harm inflicted upon others is rationalized as just punishment for their obstructions. Though reprehensible, this breed of arrogance is not uncommon in health care, given the vital importance of the work. The challenge is to avoid stooping to this level while also somehow toppling it.

"Gotcha"

"Gotcha" is a derisive accusation: "I caught you in the act of doing something wrong and now I am going to capitalize on it." The gotcha game is one of the most insidious of the signals warning you to shift into positional gear. How is the game played? Your overall record is exemplary. When weighed against your accomplishments, your mistakes are insignificant. Then you notice your reputation dissolving as minor missteps are converted into major problems. When you commit a legitimate though trivial error, you hear a loud "Gotcha" resound from your opponent. Every slip becomes an explosive complication, and you feel that you are walking through a minefield of humiliation.

What is happening? Your antagonists are building an illusory case against you. The specific points are vacuous. The issues themselves are petty. The real problem is not the poorly completed travel report, the miscommunication with a secretary, or the file that was temporarily misplaced. The real message is that they are out to ridicule and undermine you by documenting your every mistake. Your challenge is to understand their motives and methods and then mount your own campaign to put your purpose back into perspective.

Achieving that perspective is no easy matter. Your vulnerabilities and insecurities have been revealed. You feel in jeopardy. The very pettiness of the affair is insulting. If you permit yourself to believe that the poorly written travel report is evidence of your incompetence as a clinician, that the unhappy secretary reveals your inadequacy as a manager, or that the misplaced file displays your ineptitude as a planner, then you are in real trouble. You have fallen into the gotcha trap. That is the other side's ruse. Fall for it and you begin doubting yourself. You become frustrated. You get distracted. While trying to be perfect, you may miss a major thrust by your adversary.

Your challenge is to distinguish the allegations from the underlying message. The greatest danger is your own self-doubt. If you respond merely to the allegations, you become caught in the decidedly trivial pursuit that the other side has prepared for you.

What should you do? Recognize the game, document the insignificance of the allegations, and then mount your own campaign. And remember, you must be doing pretty well if others have to plunge so low to assail you.

Other Toxic Tactics

As we have said, the list of troublesome tactics is endless. You may find blackmail, extortion, threats, and coercion at your professional door. Even more painful than the hostility aimed directly at you is the cross fire directed at others with whom you work: colleagues, associates, and employees may be harassed simply because of their allegiance to you. Everyone around you may have taken sides. Your work then becomes embroiled in conflict tangential to your principal purposes. When those principal purposes begin to take a backseat to the conflict at hand, it is time to mount decisive action.

Mere acquiescence is neither preferable nor prudent. There is too much at stake, and you know that you are unwilling to bear the humiliation and the tangible losses of a positional defeat. You also know that you want to avoid tumbling to the level of your opponents. To do so would put you at even greater risk. Both professionally and personally, there is one attribute you had best be unwilling to sacrifice at any cost: your integrity. Why?

The cornerstone of negotiation is trust, that intangible trait that cannot be bought, borrowed, or manufactured. It is a quality that you carry into every negotiation, be it interest based or positional. Should you employ toxic tactics yourself, you will demean your stature in the eyes of those at the table as well as in the minds of others who are watching. Your opponents can take much from you: they can even score some victories. The one quality they cannot seize is your integrity. Your best chance of rebounding, whether from victory or defeat, is by safeguarding the foundation of your future negotiations: your integrity and the trust people have in you.

The positional game itself is not particularly difficult to pick up. We each carry preprogrammed, instinctual instructions that can guide us toward some pretty nasty tactics. In fact the real challenge of the positional game is playing as a contender while maintaining your professional credibility. That quandary is the focus of the next section: How do you prepare yourself? What is your strategy? How can you ensure that you will achieve a clean win?

Preparing for Positional Negotiation

You have already made the most important decision of positional negotiation: you have decided to use it. Let us assume your choice to be a wise one.

As with any form of negotiation, you are always preparing. You prepare for the first round. When the first round is over, you prepare for the next. Preparation requires you to collect and mobilize three essential ingredients: information, options, and choices. At each point in the process, what you acquire accumulates, and what you deduce fluctuates.

Information

You want to know whatever you can about the people on the other side. What is their strategy, and how might you outmaneuver it? What have they done in the past, and might those patterns be repeated? What motivates them, and can you appeal to those incentives? Where are their alliances, and how strong are they? What are their sources of power and influence, and can you muster enough strength to prevail? What are their options, and which are they likely to choose? The more you know, the more extensive your options and the more judicious your choices.

How do you acquire this information? There are the usual sources: documents, colleagues, and others who are familiar with your opponents. It is a matter of tracking these sources down, asking the right questions, and accurately assembling and interpreting what you have learned. These third-party sources do offer useful data, though with a bit of clever enticement, you can get the most valuable disclosures from the other side.

It is astounding what people are willing to reveal about themselves, either overtly or indirectly. Every meeting with the other side offers opportunities to collect such information. For example, at the opening of a bargaining session, you must decide whether to speak first or second. When involved in an interest-based negotiation, it is often best to speak early in order to set or reinforce the tone of the exchange. However, when involved in a positional negotiation, it is often best to go second because, initially, you should be more interested in what the other side has to say than in divulging your own strategy. People hate silence and are all too willing to blurt into the void with an unrehearsed remark. Catching them off guard, learning their concerns, and also allowing them to make statements they will later regret are actions that not only provide you with information: these tactics also make your opponents feel more vulnerable.

To assess what others are divulging, listen to more than just their literal words. Your focus needs to be on what they mean, their intentions. This message is reflected through body language: Do they look you in the eye? Do they fidget as they talk? They communicate just as much by what they don't say as by what they do say. Their tone and intonations reveal much about what lies inside.

And what do you do with this information? You let it sift through both your intellect and your intuition. You know that learning about someone else requires you to know a lot about yourself. What and whom can you trust? What is real and what is a ruse? What distortions do your own filters create? This combined information and insight helps you craft your options.

Options

Chapter Five highlighted the utility of generating a wide range of options from which to cultivate negotiated solutions. Option building is an essential exercise in all negotiation, though there are marked differences between interest-based and positional negotiation. In the former, option building is a collaborative endeavor. While going through a Walk in the Woods, the parties develop options and find mutually compatible solutions; they learn about one another, share needs, and voice concerns, all while building a constructive relationship. The outcome meets the tangible, short-term objectives as well as the long-term, integrative purposes of the parties: they reap immediate gains in the current negotiation and they anticipate continued fruitful exchanges. By contrast, in positional negotiation option building is not a mutual effort; it is a private matter. You do it on your own or with your own constituency. Your purpose is to construct a list of viable possibilities and preferences that meet your own needs, objectives, and concerns. To strengthen your position, some of your options you will reveal, others you will exaggerate, and some you will conceal. Certainly you are calculating in your disclosures, being careful not to weaken your stance. For example, in a job dispute you might broach your willingness to break with the organization because you have other offers without indicating the source of those offers or your distaste for most of them. You hide what will weaken your position; you reveal what will strengthen it.

Another significant distinction between interest-based and positional option building is the minefield you find in the latter. Your options in an interest-based negotiation usually range from fair to good to fabulous: "Just imagine what the synergy of our combined efforts could accomplish!" By its very nature, interest-based negotiation tends to be hopeful and optimistic. Conversely, positional bargaining has a dangerous edge that must be calculated into your assessment of your options.

Positional bargaining is a win-lose game, and you must appreciate the likelihood and consequences of a loss. If you lose, you could end up forfeiting your job, reputation, money, or whatever else might be on the line. To ignore the real potential for losing not only limits your strategy, it could also be the source of your defeat: "I never really considered the possibility that I wasn't going to win." It is that confidence that keeps you fighting, and it is that bravado that could distract you from gauging grave professional and personal dangers.

In a positional negotiation, the wider your range of options—the more viable and realistic, the stronger and more pragmatic they are—the greater are your prospects. Imagine yourself as a mouse in a maze: the more routes to the cheese, the better your chances are of getting the prize; and the finer your reading of the traps, the better your chances are of avoiding and escaping them.

Choices

When you are at the juncture between preparing for your positional negotiation and actually going into battle, it is time to review your options and make sure they work for you. How do you craft your preliminary choices?

Most important, you want to be clear with yourself about what it is you want to accomplish. This is the most vital yet difficult tenet of successful positional negotiation: know and live your objectives. Many positional bargainers are preoccupied with domination rather than focusing on their manifest objectives. The need to dominate may spring from a desire for revenge if there has been a past slight, real or perceived, and perhaps even before your time. So know your organization's history. Or the compulsion to dominate may arise simply from a feeling of entitlement that leads a person to try to extract every possible scintilla of value or concession possible. Such negotiators can become caught in the trap of needing to see the other side writhe in pain. They don't just want to win; they want their opponents to lose decisively and perhaps even suffer. This "punishment" not only provides personal satisfaction. In the negotiator's mind, it also vindicates and validates the rightness of his or her cause.

There are two problems with this approach. First, as previously suggested, while you are dismantling your opponents, you can be distracted from your own objectives. The mouse in the maze will never get the cheese if he forgets that the cheese is his ultimate prize. Your energies, thinking, and resources are uncontrollably diverted, and you may lose your aim and momentum. If those on the other side are wise, they will pick up on your obsession and use it against you: "You see, he is not really interested in improving services. His campaign is no more than a personal vendetta in disguise."

Second, you and those who watch you may be left with lingering doubts about whether the costs of victory were justified. Will winning in a way that is perceived by you or others as less than just come back to haunt you? Your colleagues, concerned that they may be your next victims, might congratulate you on the outside while inside they have lost respect for your professional judgment and balance. Victory that smacks of spitefulness, vengefulness, or meanness in professional circles is a high-cost proposition. You must decide if that is how you want to invest your finite personal and political resources.

The distinction between objectives and domination sets up a wrenching inner battle for the positional negotiator. It is the dilemma of choosing between reason and instinct. When your domination instinct is in control, you go for pain and punishment. When reason asserts itself, you are clear on your strategy and objective. Your focus is on what you want to accomplish and how to make it happen. You set your plan in motion and make your choices accordingly.

It is 6:00 P.M., and Dr. Nick Norton is sitting down to Sunday evening dinner. His wife has just placed a steaming bowl of his favorite—spinach fettuccine with arrabbiata sauce—in front of him when his beeper goes off. His first instinct is to ignore it: his family hates its noise, especially during dinner. "Just one minute," he apologizes, his napkin dropping on the chair as he pulls his cell phone from its holster and walks toward the privacy of the foyer.

Dr. Norton is chief of orthopedics at the Oppidania Medical Center, and this Sunday evening it is his turn to be on call. At the other end of the line is Dr. Lauren Lieber, chief resident for orthopedics. "Sorry to bother you, Dr. Norton. We just had a seventy-two-year-old woman come in with a very serious, complex hip fracture. I'm in the emergency room and have been with her for about twenty minutes. She hasn't eaten all day, appears stable, and has been cleared by her internist. It probably would be best to do her now."

Norton knows what this means. He will be going to the hospital for the surgery. It is only a matter of when. He asks a few more questions about the patient, and then asks, "Have you called about the operating room? When can we get in?"

"They're talking eight o'clock. They have two rooms going, and it's been a pretty average night."

"OK, Lauren. You get everything set up, and I'll be there by seven-thirty." Norton returns to the table and his cold plate of pasta. His wife places it in the microwave as he laments his need to return to the hospital.

Norton pulls into his reserved space in the doctor's parking lot and is in the building and into his hospital greens by 7:25, ready to talk with Lieber, review the record, and see the patient. Lieber walks up to him with a grimace on her face.

"I'm really sorry," she says. "You're going to kill me."

"Well, that depends. What's the problem?"

"There are only two operating rooms functioning tonight, and we've been bumped by the vascular team. We're set for nine o'clock. I tried to reach you, but your cell went right to voice mail."

"There are a couple of dead spots coming around the lake. I didn't even notice a message. Well, I'm not going to kill *you*, though that doesn't necessarily rule murder out entirely." Norton takes a deep breath. "It doesn't pay to go home for the one hour." Norton figures he will make the most of his presence in the hospital. He goes up to check on the condition of several of his patients on the seventh floor. He goes over the hip case with Lieber. "I'll be ready to roll at nine."

Norton is perennially early, despite his belief that the world conspires to be twenty minutes late just to irritate him. He is back to the operating room (OR) by 8:35, anxious to get going. Monday is going to be a killer day—OR cases starting at 7:30 A.M. and going all day—and he wants to get home for a good night's rest. Just as he is heading into the OR, Diane Darling, the nurse in charge of scheduling the rooms, calls him over sheepishly. ''Dr. Norton, I am so sorry. We just put an emergency C-section in your room. It shouldn't be more than an hour.''

Norton looks her straight in the eye and points his finger in her face. ''Last delay. Do you understand? I don't want to hear one more delay. The end.'' Norton angrily turns around and steams off to the surgeon's lounge. Why him, he wonders.

Two cups of coffee and one package of cookies later, he makes his way back to the nurses' station in the OR. Diane Darling looks the other way when she sees him coming. Norton notices the gesture and is ready for a fight. He likes to use a bit of humor and a firm tone when he is angry. It helps him keep in better control of himself, and it works with other people.

He affects a calm manner as he walks up to Darling's desk. ''Diane, we are all ready to go, aren't we?''

The nurse sighs. ''Oh, Dr. Norton, I am so sorry. There's a bad auto accident coming into the ER and they need your room for a tracheotomy, chest tube, and repair of facial lacerations. I have no estimate of time at this point.''

Norton decides to play it calm and firm. ''No problem. Here's what I want you to do. Call up our favorite anesthesiologist, Dr. Walter, and have him get in here to open another room. End of story.''

Darling has a sudden urge to run away. ''Well, Dr. Norton, I thought you might want me to do that, so I have already called Dr. Walter and explained the situation.'' She pauses. ''I told him about your patient, and he said it isn't an emergency. He said if you don't want to wait for the room to clear, you will just have to postpone the surgery until the morning.''

Norton is now seething. Walter, in his mind, is a typical young, lazy anesthesiologist, overly impressed with his own credentials. How could he make this decision without even the courtesy of a telephone call? It makes Norton crazy!

''Until the morning? Who the hell does he think he is?'' Norton's voice is loud enough for anyone within earshot of the station to hear it loud and clear. ''Did you explain to him that this *is* an emergency? If it wasn't, Lieber wouldn't have called me in, would she?''

''Yes, I told him all about your case.''

Norton demands Will Walter's home number and calls. There are no niceties. ''Will, what the hell is this? I've been waiting here, jerked around, since 7:30. What do you mean it's not an emergency? It's my case and if I say it's an emergency, it's an emergency.''

Walter has been through this before. ''Just what I said, Nick, it's not an emergency. If you want, you can wait it out tonight. Otherwise just do it in the morning. These things can wait.''

Norton's voice grows tenser and more brittle. He enunciates each word, so it will have maximum effect on Walter. ''I have a full schedule tomorrow, hips and knees, and nothing can be changed. So tonight's surgery happens tonight. And I am not going to sit around here anymore waiting to be bumped. You get your ass in here, and then you have two choices. Either open a third room or put a note in the chart that this is not an emergency, and you and I will meet in Dr. Fisher's office in the A.M., before my cases!"

Walter knows what Norton's ravings mean. He has been in this situation before too. The surgeons complain to Fisher, who gets involved and then always takes the surgeon's side. He does not want to hear another of Fisher's lectures about knowing when and when not to draw the line. He considers his choices and decides it is still worth one more effort.

"Nick, is this really an emergency?" he asks. "Can't you get somebody else to do it tomorrow? It's not only a matter of inconvenience; it's big bucks to get that room up and going at this hour if it's not really necessary."

Norton is losing what little patience he had left. "Will, it will be really big bucks when I stroke out. *I want you here—stat!*" The telephone recoils as Norton slams down the receiver. He is not only tired; he is infuriated that he has to go through this ordeal. Not the best way to start a week, or a case.

Later, Norton looks up at the clock in the OR as he is about to make his first incision. It is 11:42 P.M.

Developing a Positional Strategy

Having placed your impulse to brutally vanquish your opponent into a mental lockbox (allowing domination fantasies to run wild in the private den of your imagination is a healthy way to satisfy those urges), you can turn to step one in developing your positional strategy: focus on what you want to accomplish. The more coherent your list of objectives, the more reasoned your choices, the more vigorous the support from your allies, and the more explicit your target, the better will be your chances of winning. Again, this is a win-lose game, and you want to do what you can to enhance your chances of winning.

Your professional negotiations will likely revolve around two categories of benefit. The first involves exchanges of tangibles: salary, preferred assignment or shift, space, and equipment as well as the substantive information needed for you to do your work. The second involves the less tangible professional recognition and status: from career advancement and promotion to avoidance of censure or accusations of wrongdoing.

Whether your positional negotiation is about tangibles, intangibles, or some combination of these, your task is to find and establish a standard measure, preferably one favorable to you. This standard allows you to compare your position against a commonly acceptable and reasonable gauge. Your game plan is to employ that standard to advocate your position. For example, in a contract fee negotiation, establish the usual range for professionals with your qualifications, and then demonstrate how your unique added value and experience justify the same standard or a higher amount.

There are three benchmarks to calibrate as you plan your positional strategy. Your *target range* is what you reasonably hope to accomplish. Your *high range* is the inflated stipulations you open with and are willing to concede in order to make the deal. And your *low range* defines the point at which you leave the negotiation to pursue other offensive or defensive alternatives.

Setting the Target Range

Start with your target range. For the sake of illustration, imagine that you want to sell your car for $2,000. You have researched the book value of the auto, the market demand for the vehicle, and the relevance of the time of year. It is May and students are looking for summer transportation, the amount you want is reasonable, and you are confident that you can find a buyer willing to pay the price.

As you formulate your target range, assess what is negotiable and what is not. Be clear on the scope of issues and their ramifications. Know that what you have staked out is achievable.

In American culture, cars—especially used cars—are on the list of negotiable items. Each culture and organization has its own list of negotiable and non-negotiable items. Spaghetti in a grocery store, salary in a governmental agency, emergency medical care in a hospital: all are relatively nonnegotiable items in this country. Cashiers are not authorized to haggle over the price of groceries. Public agencies offer salaries established by a grading system with little flexibility for individual circumstances. And it would be unethical to discuss billing during a life-or-death situation in a hospital. Conversely, items such as cars and houses and also salaries in private organizations are permissible items to negotiate. Similarly, department budgets, office space, and institutional policies and procedures are legitimate negotiable items. You do not want to bargain or advocate for matters that are inalterably nonnegotiable, because it is a waste of time and effort and it makes you appear uninformed.

What distinguishes the negotiable from the nonnegotiable, the definitive from the disputable? An object or service without an absolute, recognized value is open for deal making, as is an issue without a conclusive, agreed-upon outcome. The purpose of bargaining is to establish an acceptable value and a deal. Placing an object into a category with a set of standard values—for example, the book value of cars—is the essence of negotiation. Likewise, the cost of medical services can be set on the basis of generally accepted community billing rates or a global payment system. And a public health matter can be debated based on data and the experience of successfully or unsuccessfully addressing it elsewhere. The question is whether the standard value or agreed-upon outcome is convincing or applicable. Do car buyers endorse the recommendation of book value, or are such values perceived as tilted in favor of sellers? Are community billing rates seen as reasonable, or are they seen as inflated by providers? And is the public health experience elsewhere comparable to the conditions seen locally?

Similarly, when you have been accused of a personal or professional transgression, what standard is used to determine whether you have committed the offense? What is the accusation, and by what standard is your act considered wrongful? Is there valid evidence against you, and does it prove your culpability? Is there congruence between the accusation of negligence, liability, or mismanagement and the acts committed? Furthermore, were there mitigating circumstances that must be taken into account as the charges are assessed? How will the problem be judged, and what are the implications for all involved?

The distinction between what is and is not negotiable likewise applies to questions of professional behavior. Sexual misconduct, gross financial embezzlement, and actions intentionally harmful to patients all call for disciplinary action against the offender: the question is only how severe that action will be. Continued patient contact is likely out of the question. However, minor infractions taken as major offenses can also fall within the purview of positional negotiation. You must clarify that a simple miscommunication, misunderstanding, or miscalculation does not belong in that category of condemnable violations.

Although the courts may subscribe to the precept "innocent until proven guilty," in the councils of professional practice, such equanimity is rare. Once you have been branded by the arbiters of public opinion and gossip, that judgment could have devastating implications for your career. Just as you must establish your target range for a car sale, you must be deliberate about what you hope to accomplish in response to a professional accusation. What is your victory?

Likewise, if you are advocating for professional promotion, a salary increase, or other advancement, what is the basis of your position? What standards have you chosen against which to gauge your requests: Are they reasonable and recognized? Do others value your accomplishments as much as you do? What tangible benefits have you delivered, and how might your continued success benefit the organization?

Whether it is a purchase and sale agreement, a professional dispute, or an organizational negotiation, test your target range against the scale of reasonableness. If your target range is not tenable, you are setting your own trap through greed, disappointment, and miscalculation, invoking your own defeat before you even begin the fight. You will have given your negotiating counterpart an easy, and valid, reason for closing negotiations without your desired outcome achieved. Assess the necessary considerations and take aim for an objective that is both feasible and satisfying. Your objectives should be meticulous, resourceful, and street-smart: one triumph can lead to your next victory.

Setting the High Range

Your target range is private: you keep it to yourself or share it only with trusted compatriots. Your high range, however, is public. It is what you say you want in your opening bid. Incorporated into this initial proposition is room to move, a cushion. Why and how do you create this latitude?

Positional negotiation is a game. Unlike organized sports, in which explicit rules determine the winner and loser, in positional negotiation you determine your own criteria for winning. Thus it is possible for the other side to think you have lost when you know that you have won. How can this be?

Between your target range and your opening bid, you place one set of requests that you would love to have and another set that you are willing to concede. In the give-and-get of negotiation, you give up what you did not care about getting in the first place. In the face of your "concessions," the other side is motivated to come to an agreement. With this ruse, the other side may feel that you caved in when in fact you got everything you wanted. Note that the other side will likely be engaged in the same behavior.

There is an art to setting your high range. On the one hand, if it is too high you will appear unreasonable, and the other side will score points against you. For example, if I advertise my $2,000 car for $4,000, I leave plenty of room to move down. The problem of course is that the people who come to view the car will be in the market for a vehicle of much higher value than my junk heap. They want a car worth about $4,000 to $5,000 in caliber and quality. I will have attracted the wrong buyers and my advertising investment and time will have been for naught. No concession on the price will convince these buyers to purchase my car. Similarly, if you are negotiating for building space to house your department, insisting on a whole floor when you are likely to get little more than a wing makes you appear unreasonable and ridiculous. Your request will appear outrageous and your competitors for space will tout the folly of your miscalculation. And finally, if you claim zero responsibility for a professional misdeed in which you did have some culpability, you set yourself up to have the book thrown at you. If your opening bid is beyond reason, you sacrifice your credibility and give the other side command of the shots—not a desirable situation.

On the other hand, if your opening bid is too close to your target range, you afford yourself little room to move and, with it, you hold meager leverage. As a result, even if the people on the other side obtain what is in fact a favorable outcome, they will feel cheated if they had anticipated some concessions and you offered few or none. This is an enigma to the interest-based negotiator who does not comprehend the positional game: the other party always wants to think he or she got a good deal. This is the logic of the many antiques dealers who mark an item at one price and fully expect to sell it for 10 or 15 percent less. They know that many customers like to haggle over the price for antiques and gain satisfaction from telling their friends about the hard bargain they drove and the great deal they thus secured. Furthermore, if your opening bid is too close to your target range, and you are forced to give concessions, your outcome may be below what you hoped to achieve. You will have needlessly negotiated from a deficit position.

Someplace between too high and too low is the sweet spot for your opening bid. How do you set it? Short of common sense and research, there is no universal rule of thumb. Much of your calculation will rely on context, such as the generally accepted and unwritten rules of the organization culture in which you work. For example, at budget time it might be generally known that in anticipation of a cut, everyone inflates his or her proposal by 10 percent. It is part of the ritual of the apportionment process. To request only the budget you really need will leave you with a shortfall. To request 30 percent over your target makes you appear greedy and may raise questions about your managerial competence.

The difference between the good negotiator and the conqueror is that the latter wants it all. He is not willing to concede anything. That stance tends to drag the negotiation process out endlessly or to stifle it with onerous demands. In the first instance you seek the win, which you can achieve through negotiation, and in the second you seek the conquest, which generates new enemies and antipathy and which might eventually sow the seeds of your own defeat.

Choosing the right opening bid is a matter of strategy. And who knows? Perhaps savvy and luck, resourcefully combined, will yield you a tidy surplus.

Setting the Low Range

On one end you calculate your high range, an opening bid that gives you room to move. On the other end you establish your low range, a point beyond which you are unwilling to concede. In the case of the auto, for example, the low range is the price below which you are unwilling to sell. If your target is $2,000 and your opening price is $2,500, you might set $1,500 as your bottom price. You presume there must be someone out there willing to spend at least that much for the car. If your first customer offers not a penny over $1,200, you decline the offer, confident that someone else will bring a better price. In health care negotiations the low range could be defined by staff working conditions, patient care decisions, or service reimbursement rates beyond which you are unwilling to concede. For example, you might be unwilling to accept more than six patients to one nurse in your hospital unit, unwilling to allow restraints to be imposed on nursing home patients who are usually competent, or unwilling to accept rates of reimbursement that are below your actual cost of providing care.

Your low range defines what Fisher, Ury, and Patton (1991) describe as your BATNA, your "best alternative to a negotiated agreement." Your BATNA determines the point at which you walk from the negotiation table. When the other side is making meager and or otherwise unacceptable offers, the better alternative may be resigning and taking a new job, going on strike, going to the media, or filing a lawsuit. Before you put your BATNA on the table, you should already have that better alternative in hand. For example, before threatening resignation you should have another firm job offer available to you: you will be taken more seriously. Exercising your BATNA means disengaging yourself—at least for the time being—from constructive, solution-oriented discussion. Your BATNA could be passive: you simply leave the scene or do not show up for a meeting. If you are a valued staff member or colleague, your departure or absence inflicts a high personal and professional price on the other side. Ideally you will reveal your better option (such as that great job offer at a competing institution) just before you act on it. Your BATNA may also be aggressive, such as having an attorney in the wings ready to press a legal challenge to the other side.

There are two important reasons for appraising your bottom line and setting your low range early in the process. First, you do not want to remain at the table when the other side has transgressed into what you consider professionally, morally, or pragmatically repugnant tactics or demands. Many negotiators stay too long, hoping they can somehow convince the other side to change its position. Wake up! Their position is clear: you just don't get it! For you to endure conditions that the other side knows you find unacceptable is a strategic mistake. You weaken your own position when the parties on the other side find you are willing to suffer their taunts graciously. You will have issued an invitation for punishment, and if they are evil enough, they will have a good time with you. Kritek (1994) refers to the importance of leaving the table with your dignity intact. When you stake out your bottom line before you get there, you are less likely to get snagged in the spiral of an escalating assault.

Second, when you have anticipated your low range, you are strategically best able to cope with the pressures of bargaining. Some negotiators panic at the mere thought of making a concession, even a minor one. In their minds it is a sign of weakness to give up anything, no matter how paltry. Because they have not clarified for themselves what is important and what is not, they are more likely to get trigger-happy and reach too soon for their BATNA. They stomp out of the room before giving negotiation a fair try. This is a strategic mistake.

If you are altogether inflexible and threaten to pull out your BATNA as soon as you meet any resistance, you cue the other side into pushing your panic button. If you appear too desperate to leave, the other side might just call your bluff and then flaunt the rigidity and unreasonableness of your position. Leaving the table prematurely creates the impression that you are interested only in domination. It is not sportsmanlike. You render yourself too easy to dismiss.

As you contemplate your low range, you also discover your own bottom line of process preferences and substantive principles. Your process preferences constitute your own code of negotiation. There are some negotiators who are ready, with proper warning, to walk from the table when the time is right. There are others who, having given the other side proper warning, maintain that persistence at the negotiation table is the only way to settle differences. These people will continue collaborating, talking, or conceding, no matter the cost. They view walking, striking, attacking, or suing as a violation of their philosophy. They are opposed to exercising any BATNA. This unwillingness ultimately—and unfortunately—may impair their negotiation effectiveness. If the parties on the other side detect this attitude, they just might boost their goading, knowing that there is no limit to what they can pull off. By ruling out any BATNA, you weaken your negotiation effectiveness.

Your substantive principles refer to your own code of professional ethics: What are you unwilling to tolerate? Are you willing to pay the price for exercising your BATNA when faced with wrenching moral dilemmas, professional improprieties, or personal misbehavior? At what point are conditions so deplorable that you are willing to accept the financial uncertainty of unemployment, the professional risks of a public scandal, or the high costs of a court battle? Ample experience has proven that not every dispute can be resolved through negotiation. Where do you draw your line?

When it comes to identifying and exercising negotiation BATNA, there are two primary types: the perseverers and the bolters. A perseverer might say, "If we could only improve our relationship, we could find a solution to this problem." There is a reluctance to declare a BATNA, no matter the cost. Conversely, a bolter might conclude, "I'll leave right now and show them that I can't be pushed around." There is an enthusiasm among bolters to jump at the BATNA, no matter the situation. Whatever your own tendency, combining self-awareness with strategic decision making improves the chances that you will neither stay too long nor leave too fast.

Remember, there are a range of options to consider as you plan your BATNA; time and energy devoted to planning your better alternatives is a worthy investment; if nothing else it can improve your sense of negotiation security. Using BATNA effectively requires both courage and creative thinking. Mahatma Gandhi, Martin Luther King Jr., and other leaders advocated non-violence at times when followers were all too eager to adopt more destructive tactics. A work slowdown is less severe than a strike, as are a deluge of letters of support, a sympathetic news article, and a run to the board of directors. Whatever strategic method you choose, it is essential that you do not in the process lose your most important asset: the supporters and allies who legitimize the actions you are taking.

Balancing High, Low, and Target Ranges

How are these three strategic ranges used in practice? In positional negotiation, you open the bargaining by associating the item in question with a value that is slightly outside your desired end point. The car seller might point to the pristine appearance of the car to justify its slightly above book value price. The buyer might counter that the unusually high odometer reading in fact places it slightly below book value. As there is no absolute value for the used car, they go back and forth over the relative merits of appearance versus performance. Each emphasizes his own claim while privately considering the merits of the other's arguments: yes, the buyer lusts at the thought of driving that red convertible, top down, on a sunny day; and true, the seller reckons he did get a lot of use from this now well-worn vehicle. Whether they come to an agreement depends on whether, amid all the objective and subjective information, they can find a value that falls into the acceptable range for each. What tactics do they use to get there?

"Dumb-ass fool. I hope she gets what she deserves. We've been putting up with that crap for years, and we don't fall apart every time some doctor gives us a look." Cathy Crow seems to be only half-conscious of what she is saying as she unscrews the top of her coffee thermos. Her eyes follow the steam from the coffee as she pours it into her cup. She is tired and eager for the caffeine that will return her pep.

Pauline Patrick glances to her side, more focused on getting her sandwich unwrapped. Five nurses on the Six West general medical floor are taking their dinner break and discussing the latest gossip in the Harriford-Cummings "affair," as it has ironically become known. Patrick has not signed on to the disgust some nurses are expressing for Harriford. She can see something on both sides.

Sylvia Sheffield looks over to Crow with a wry, experienced smile. Sheffield is nearly sixty years old and has watched all manner of hullabaloo about nursing come and go. She gives it all little concern. She knows what the job requires and has little patience for all the haggling that goes on. "Actually, I think Cummings is a good-looking young man," she says. "I wouldn't mind it if he chatted me up a bit." Sheffield garners the glances and smiles from Crow and Patrick that she was hoping for.

Judy Jameson stares at the three of them at the far end of the table. She cannot believe what she is hearing. She is frozen in rage. Finally she blurts out. "I can't believe it. How could you say such a thing?" She speaks directly to Crow. She has written off Sheffield's comment.

Crow is quick, almost as if she were expecting—even prodding—Jameson. "Well, look who's getting hot under the collar. What's the problem, Judy? Rejected because he didn't go for you?" Crow's ridiculing agitates Jameson no end.

Jameson grits her teeth. She speaks slowly and deliberately. "Cathy, don't you have any respect for nursing and for what we do? When Cummings violated Heather, he violated all of us, personally and professionally. If we don't stand behind her on this, then"—she pauses, not certain how grandiose to make her next statement—"then we are compromising ourselves. Then what Cummings did to Heather is nothing compared to what we are doing to ourselves."

Crow relishes Jameson's fiery reaction. "Oh, come on, Judy. What are we doing to ourselves? Get off your soap box. Cummings made a pass at Heather, and she misinterpreted it. If I made such a fuss every time that happened to me"—she mimics Jameson's dramatic pause—"why, I wouldn't get any nursing done."

Crow's sarcasm presses every one of Jameson's buttons. She points her finger straight at Crow. "You call what *you* do nursing? You have an attitude problem, Cathy, and that's not what nursing is all about."

Crow flares in anger. "You puny little thing. Don't you question my nursing or my attitude about nursing. My mom was a nurse, and my sister is a nurse, and you don't make fun of nursing around me. All I'm saying is that Heather made a stupid move and it makes us all look bad."

Debby D'Alfonso is sitting quietly through the whole conversation, afraid to say anything but agreeing in her heart with Jameson. There is a heavy, lingering silence in the air after Crow's outburst. Finally, D'Alfonso speaks, "I think you guys missed the point. If Heather feels she was violated, she *was* violated. And I don't think any woman should have to put up with that—I don't care if she is a nurse or a doctor or a housewife. And it's all the worse because Heather was doing what we do all the time. She was sending out a warning cue to a doctor who wasn't paying attention. And his fixation on Heather instead of the patient was going to cost that patient a lot of suffering, if not worse. That, to my mind, is the crux of the issue, and I think it should be respected as that. No more and no less."

Crow and Jameson are both feeling rage mixed with a measure of foolishness. Again there is silence. This is a sensitive topic, and the incident involving Harriford is a tough issue. Each nurse is feeling a blend of what she feels is acceptable and is unacceptable about sexual overtures and doctor-nurse relations, combined with her own personal feelings about Harriford.

Sheffield has traditionally been the one to smooth things over when controversy riles the nurses on Six West. It has always been her role in her family, and it was the role she plays at work. She tries to change the mood. "Look, it's no matter in the long run. Heather will come back just the way she has; Cummins will probably get his wrist slapped publicly while the guys slap his back when we're not around. This has been going on since before you were born, dearies." She sighs, a measure of weathered experience. "Just used to be that we had more of a sense of humor about the whole thing."

Jameson is not mollified. She likes Sheffield and realizes she is from an older generation that had been less empowered about these issues. Nonetheless, she cannot let the remark go unchallenged. "There is nothing funny about what happened to Heather, Sylvia. And there is nothing funny about what happens to other women, women who work in this hospital and women that are brought into this hospital on a stretcher. We have to start drawing the line, and I respect Heather for having the courage to do it. She deserves at least our support, if not a whole lot more."

Crow lifts her hands and starts clapping. The clapping lasts for an endless moment. Everyone is waiting to see what Crow says. "So what do we do, start giving out medals? Great. Heather made a big deal about something that goes on all the time. And it's not like he groped her. That's the problem, Judy. You've got the whole thing confused. You don't know what real harassment is. If you cry wolf every time a doctor gets a little flirtatious, then when the real stuff hits, nobody's going to be paying attention."

D'Alfonso jumps in before Jameson can respond. "Cathy, you're not hearing what Judy is saying. Are you suggesting that all this pushing around we have to put up with is a good thing?"

Crow is quick. Her voice is tense, and she raises her hand to point at D'Alfonso. "No, I never said it was a good thing—" She stops as she catches a glimpse of Heather Harriford approaching.

Harriford has been with Mrs. Hayward's family. Mrs. Hayward's condition has deteriorated further. Her weight is down; she is lethargic. Her family are gathered in a hushed room down the hall. They are distressed and need a great deal of care and attention. They quiz Harriford often about whether their mother is experiencing pain or other discomfort. There is a lot of crying accompanied by hugs of support. Having established a good relationship with Harriford, the family finds a great deal of comfort in her presence. She's begun to be able to read their feelings before they even speak. She had postponed her dinner break in order to tend to the needs that she sensed among them.

Now finally, after she has done what she can for Mrs. Haywards's family, Harriford walks briskly into the nurses' lounge. She is emotionally drained, though invigorated. The time she spent with Mrs. Hayward's family has helped her to forget everything else that is going on at work. She plops a sandwich and a diet soda on the table. She looks around the strangely quiet room. No one makes eye contact and the "other stuff" comes roaring back to her mind. "Let me guess. You were discussing the weather. I know, all these warm days we've been having. Could it be climate change?"

D'Alfonso sometimes gets carried away with the obvious. She hates awkward silences. "OK, busted. We were discussing this whole mess with you and Dr. Cummings. I think it's fair to say that there is a good deal of arguing going on about the whole thing."

Harriford shakes her head wearily. "Let me guess. Cathy, you think I should have gone to bed with him. Best thing for a nurse's financial future is to bag a doc, right?" Harriford knows exactly what she is doing with this comment. She and Crow come from very different backgrounds. Harriford had a middle-class upbringing, finished her nursing training at a major university, and is applying for entry to an advanced-practice master's program. Crow came from a working-class background, and even her community college degree was a first for her family. The animosity between them runs deep, and this incident with Dr. Cummings is just another hook on which to hang their feuding.

"What are you implying?" Crow shoots back. She does not wait for an answer. "Let me tell you one thing, cutie pie. I was around here long before you could spell 'hospital,' and I'll be here long after you get your next fancy degree. And I have to survive in this place. And survival is not about complaining every time some Tom, Dick, or Harry looks you over. What you are doing is helping no one but yourself. I don't know what the hell you're hoping to accomplish, but you can get off your high horse about doing something for the rest of us. You are nothing but a pain in the ass, and don't you forget it!"

As tough as it is to hear Crow out, Harriford is ready for this onslaught. She has known it was coming. She stares Crow down and doesn't say a thing. Sheffield speaks through her stare. "Now, now—enough, the two of you. It's a shame that this is dividing us so." Sheffield pauses, as if what she has said was as revealing to herself as it may have been to others. She continues. "Actually, we won't work well together if this divides us." Her afterthought hangs in the air as she packs away the remains of her dinner. "Well, it's back to the salt mine. I've got to get to work."

Crow also cleans up the remains of her meal and shoves her chair noisily back against the table before marching defiantly out of the room. Patrick follows, offering Harriford a sympathetic look as she races after Crow.

Harriford unwraps her sandwich and meets Jameson's and D'Alfonso's sympathetic looks. "Now, isn't that a great way to start a break," she says. She looks down at her tuna on wheat and lets her hands go limp. She's no longer hungry. Jameson and D'Alfonso stay a few minutes to lend comfort and support before they also have to return to their patients.

Harriford is left in the brightly lit room feeling alone and defeated. "What good does integrity do you at a time like this?" she thinks to herself.

Combining Tactics and Strategy

Negotiation is the art of persuasion. In the case of interest-based negotiation, the carrot of mutual benefit and the potential for future gain motivates both parties to make rational choices. In the case of positional negotiation, it is the stick of leverage that prods other parties toward the direction you desire. You pose a convincing argument by imposing your power, influence, and clout upon the other side's deliberations. Your positional tactics define how you do this.

Basic to the development of your positional tactics are perceptions. It is the perceptions you foster, embellish, and sway that convince the other side. Just as there is no absolute value for an item in a positional negotiation, there is also no absolute distinction between what is real and what is merely perceived. You may believe that you have great power within your organization. However, if the other side perceives you to be weak, then you have little clout during your negotiation. Likewise, your real organizational influence may be marginal. However, if those on the other side believe you hold the key to their future success or failure, then your bargaining power is greatly enhanced.

The use of perception to fortify one's position is a common ploy of positional bargaining. In military conflicts, for example, an army magnifies the apparent size of its force; in legal disputes, one side exaggerates the size and legitimacy of its claim; and in professional negotiations, one party magnifies the consequences that a budget reduction will have upon it. The key is not the actual size of the army, amount of the lawsuit, or consequence of the cutback. The key is what those on the other side believe and what action they take as a result. Positional tactics are used to create the perceptions necessary to stimulate the hoped-for reaction from the other side.

This tenet of positional bargaining raises an awkward ethical question: do the ends always justify the means? The answer is no. It depends on the context. A tactic that is morally correct in one instance may be immoral in another. Having exhausted other avenues to address the problem, going to a government agency that has prosecutorial powers with a report about patient abuse could be appropriate as you balance ends and means. To use the same tactic for an internal professional dispute would be improper. The responsible alignment of ends and means must be assessed for every negotiation. One can be a successful positional negotiator while remaining within the bounds of what is considered appropriate professional and personal conduct. Two alleged rules of the British diplomatic corps offer a guide: "Never lie and never tell the whole truth."

How does one create the necessary perceptions and desired reactions in one's opponent? Following is a sampling of positional tactics to inspire your thinking. Again, use the reservoir of your imagination to construct a scheme appropriate to your situation.

Learn Their Strategy

International negotiation is marked by the intrigue of intelligence agencies who spy on the workings of their opponents. Apart from the cinematic romance associated with these operations, they illustrate a fundamental premise of positional bargaining. The more you know about the parties on the other side, the more effective your own strategy will be. What are their target, high, and low ranges? To maximize your gains, you want your opening bid to be as close to their low range as possible. What perceptions are they trying to manufacture and how concerned should you be about them? You do not want to misread what could be a real threat. And how do they perceive the signals you are sending them? If they do not take you seriously, you may have to raise the stakes.

You only abet their cause if you violate the law or organizational policy to uncover their strategy. Nonetheless there are a number of perfectly legal and proper ways to learn what the other side is thinking. Going out to lunch with the right people; tracing public memos; getting the inside scoop from trusted colleagues; reviewing your opponents' past behavior to predict future patterns—such tactics can provide useful information to help you discern what they are doing and to anticipate what they will do next.

Set Up a Boomerang Effect

Having assessed your opponents' strategy, you have the opportunity to get one step ahead of them. Once you know their options and choices, defeat them by gently closing those choices so that they are adversely painted into their own corner. If you learn that they are on their way to the director to blast you, get there first with your own version of the story. By the time they get to the boss to launch their offensive, the boss will already be sympathetic to your version of the story. If someone plans to embarrass you at a meeting with a malicious accusation, privately warn the other participants beforehand about the regrettable performance they are about to witness. Your opponent will look like a fool. If people in another department are about to steal some of your office space, contract for customized renovations and then leave them holding the bill. Like a bullfighter, you want to outsmart the opposition by fostering illusions that provoke your opponents to attack you in such a way that you sustain no injury.

These calculated, proactive moves must be taken with great caution. If your opponent does not show up at the director's door, does not bring forth the accusation, or does not go for a territorial grab, you are left looking an even greater fool. Remember, they are playing the same game.

Employ Diversionary Tactics

Imagine that you are confronted with two issues: issue A and issue B. Issue A is of vital importance to you. Issue B is of secondary importance. Upon which one do you focus initial public attention?

Many people respond, "Issue A—you fight for your priorities." In fact, the better choice may be issue B if issue B is of vital importance to your counterparts. To achieve a win on issue A you feign a great interest in issue B, making it look as though it is important to you too. Then, during your negotiation, you graciously concede on issue B, perhaps with a certain amount of fanfare and with a low-key request for a reciprocal concession on issue A from your counterpart. You appear to be magnanimous. In return, and for a paltry price from your perspective, you gain success on what is really important. Issue B is usually the increment that separates your target range from your high range. As you retreat from your initial proposition, you will create the perception of having made a compromise, though all along you have adhered to what is essential for you.

Conversation ebbs and flows in the physicians' lounge as new people come and go, different combinations gather, and topics meld from one to another. Someone walks in to make a call, grab a cup of coffee, take a snooze, or just relax for a few minutes on the inviting chairs and couches. Every so often a particular issue hangs in the room, moving from one group to the next. The Cummings affair has quickly become one of those lingering topics. Four male physicians are alone in the corner by the soda machine, animatedly debating the matter.

"Cummings got screwed." Dr. Steve Schilling, a second-year resident, makes his point while waving a half-eaten apple in the air. "What did he do? Look at some nurse's boobs? I mean, this place would turn into a convent if they knocked a guy every time he checked out the territory. Give me a break."

Another second-year resident, Dr. Cliff Clemens, agrees. "The screwy thing is that they let it get so out of hand. They are talking about disciplining him. What the hell?"

Uncomfortable with the conversation, Dr. Charlie Collins watches the two of them and wonders if this is an instance when it is worth violating the macho code. On the one hand, suggesting that there may be a different view of the incident would definitely run counter to the dictums of male solidarity. On the other hand, he isn't sure he can live with himself if he doesn't say something. "I disagree. I think Cummings deserves to be called on this."

"You think Cummings should be penalized?" Schilling asks quizzically, as if he assumed Collins was joking. He is incredulous. "Come on, what did he do that any of us wouldn't? It was a friendly touch to her shoulders and arms. He maybe glanced at her breasts. You call that sexual harassment?"

"That wasn't the whole problem, and you know it, Steve. He was pushing morphine incorrectly for a patient as part of this game he was playing with Harriford. You want to ask a nurse out? Great. But that stuff can never get in the way of patient care. I've seen Cummings operate before. He was bound to eventually cross the line, and she simply called him on it."

Ken Kavanaugh, chief of the intensive care unit, occupies the fourth side of the box of couches. He lounges with one leg folded over the arm of his couch. Kavanaugh likes to come into the lounge periodically, even though he has his own office, just to get a pulse on the place. As the oldest of the foursome, Kavanaugh had decided to listen before he speaks; now he's ready to join the discussion. "Collins is right. What Cummings did was wrong. First, he crossed the line with Heather Harriford. Every woman sets her own line, and even if what he did is OK with one woman, it doesn't mean it's OK with another. Heather was doing her job, and coming on to her was wrong, no doubt about it." Kavanaugh pauses to draw a distinction between his points. "The other thing, about the medication. He should have been more careful, and Heather was saving his ass. He was too proud to admit it, so he tried to change the topic by playing Dr. Tough. I'm sorry if this is not cool. There is social touching and there is sexual touching, and from what I heard of what went on, he pushed beyond mere friendly touching. I'm not saying that they should take away his license. They should do something, though.''

As the senior physician in the group, Kavanaugh carries a lot of weight. Schilling can't drop the topic though. ''OK, Ken, so where do *we* draw the line? What about the whole role of physicians here? If everyone is going around second-guessing doctors, then what's our use? I think we have to set an example with Chuck. If we are soft on this one, every nurse in this hospital is going to be filing a report every time we check out what's written on her T-shirt or complement her on nice earrings.''

Clemens jumps in to support his friend. ''It's not just the so-called harassment. We have to draw the line on nursing, Ken.'' Cliff was hoping to appeal to a common denominator and turn Kavanaugh around. ''Everybody is trying to take a chunk out of medical practice, and I don't think we should give in. If we don't stick together, they'll divide and conquer. We have to think about that too.''

Kavanaugh can't believe what he is hearing. He thought these young guys would be more aware. He decides to play the mentor role: he can't help it. ''First off, women have a right to send a message and have it respected. That goes no matter where they are: in the hospital, on a date, or in public. Heather stepped away from him. That was his cue, and he ignored it. If the cue is clear and you ignore it, you're on thin ice and you open yourself up to legitimate accusation. Second, I think it's great for people to meet here and get together. Great. Just don't do it on company time, and don't mix it up with doing your job. Meet after your shift, go out, do whatever you want. Just don't mix your come-ons with your responsibilities. Finally, Heather was giving Chuck a clear message about a mistake he was about to make. Never, ever ignore a warning sign if someone is flashing it for you. It could be a nurse, a patient, a family member, or a colleague. That warning could save your career, to say nothing of your patient's life. Don't let your ego take control so that you feel some macho compulsion to ignore the warning. Check out what's being said, why, what you may have missed. Only after you are completely sure do you go ahead. It's like those warning lights on airplanes. The pilot doesn't ignore the light, even if it's only a problem with a broken bulb.'' Kavanaugh stops to take a breath and suddenly hears someone behind him clapping. He turns around to find Dr. Beatrice Benson beaming.

''Good job, Ken. I like it.'' She is smiling. Kavanaugh blushes.

''We were just debating this whole Cummings thing,'' Kavanaugh explains, somewhat embarrassed now about his passionate speech.

Beatrice plops herself down next to Kavanaugh. ''What's to debate? The guy's a jerk.''

''Well, there's not a unanimous vote for that sentiment.'' Collins gestures to Schilling and Clemens.

Benson turns to them. "What?"

Schilling opens up somewhat cautiously. "I just don't think the guy should be fired. I think everybody is making too big a thing about what Chuck did. That's all."

Benson turns to Kavanaugh and points a thumb at the others. "Where were these guys when the women's movement was born?"

Clemens feels the steam blowing out of their argument. Nonetheless, he can't stand not defending himself. "I think it's unfair holding doctors to a different standard than everybody else. What Cummings did was not that terrible."

Kavanaugh lifts up out of his chair to make the point. "There, you've got it, Clemens. But you're wrong. It *is* fair to hold doctors to another standard. We are involved in the most intimate aspects of our patients' lives and bodies and emotions. That is a trust that society places in us. That is something you take with you everywhere you go, because now that you've got that MD behind your name, society always thinks of you as a doctor. Always, every minute. Yeah, that is a burden. And it's because you are carrying that burden that society is willing to pay you a decent salary and give you an extra measure of respect. Cummings is learning that lesson the hard way. Do yourself a favor; pick up the advice before you find yourself walking in his shoes."

With that someone notes the time, and everyone begins to peel off to go someplace else. Benson pats Kavanaugh on the back and shoots him a smile as he gets up from the couch.

For example, your organization acquires a new office building. As space in the building is being apportioned, your concern is more with location than with square footage. You want to be close to other departments, to patients, and to amenities for your staff. The primary point of contention among the various departments, however, is square footage: everyone is arguing that his or her department has unique requirements and requires a lot of space. You too sing these blues—and then offer a concession. You will accept a smaller space than you would prefer in exchange for a better location. If the administration is having headaches over excessive demands for space, your concession could win you points and the location you desire.

Create Leverage

There are some issues about which the other parties care and some about which they do not. Focus on the former. What motivates the other parties? What incentives would prompt them to shift? Once you understand what can induce them, create and demonstrate a capacity to influence those very outcomes. In so doing you raise the stakes for anyone not complying with your wishes. You have created real choices, with the potential for uncomfortable consequences. In the process, you have devised leverage: the power of persuasion.

For example, in the course of a budgetary dispute at a public hospital, you learn that a significant sum of money has recently been diverted into an unusually generous administrative line item. These funds have, in fact, been generated by your department and are necessary for the continuation of services to vulnerable populations. The bargaining has become positional. You know that the commissioner of the local public health agency that oversees the hospital, a relative neophyte, is particularly sensitive to bad publicity because of his tenuous political appointment. Your reputation is long-standing and solid. At some point during the negotiations, you gently comment on the interest that the mayor might have in this gross misappropriation of funds. Later in the conversation, while on a different topic, you let it drop that an adviser to the mayor, a close personal friend, is coming to your home for dinner. You have pinpointed one of the commissioner's primary anxieties, and you have demonstrated your capacity to influence that motivator. Chances are that your budget will be restored before the mayoral adviser arrives for dinner.

Sow Info Bits

There is an old military trick that might inspire useful positional maneuvering on your part. Consider the dilemma of a small group of soldiers positioned at the top of one side of a wide valley and facing a full battalion at the top of the other side. There is little hope that reinforcements will arrive before dawn. They want neither to surrender their position nor to fight the battle, which they would surely lose. What can they do?

Once darkness falls, they drive their few trucks quietly and without lights down from their position on the hill. At the bottom of the hill, the drivers turn the trucks around and switch on their lights. They then ascend the hill noisily. Once at the top they turn off their lights and drive back down. This continues and is watched by the other side all night. The opposing army, convinced that they now face a full legion, decides not to attack.

Whether you create a perception of power by walking through the corridors with someone of great stature, having your name appear frequently in the press, or touting your professional accomplishments, the impressions you create and employ will be carefully watched by your opponents. What they do will be influenced greatly by what they perceive. Carefully orchestrating those perceptions to your advantage is a potent ploy of positional negotiation.

Dr. Ted Tuckerman has seen it all in his thirty years of internal medicine practice: the aches, the pains, the discomforts. He has a good reputation as a careful doctor, which he carefully guards. The day that changed his practice happened slightly over one year ago.

Mrs. Betty Brown had been a patient of his for nearly ten years. A grocery store clerk, she seemed to live for her ailments. She was a complainer, and Dr. Tuckerman imagined that she spent her time with her friends recounting, in great detail, the minutiae of each of her visits with him. Nonetheless, Tuckerman had grown fond of Mrs. Brown, who brought a poppy seed cake into the office every holiday.

It was three years ago when the trouble began, just after a particularly frigid and inclement spell of winter. Mrs. Brown complained of dizziness and colds. She was enrolled in a managed care plan, which she had joined through the supermarket chain where she worked. It was a frugal plan, and it was particularly careful about limiting what were considered unnecessary tests and referrals. At the time Tuckerman had assumed that her complaints were just another of her bouts with frequent colds. He encouraged Mrs. Brown to put them into perspective and not be too worried. He was reluctant to go through the hassle of sending her for another full workup for naught.

It was three months later, in the middle of May, when the complaints had not abated, that Tuckerman finally became concerned. Her condition had deteriorated, and she was having trouble breathing. She had never been a smoker, though on questioning, Tuckerman learned that her late husband had been a pack-a-day smoker throughout their marriage.

The X-rays came back with what Tuckerman had most dreaded. Mrs. Brown was suffering from a progressed case of lung cancer. At this point even aggressive treatment would give her only a few more weeks. Against the wishes of her family, Mrs. Brown decided to forgo chemotherapy. She returned to her home with hospice support and died two weeks later.

It was thirteen months later that the letter arrived from the state board of medical registration. Mrs. Brown's daughter, Leslie Long, had filed a complaint against him with the board. The complaint alleged that because of his negligence, her mother had suffered a cruel death that could have been averted had he conducted tests earlier. Ms. Long had written the board a long letter detailing Mrs. Brown's medical history, her illness prior to the diagnosis, and her painful death. It described her centrality to the family and the deep loss they had experienced since her passing. There was nothing positive in the letter: it neglected to mention anything about the many years of exemplary care Dr. Tuckerman had given Mrs. Brown. It was a stinging attack. It ended with a plea for the board to remove his license to practice medicine. The family could not endure the possibility that someone else might have to suffer as their mother had.

For Tuckerman, the letter was a nightmare. Now he sits moribund in the office of his attorney, Larry Levine. Levine is matter-of-fact about the situation. He has successfully walked other physicians through similar problems many times.

"So, tell me everything you can about this Mrs. Brown," Levine asks. "Was she a whiner?"

Tuckerman speaks glumly. "She was difficult. Whenever she came in, she had an endless list of aches and pains for me. I listened patiently to each, though I couldn't take every one seriously: I would have spent her whole plan's yearly budget on senseless procedures. The trouble, of course, was that there was the danger that I would miss something. And as it turned out, I did. Nothing much more to it than that."

"Ted, Ted, you've got an attitude problem." Levine pauses to consider what can bring Tuckerman to his senses. He gets up from behind his massive mahogany desk to sit closer to his client. "I have a question for you, Ted. Are you still planning to continue your practice of medicine?"

Tuckerman looks incredulous. "What kind of a thing is that to say? Of course I want to continue my practice. That's what I hired you to guarantee me."

Levine smiles as if he had just won a small victory. "OK, Ted, I'll do that. But I'll need your help. You see, we're fighting a good-guys-versus-bad-guys battle here. Right now, you're the bad guy. We've got to turn you back into the good guy who made a reasonable miscalculation—if that—all in the name of good yet prudent medicine. Do you understand?"

Tuckerman feels like a small boy who has just been reprimanded by a teacher. His reply is reluctant: "Yes, I understand."

On the one hand, part of the problem for Tuckerman is that in fact he does feel a bit like the bad guy. This incident has shattered his confidence and his faith in his own medical judgment. Just as Ms. Long's letter has neglected the many achievements of his career, so too has his own current perspective erased those achievements. He does feel guilty. Not guilty enough to abandon his career, yet guilty enough to believe that he somehow contributed to Mrs. Brown's demise, or at least deprived her of a chance for prolonging her life.

On the other hand he has another mix of feelings adding to his sense of confusion; these feelings involve his wife, his kids in college, his mortgage, his career, and his future. He certainly does not want to sacrifice all he has worked so hard to build. When he looks at this mess from that perspective, he reminds himself that in the overall scheme of things, this was a legitimate oversight. His wife has reminded him of that too, as have the few close friends in whom he has confided about this catastrophe.

So here he sits in his attorney's office, preparing a reply to the medical registration board's request for a response to Leslie Long's complaint. He has brought a sequential description of the medical facts, the necessary records, and his own draft of a letter. Levine assures him that he will look over the file and prepare an appropriate retort for submission to the board.

As the meeting comes to a close, Levine rises up and confidently puts out his hand to Tuckerman for a good-bye handshake. "Remember, Ted, you are a great doctor. When we are done with this, I am certain that you'll be looking here at little more than a blip in your career, not its demise. You hear me?"

Tuckerman, staring at the ground, nods glumly. "That was a pretty rough letter, Larry." He looks up at his attorney. "Yeah, Larry, I hear you."

Dr. Tuckerman's official reply to the board outlines his actions and justifications. It asserts that over the years he had seen her, Mrs. Brown had been given excellent care. It concludes that lung cancer, a devastating and swift disease, would have claimed her even if it had been detected somewhat earlier. He expresses his regard for Ms. Long's mother and his own sense of loss upon her death.

As he signs, seals, and sends off the letter, his fears grow. He has seen what had happened to friends. He knows that the competitive marketplace for doctors, being what it is, could turn this black mark on his record, as minor as it might be, into a fatal flaw.

It is now just a matter of waiting.

Engage in Reasonable Mischief

There are endless possibilities for making the other side uncomfortable. Cultivate fear by having others plant incendiary comments. Negate your opponents' actions by convincing others of the insignificance of what they are doing. Undermine them by appealing to superiors, subordinates, and colleagues. Foster the general impression that even associating with the other side casts someone in an unfavorable light. Surround them with tactics until they give in. If you must, undermine the very ground on which they stand.

Consider Threats; Duel If Necessary

The tactics discussed in this chapter are devious by their very nature. Your aim is to manipulate the professional and personal habitat in which your opponents function: all that surrounds them turns hostile. The advantage of this strategy is that it is not you who carries the smoking gun. Altering perceptions with reasonable mischief is a sublime way to force the issue. The general consensus turns against the other parties as their professional assets slip away.

At some point, however, these circuitous maneuvers may not be enough. You may have to mount your own scheme to destroy your opponents outright, by whatever means necessary.

The customary rules of warfare—whether for military or professional conflict and conduct—require fair warning before launching an attack. If the warning is taken seriously, you may be able to attain your objectives without engaging in the messy business of open conflict. In most cases you are better off if you can win without going to battle.

Make your threat known to the other side: explicitly outline the choices and consequences they face. There are three necessary ingredients for an effective threat. First, your opponents must be convinced that you have the will to go through with your scheme. If not, they will call your bluff, hoping to make you appear to be a wimp. Second, they must be convinced that you have the means to implement your plans. If not, they will allow you to attack, confident that they will defeat you in battle. And third, when they do not conform to your demands, you must carry through with your threat. If not, they may try to stall or deplete you into defeat.

A successful threat affords you a win without encumbering you with the costs, whether they be financial, the expenditure of time and effort, or the potential for public ridicule. A threat, when successful, is less dangerous than exposing yourself to the perils of battle. And if your threat does not succeed and you must proceed to a duel, do what you must to win.

What If You Can't Win?

There is a popular misconception that if you cannot score a win you are doomed to enduring a loss. Among those who hold this view, a lamentable lack of imagination presumes that the opposite of triumph is defeat. Is there another option?

Of course! If you absolutely cannot win at the game you are playing, change the game. There are a number of ways to do this. One method is to start playing football while your opponents are still playing baseball. If the fans in the stands show up to see football your opponents will look quite silly. Turn a losing budget battle into a race for public recognition—get your name and that of your program prominently featured in local media outlets—and deposit the accolades into the bank for later withdrawal. Do an absolutely positively great job at what you are doing, acquiring admirers and supporters as you excel above the seeming pettiness of others. Another method is simply to leave the field with your ball. If your opponents continue to compete even without the ball, they will appear to be motivated more by the fight than by the real issues at hand. If you are locked into a losing battle for control of your organization's overall operations, preserve your professional autonomy and demonstrate a greater interest in achievement than in domination. You can simply start playing on a different field altogether.

If your opponents seek your defeat within the organization, find a better job elsewhere and convey your talents and resources to a more hospitable arena. Your departure and subsequent accomplishments in that more attractive setting will offer those on the other side little more than a hollow win. After all, theirs is not much of a win if you elude the game and find more rewarding endeavors.

Finally, if there is no way to salvage the situation, know when to accept a loss and move on. There is no need to allow your opponents the vicious pleasure of watching you writhe in defeat.

A Clean Win

Just as there is a proper way to lose, there is a proper way to win. Earlier in this chapter, the notion of achieving a *clean win* was introduced. Many people are startled when their win reverses, turning into a loss. Their tactics and strategies may have won them the battle. However, in the long run the damage they have done to their reputation, their resources, and their own self-esteem makes them casualties of their own war.

The clean win is based on clean tactics and clean outcomes. It is a win that is fair, just, equitable, and honest. It is an outcome that mixes wisdom and compassion with triumph and good fortune. It is a victory that preserves ethical principles and virtue.

Certainly, there is a temptation to gloat over the loser. Just as you may have allowed yourself private fantasies in order to contain your urges to destroy the other parties, so too should you check any impulses to torment them after your win. Know when to let go. To attain your objectives, you need not annihilate your adversaries. You have outsmarted them—that is enough. If you instill in them the need for revenge or retribution, you will start a cycle that will condemn you to repeat positional battles when what you want is to move future interactions to the more positive realm of interest-based negotiation.

Mixed Models

In order to clarify the difference between them, this chapter has treated interest-based negotiation and positional negotiation as two distinct models. In reality, you are likely to combine and intersperse the two in your negotiations. For example, the tone of a discussion with representatives of another organization is likely to be collaborative for the most part. However, if you detect that they are playing games or being needlessly reticent, you might employ a few rounds of positional bargaining. In so doing you demonstrate your capability and willingness to play hardball when you must. Curiously enough, a temporary positional stance is sometimes the most potent way to persuade other negotiators to adopt or readopt an interest-based tone.

As you shape your mix of strategies, strive for a suitable fit. Connect persuasive strategies to the specific circumstances of your negotiation. Mold that pathway by clarifying your own objectives, understanding those of the other side, and recognizing the general context in which you are negotiating: assess your picture, the others' picture, and the big picture. The process itself is pliable. Each frame evolves as the negotiation unfolds. With each step and each shift, test the waters, guiding your statements and tactics to assess reactions and explore alternatives. Proceed in small steps. If something works, move with it. When you are tripped up, attend to the cues your opponents are sending out and readjust your tactics accordingly.

Just as a carpenter has a toolbox of proven implements for varied situations, a negotiator has a set of good options that can be exercised to drive the back-and-forth of the bargaining. As the old saying goes, if you only have a hammer, every problem looks like a nail. If, however, your negotiation toolbox boasts a variety of tools, you will be able to draw from that wide range of options and strategies. If you know how and when to use each one, you will be able to create the best fit between task and tactics. Use the right strategy at the right time and your negotiation will come together like a piece of fine furniture under the hands of an expert woodworker. Use that same strategy at the wrong time and the outcome may look more like an amateur shop project. Crafting the right fit requires insight, courage, and perseverance. You must be willing to take risks.

You should also be aware that you will sometimes make mistakes, and you must have the common sense to learn from them when you do. Your insights will derive not only from your professional experience. More important, you will gain immensely from your accrued wisdom and your willingness to learn from both failure and success.

Conclusion

In this book on interest-based negotiation, this chapter is an anomoly. It was a challenge to write. And for you, the reader, some of the passages likely evoked visceral reactions. Why did we include this perspective?

If you are to be an all-around, effective negotiator, it is vital that you know and understand positional negotiation: its design, methods, and consequences. First, you will be better able to spot when others are using it against you. This is particularly important when you work with those who talk interests and play positional.

Second, you will know when to use it and when not to—perhaps the most difficult choice to make in negotiations. It is the do-gooder impulse characteristic of many in health care that makes this choice so complex. Some advocates, self-righteous in their cause, are too swift to adopt positional negotiation. Their mission can then be lost in the fray of what they perceive as a battle; they create enemies and lose allies. Others are too reluctant to use positional strategies, eschewing these contemptible maneuvers that their goals demand. Their purpose ends up being sacrificed to their unwillingness to fight for it.

As a rule of thumb, deploy the techniques of interest-based negotiation three times. If, after the attempt, the other party remains a positional bargainer, then you should feel free to engage as one as well. Being an enlightened negotiator does not require that you sacrifice your interests solely in order to remain true to a negotiating model.

Finally, in reading this chapter you may have discovered parts of yourself that you in fact do not relish. Are there times when you are instinctively positional when a battle is not necessary? Are there times when you give up on what you know to be right because you cannot face a positional struggle? To enhance your negotiating effectiveness, you may want to transform both your style and your strategy. Knowing yourself, recognizing all your preferences and instincts, likeable or not, is step one in making that shift.

CHAPTER 9

MEDIATION, ARBITRATION, AND DISPUTE RESOLUTION

DISAGREEMENTS AND differences are common in the frenetic work of health care. Most disagreements are routinely resolved through direct negotiation: people talk through the issues and eventually reach a solution. Nonetheless, the disputes you most likely remember are those that were not so easily settled. These are the conflicts that painfully escalated so that others became involved in waging or resolving the disagreements: colleagues who took sides, supervisors who entered the fray, attorneys who were retained to represent the contenders. Once these others were recruited, the fighting surged to vicious, passionate, and vindictive battle. What are the options in such a situation?

Escalating conflict ignites a storehouse of weapons: engaging more senior colleagues or a union representative, starting litigation, adopting full-scale confrontation, and even using violence, to name but a few of the methods and consequences. Many such conflicts soar seemingly out of control as they become high-stakes contests. The parties become so distant and combative that their only signals to one another are bombshells: a subpoena, a defamatory article in the press, a devastating threat, a shattering blow to the other party's reputation. Fearing defeat, the parties take cues from one another: "Get them before they get you." Each new signal provokes a fresh assault, causing the conflict to surge into its next hostile offensive.

There are other choices. *Alternative dispute resolution*, or ADR, refers to a range of interventions intended to take the place of these impulses toward escalation. *Arbitration* and *mediation* are the most common forms of ADR. Their purpose is to interrupt the escalation by offering the parties a structured, monitored framework in which to air and possibly resolve their dispute.

ADR has roots in a number of arenas. Legal reformers, seeking alternatives to the long waits, high costs, and contentious framework of the judicial system, created the *multidoor courthouse*, which offers mediation and arbitration as alternatives to litigation (Goldberg, Green, & Sander, 1985). Labor organizers began using mediation years ago to resolve bitter labor disputes, and the federal government's mediation service is now regularly called on before and during strikes. Out of the 1960s' community justice movement have come neighborhood dispute-resolution centers, established to resolve tenant-landlord conflicts, fights between high school gangs, and disagreements over land use. Divorce mediation has become a popular avenue for settling potentially divisive family conflicts, and in the international arena, mediation and citizen diplomacy are used to ease tensions between nations (U.S. Department of State, Foreign Service Institute, 1987; Kelman, 1995).

ADR methods can be applied to health care conflict resolution in a number of ways (see Slaikeu, 1989; Dauer, 1993; Robson & Morrison, 2003; Szmania, Johnson, & Mulligan, 2008). ADR is employed to manage classic legal disputes, including malpractice and employment cases, complex organizational and professional problems, patient care–related issues, and family relations conflicts. A growing number of managed care organizations and hospitals, looking to avoid litigation, require patients to sign agreements specifying that disputes arising in the course of their treatment will be handled through ADR. Similar provisions are being incorporated into staff contracts and interorganizational agreements. In Massachusetts the state medical board for some time operated a voluntary mediation program to provide patients who filed a complaint against a physician with the opportunity to seek resolution through mediation. At the Montefiore Medical Center in New York, a mediation model has been developed and tested for its effectiveness in resolving bioethical disputes (Dubler & Marcus, 1994). This and similar models are being incorporated nationwide to resolve complex patient care disputes. In Washington, D.C., the American Bar Association has developed a program to build mediation into nursing home dispute resolution.

What is the value in making a dispute resolution alternative available, especially in the high-stakes and emotionally charged arena of health care? What are the options for interrupting the escalation and resolving the dispute before it spirals further into mutually destructive conflict? How do you encourage the disputants to begin talking?

Guiding the Parties to the Table

Parties involved in an adversarial, high-stakes dispute often become focused on one objective: victory over their contenders. Whether it is a malpractice issue, a conflict between departments in a medical center, or an internal staff dispute in a health clinic, each side sets its objectives and gauges its progress in achieving defeat of the other side. Conflict can become a matter of obsession as time, costs, and distractions accumulate for each side.

The burden of conflict affects more than just the primary parties to the dispute. In a nursing strike for example, the pressures are borne not only by the nurses themselves. The conflict also affects secondary parties—those people left behind to do the work that must still be accomplished. The conflict's effects are also endured by the tertiary parties: the underserviced patients and the members of the general community who wonder if hospital care will be available should they be in need.

What pressures could shift the attention of battling parties toward a possible settlement? At times such pressures may come from secondary and tertiary players who encourage or persuade the opposing sides to talk. A weary hospital staff member approaches the picket line and compassionately describes the dire consequences of the strike for the patients, questioning whether the job action is worth the real human cost. The media rebuke the hospital's leaders for imposing the working conditions that led to the strike, admonishing them for neglecting their public responsibility and for placing the community at risk. Hospital trustees question the CEO just as nurses on the picket line confront their union representatives, each imploring the frontline negotiators to engage in earnest.

Similarly, a supervisor, judge, colleague, or spouse might spark the impetus to settle. Such pleas represent a wake-up call, a perspective from someone who is less invested emotionally in the fight and who can therefore see its boundless costs and its finite benefits. In a high-intensity dispute, only rarely do the parties reach this realization on their own. There is a reluctance to acknowledge the desire to settle, as it creates the appearance of capitulation or might be interpreted as a sign of waning energy and therefore a signal of vulnerability. By contrast, if the inducement comes from an outside source, a third party such as a mutual friend or an impartial authority, the disputants are relieved of the illusion of surrender. In the process of being eased to the negotiation table, each side, either implicitly or explicitly, begins to reconsider its objectives and tactics.

This bystander to the dispute must be able to win the confidence of both sides in order to ease them, one step at a time, from battle toward conciliation. Without this attention, one inflammatory remark by either side can propel both back into their hostilities.

Talking is a tenuous process. It is fraught with danger: you could say too much; you could give the wrong impression; the other side could pummel you when you are vulnerable; your regrets about the meeting could overwhelm you; you could be provoked into lashing out, verbally or physically, toward the other side. An outsider can help keep these passions in check and retain the disputants' willingness to talk.

In the process of allowing themselves to be eased to the negotiation table, the parties to the conflict begin to reconsider their objectives and tactics. The turning point emerges when those involved, separately though somewhat simultaneously, realistically assess the costs, risks, and potential benefits associated with their shared dispute. It is a sobering moment. It has built within it some mix of humiliation, defeat, fear, bravado, and vulnerability. The mounting downsides of the dispute are no longer tolerable and the drive to escalate evaporates. The delusion of reaping substantial benefits wanes as the realization of the dispute's real costs looms. It is time to roll back the cannons. It is time to talk. How can this negotiation be initiated?

The acknowledgment of a willingness to talk is a subtle though important signal. There are some who resist the shift: they regard talking as a mark of weakness. It is and it is not. The distinction is important. It certainly is a suspension of the escalation. It surely need not be a surrender of the concerns, principles, or objectives that carried the parties into conflict. After all, resolution emerges only if a way can be found to honor and reasonably satisfy those considerations. Talking through the issues can offer a form of persuasion different from fighting. Guiding the disputants through this distinction is crucial. The suspension of hostilities is not capitulation. The willingness to talk simply opens a new option for engaging the conflict.

For some it is hard to accept negotiation. In their minds intimidation is the only firm form of persuasion. It is what they understand and what they know to do. Their worldview is one of winners and losers. They "win" only by fighting hard and significantly harming or destroying the other side. They believe the adversarial method is the best, if not the only, means to reap true justice. Life, like health care, is, however, not a game of football. Barreling toward a single all-important objective and pummeling others along the way does not enhance necessary collaboration. Even members of one's own team may be aghast at such offensive maneuvers. Those who are adversarial by nature must be convinced that resolution usually emerges from a balance between the sides. A third-party neutral or trusted bystander can help opposing parties to accomplish this transformation, legitimizing an alternative that is better than continuing the fight.

Whether the negotiation is voluntary or mandatory (such as when the parties are contractually bound to first use ADR or are ordered by a judge to an ADR procedure), the decision to attempt the use of arbitration or mediation does not foretell the settlement itself. It simply demonstrates a willingness to explore the options. ADR reveals the prospect that pursuit of resolution does not have to be a destructive contest. It exposes the high financial and social costs of the adversarial method. It reframes the dispute and offers a process for bringing it to conclusion.

Getting the parties to engage one another at the negotiation table is a major hurdle. Beyond that, getting them to settle presents another set of issues. The purpose of this chapter is to introduce you briefly to alternative dispute resolution methods. The focus is on mediation, because mediation will be most immediately useful to you in resolving the everyday issues that you find in your workplace. Because the intent of mediation is, in part, to bring interest-based negotiation to the fore, the methods discussed here are also instructive for your own general negotiation and dispute resolution endeavors.

Defining Negotiation, Arbitration, and Mediation

Alternative dispute resolution entails the use of an impartial person whose purpose is to help the disputants reach a resolution (see Crowley, 1994; Singer, 1994). By definition this neutral third party has no direct stake in the substantive outcome of the settlement. The impartial person's prime focus is in guiding the parties through a series of steps from conflict to resolution. His or her detachment and lack of bias reduces the disputants' suspicions and helps these parties to invest the necessary trust and confidence in the process. The task of the neutral person involves establishing that confidence, forming an understanding of the issues, and then forging a strategy and path for resolving the dispute.

The most important distinction to be made among negotiation, arbitration, and mediation concerns partisanship. As a negotiator, you are naturally partisan. You advocate your own interests or those of your constituency. Because you have a stake in the outcome, it is presumed that you are biased on your own behalf. You are predisposed to assess the scenario through a subjective lens, as are the other negotiators, and you are naturally partial to solutions that are in your favor. Even as you ponder and acknowledge the issues from other perspectives, you are predisposed to meeting your own objectives.

Conversely, in arbitration and mediation, a neutral third party is introduced into a dispute precisely for his or her lack of partisanship. When the parties are locked in conflict, the neutral party is able to offer an objective analysis of the issues, a new set of eyes for considering options, and a process for resolution that disputants view as just and balanced. ADR methods work best when the parties desire settlement and when they believe the neutral person to be honorable and objective in handling the dispute. That confidence is fundamental to approval of both the steps along the way and the outcome derived from them.

Yet partisanship also distinguishes arbitration and mediation. As just described, the negotiator begins as a partisan and remains a partisan throughout. The *arbitrator* begins a case as a nonpartisan. However, as the role of the arbitrator is to recommend or determine a settlement, the arbitrator eventually reaches a decision in favor of one side or the other, assuming a partisan tone in the process. The *mediator*, in a very important distinction, begins as a nonpartisan and remains so throughout.

Arbitration is often viewed as a better option than litigation; the latter is governed by the rules and lengthy processes of the courts, which are also public and which at times operate on the unpredictable whims of a judge. In arbitration, the parties advocate their positions to the arbitrator, each hoping that issues in the case will be judged in his or her favor. After hearing the arguments of the disputants, the arbitrator issues a determination. When the parties choose binding arbitration, they are contractually obligated to abide by the ruling. If they violate the terms of the settlement, they face the consequences delineated beforehand in the arbitration contract. In nonbinding arbitration the arbitrator's ruling is offered only as an opinion. It remains for the parties to negotiate a mutually acceptable settlement, using the arbitrator's opinion as a benchmark. The advantage of binding over nonbinding arbitration is that the case usually ends with the ruling, thus limiting the expense and time invested in the dispute. The disadvantage is that the parties lose control of the outcome and the possibility of negotiating with others at the table.

Many workplace grievance procedures and patient coverage disputes contractually mandate the use of arbitration in the event of a dispute, in order to significantly reduce the use of expensive litigation. A grievance is submitted by an employee and appraised through a hearing process. An individual reviewer or a representative panel hears the case and issues a decision. Depending on the grievance procedures in place, that determination may be final or it may be open to appeal if it meets specified criteria.

In mediation a neutral third party helps disputants find and agree to an acceptable resolution of their conflict by way of a private and confidential process. A mediator does not issue a ruling. The purpose of mediation is to guide the parties step by step through a process for reaching a settlement (Folberg & Taylor, 1984). The mediator does not act as a judge and has no power to impose an outcome upon the parties. Rather, the mediator facilitates the conversation between the parties, helping them to better understand their options, the choices, and the consequences of each. The mediator is a catalyst for settlement, not an advocate for one party over another. The outcome of mediation is determined by the parties: they each have the authority to reject or accept the offers presented to them.

Disputants choose arbitration over litigation when they want to settle their dispute without the complications of a courtroom battle. They confer to the arbitrator control of both process and outcome. Disputants choose mediation over arbitration when they want to maintain greater control over the settlement itself. They confer to the mediator control of the process, and they maintain control of the outcome. Disputants choose negotiation over mediation when they want to settle on their own, without an outside intervener. They control both process and outcome.

Using Mediation to Resolve Health Care Disputes

This chapter highlights mediation. (For further discussions of mediation methods and practices, see, for example, Moore, 1986; Laue, 1987; Kressel, Pruitt, & Associates, 1989; Folger & Bush, 1994.) This process offers a readily adaptable and constructive framework for resolving health care disputes. Its methods can be adjusted to facilitate the complex process of convening key stakeholders in a meaningful, defined, and pragmatic manner. Because control of the outcome itself remains with the parties to the dispute, the process attends to their varying roles, stakes, interests, authority, purposes, and expectations in reaching a mutually acceptable outcome. Given the need to balance these many considerations, the flexibility and inclusiveness of mediation is critical to its success.

Dispute resolution is in fact a routine aspect of health care work. On a regular basis, health care professionals facilitate agreement among a complex web of issues and people. In most cases this reconciliation is accomplished without particular attention to the process by which it is performed. The mediation framework offers a set of systematic methods for assessing and settling existing and anticipated conflicts. Mediation can be incorporated into a health care organization's processes so that it is easily accessible—as part of a broadly available internal dispute resolution system—offering parties a safe meeting ground for fairly discussing and resolving their differences.

Mediation is most advantageous when applied in a manner that conforms to the nature of the dispute, the proclivities of the people, and the conditions that frame the range of possible solutions. Two forms of mediation—with different frames of reference—apply to health care situations: formal and informal mediation.

In the process of *formal mediation*, the impartial facilitator is explicit about the parties' being brought together for the purpose of mediation. The neutral facilitator is an outsider and is recognized by all parties as an acceptable mediator for the case. He or she establishes the process at the outset, describing the roles, rules, and steps necessary to find settlement. The parties acknowledge their involvement in a mediated dispute-resolution process. Going through this civil set of procedures is particularly helpful when the dispute has reached the stage of inflamed emotions and adversarial interactions. The structure itself calms tensions and creates a venue for constructive negotiation.

Familiarity with the professional context of the dispute, be it a commercial, environmental, or health care disagreement, can be an advantage for the mediator, though it is not an absolute requirement and may sometimes even be an obstacle. A fundamental familiarity with the subject matter allows the mediator to legitimately and knowledgeably ask appropriate questions of the parties, focus attention on the primary issues, and adeptly advance the parties to a feasible resolution. Nonpartisan health care professionals, for example, can successfully serve as mediators as long as they are perceived as neutral and behave as such. That perception is critical to the effectiveness of the process. For example, in patient-physician disputes, a physician as mediator or co-mediator is a boon to understanding issues, involving the parties, and forging resolution. At the same time, a patient might feel that the presence of a physician as mediator tilts the process in favor of the doctor. In this scenario a health care manager, a lawyer who specializes in medical cases, or a nurse may be more agreeable to both parties.

How can you secure an outside mediator to help battling parties to resolve a dispute? The Internet is of course a useful source for scanning the field. Mediation and arbitration services and solo practitioners, some specializing in health care, can be found across the country. In addition, courts offer ADR programs as do law firms. Federal agencies can provide mediators to help resolve major labor disputes. You should confirm the credentials of the proposed mediator. Among the more important criteria for recruiting a mediator are the acceptability, neutrality, and legitimacy of his or her impartiality to each of the disputants.

Disputes most likely to call upon formal mediation are those in which there is a clear and tangible cost to nonresolution, such as when the anticipated extravagant expenses of a protracted legal dispute propel the parties to a more low-cost, private process. These may include malpractice disputes, conflicts over physicians' hospital privileges labor disputes, or disputes over institutional jurisdiction, to name a few.

By contrast, *informal mediation* incorporates the methods of formal mediation without the formal structure, applying these methods liberally to meet the particular circumstances of the dispute at hand. Formal mediation is a structured process, with clearly defined roles and expectations. The mediator sets and maintains this framework, directing the parties from exploration of the issues to option building and settlement. For example, during formal mediation, the mediator opens the session with an introduction that explains the process, the voluntary nature of the parties' involvement, and the meaning of his or her neutral role. However, in the circumstances typically encountered by a bioethicist for example, a formal discourse about mediation will likely be seen as irrelevant, given the highly charged emotional questions facing those involved. An ethicist entering an intensive care unit to help resolve a disagreement about a do not resuscitate order had best not lecture the parties about the methods and processes of mediation. Instead, he can use the formal framework as a guide as he adapts the process to the circumstances of the dispute. Thus informal mediation is particularly useful for resolving immediate, in-house issues as they arise in a health care organization. Bioethical conflicts, staff disagreements, interprofessional disputes, policy issues, and matters that arise between family members, patients, and staff are typical of the day-to-day disputes that can benefit from the flexible application of mediation methods.

There are legitimate problems and pitfalls in the use of informal mediation and if they become an obstacle to resolution, they must be dealt with. Foremost is the problem of neutrality. When issues that lend themselves to informal mediation arise, usually no one has the time, resources, or willingness to call upon an outside neutral party to intervene in the case. In these instances an individual with the training and recognition to mediate from within can be an invaluable resource for the institution and those associated with it. However, in certain situations a mediator employed by an institution will not pass the test of pure neutrality. For example, she might be asked to mediate a dispute between a patient's family and the hospital regarding the patient's discharge to a nursing home when the family objects and the hospital is pressing the action to relieve itself of a costly financial burden. It would be disingenuous for her to present herself as impartial if her boss dispatches her to the assignment with the proviso, "And just make sure the patient is out of here pronto when you're done!" She can help resolve the problem using her mediation skills, *and* she is not a neutral in this case, especially if she wants to keep her job.

Loyalties and preconceived notions may also complicate the practice of informal mediation. If you are asked to informally mediate a dispute between a nurse supervisor and a physician on a medical floor, you may be too familiar with and affected by that physician's boisterous behavior to enter the fray unbiased. Similarly, the disputants may know too much about you to trust your objectivity. If your reputation is one of favoring one side or the other, or if your allegiance to the agenda of your boss is mistrusted, your influence as an informal mediator may be compromised.

In spite of these problems with informal mediation, it does offer a practical and systematic avenue for resolving the myriad disputes common to health care organizations. However, the best way to describe and understand the mediation process itself is from the perspective of its more formal practice. Following is an illustration of mediation as a formal process, with recommendations for adapting the process to the realities of health care decision making.

The Long-Tuckerman case is reviewed by the state medical board. A staff member investigates the complaint, looking into the care given to Mrs. Brown and Dr. Tuckerman's overall medical record. Although it is felt that the doctor had made a miscalculation in this case, the board decides not to take disciplinary action against him. Such action could have included temporary suspension or full confiscation of his license to practice medicine. The board generally restricts such unilateral action to more serious cases, of which there are a significant number in the state. This case does not meet the criteria for such action, especially in light of the physician's general record.

Nonetheless, the board does not want to fully dismiss the case. It decides to refer the parties to the board's voluntary mediation program. The chief investigative officer for the case calls both Leslie Long and Ted Tuckerman to describe the program and to inquire about their interest in meeting to see if a resolution might be possible. The investigator explains that if a mutually agreeable solution can be reached, then, with the consent of both parties, the case can be removed from the board's public files. The board will keep a record that the case has been settled. If the case is not settled, it will remain an open case on file with the board. This system offers some leverage to the complainant, to better level the negotiation table and offers an incentive to the physician to participate and be amenable to settlement. If the complainant's demands are unreasonable, the physician is under no obligation to accept them.

Long and Tuckerman both agree to meet with a mediator. Tuckerman asks about bringing his attorney. The board staff member he talks to says he may do so if he insists. She recommends against it, however, as the presence of an attorney tends to make a discussion slightly more adversarial than it would be if only the disputants themselves were present. Tuckerman discusses the question with his attorney, who recommends that he give mediation a try without the presence of counsel.

The case is referred to a local mediation agency with a state contract to provide the service. The agency's independence from the state medical board enhances the neutrality and confidentiality of the process. The agency is able to schedule the mediation without a long delay.

On the day of mediation, Bob Bennett, an experienced mediator with the agency, welcomes Long and Tuckerman into the mediation room. He introduces himself and takes his place at one end of the conference table. Long and Tuckerman sit on either side, facing one another.

"First, I want to thank you each for coming here to discuss the complaint brought through the board of medical registration," Bennett begins. "I have spoken with each of you about the issue and explained that, unlike litigation or arbitration, in which a judge, jury, or arbitrator decides the outcome of a dispute, in mediation the development and acceptance of the settlement is up to you. We will explore the issues together, considering the options for reaching a resolution you both can accept. Then *you* decide whether you are going to accept the outcome. That outcome is not imposed upon you. You create it, and you decide whether to accept it."

"Your presence here acknowledges that you are open to using mediation to explore the possibility of coming to some sort of settlement," Bennett continues.

Long and Tuckerman nod their assent.

"That of course does not mean that you will each get everything you want," Bennett continues, with a gentle smile. "If the settlement is one that both parties can accept, it usually means that there has been a good deal of listening and understanding, along with some give-and-take in order to reach agreement. That is, the settlement has to be acceptable to you as well as to the person sitting across the table."

He explains that the role of the mediator is to help them move through the steps of listening, understanding, developing options, and coming to an agreement. He clarifies that his role is not to tell them how to settle their differences.

"At times, I will help you better understand your choices," he says. "The acceptance of the choices and the consequences, though, is totally up to you. I am not here as a judge: creating and accepting the settlement is your task."

He assures them that each will get a chance to tell his or her story and air his or her feelings about what happened. He outlines some of the other ground rules. At times they will meet together in this room; at other times he may need to speak privately with one or both of them. Then the other person will wait in the adjoining room. It is perfectly acceptable to share confidences with the mediator. They are both here on a voluntary basis, and either of them can call off the talks if not satisfied with the progress. If they are satisfied with the results of this mediation, the process will conclude with the preparation of a written agreement that responds to the needs and interests of both parties.

"As I mentioned on the phone, the process itself is confidential," Bennett counsels. "Obviously, the three of us sitting here are not in the public glare of a courtroom. We are also not operating under the direct rubric of the board. I am obligated only to report back whether or not we reached settlement: yes or no. I must also remind you that under the laws of this state, whatever is said here cannot be entered into a courtroom hearing. As a mediator, I cannot be called into court to testify should this conflict get to that point. These protections have been enacted in the hope that they will encourage people to resolve their disputes honestly and directly with one another, well before they get to the courtroom. Therefore, I hope you will each use this opportunity to genuinely express what is on your mind, to hear what the other person is saying, and to sincerely explore this opportunity for settlement. One last but important ground rule: I ask that one person speak at a time. It is vital that we hear and heed what is being said. Are there any questions?"

Both Long and Tuckerman shake their heads.

Bennett says, "Oh, I have one. Do you prefer first or last names?" He hopes they will be comfortable with the greater informality of first names. He looks to Long, who says, "Leslie is fine with me." Tuckerman too agrees to be called Ted.

"Fine," Bennett says. "First, I would like some background. Leslie, you initiated the complaint. Could you please tell me what led to the filing?"

Leslie Long relates her story, her voice full of emotion. Her emphasis is not on the medical facts, though she makes reference to the fact that Tuckerman missed the beginnings of the cancer. She speaks more of what her mother meant to her. The implication is that Tuckerman is guilty of killing her mother. Bennett listens carefully, nodding to indicate his active concern for Long and periodically looking over to Tuckerman to assess his reaction.

When she finishes, Bennett synthesizes her comments: "Leslie, if I understand what you are saying, you feel that Ted missed some important diagnostic indicators that, had they been found earlier, could have saved your mother's life. Is that correct?"

"Yes, that captures how I feel."

Bennett next turns to Tuckerman. "Ted, tell me your view of what happened."

Tuckerman speaks directly to Long. "Leslie, first I want you to know how much I cared for your mother. I also want you to know that I too felt a sense of loss at her passing. As I'm sure you know, I was her physician for ten years. Not a holiday passed without her bringing in a poppy seed cake."

Long turns to the mediator to explain. "Mom made the best poppy seed cake in the world."

Tuckerman continues, "Now, when you're a doctor you have to make a lot of tough judgment calls. I don't think I would be telling you anything new to say that your mom was very concerned about her health."

There is a moment of silence. Finally, Long speaks. "Actually, Dr. Tuckerman, you're being kind with that. Mom was obsessed with her health. Whenever she had a visit with you, she would call me up to tell me every gory detail: the pills, the aches, the pains, the tests. There were times, love her, that I felt like putting down the phone and then coming back twenty minutes later when she was done. She was a little bit of the martyr in that way."

Tuckerman listens intently and then continues. "Well, I won't disagree with you on that. Now, as a physician, I am sometimes in a tight situation. I have to weigh very carefully the tests I order for each patient. I always want to be as careful as possible on the one hand. On the other hand there is a lot of pressure to be prudent about health costs and tests can carry risks of their own. That is what I have to balance. Since you didn't put down the telephone when your Mom called, you know that she got a lot of attention and a lot of tests and whatever medications we thought could cure her, whatever the ailment."

"I'm not saying, Dr. Tuckerman, that you didn't give her good care for all those years. All I'm saying is that in the crunch, when it really counted, you weren't there. You didn't come through, and it killed Mom," Long's voice cracks slightly as she holds back tears.

Bennett watches Tuckerman tense up. He decides to cool down the situation and turns to Long. "Leslie, to say to a doctor that he killed his patient is a pretty hard accusation. Are you sure that is what you mean?"

"She's dead, isn't she?" Her voice is strident. "And Dr. Tuckerman was her doctor, wasn't he? What do you call it?"

Bennett looks at Tuckerman. "Ted, I'm not an expert on cancer, though I know a bit from personal experience about lung cancer. Could you explain the disease to us?" Bennett is hoping that the pointed question will help refocus Tuckerman and get him out of the basement. The mediator can see that the physician is seething from the implication that he had somehow murdered his patient.

Tuckerman takes a deep breath. "Lung cancer is in fact an insidious disease. In some forms it comes on very quickly, and it is deadly. Even though there has been tremendous progress in recent years with many patients responding well to treatment, it is still a very difficult form of cancer to treat. Your mother had a particularly bad case. Even if we had caught it slightly earlier, it is unlikely that the outcome would have varied by much. She had been exposed to a lot of secondary smoke, even though she wasn't a smoker herself. The problem was that the symptoms that would have alerted us to the lung cancer in some ways were masquerading as a common cold. Those colds were a pretty usual winter occurrence for your mom."

Bennett allows Tuckerman's comment to sink in for a few moments. He watches Long carefully. "What do Ted's comments mean for you, Leslie?"

Long folds a tissue in her hands. "I don't know. Given her age and that she had lung cancer, I guess it was inevitable that she was going to die eventually. I just can't buy that Dr. Tuckerman, I mean Ted, wasn't negligent for not being more careful about checking for it."

Bennett sees that once again Tuckerman looks as if he is about to explode. "I think this would be a good time for a private session," Bennett says. "I would like to speak to each of you privately. Ted, I would like to start with you. Leslie, could you go out to the waiting room for a few minutes?" Long agrees and leaves the room.

Once the door is closed, Tuckerman stands up and lets loose. "Look, Bob, you're a real nice guy and all, but this simply is not going to work. She has it stuck in her mind that I killed her mom, and no amount of gibberish is going to change that." He chops the air with his open hand to emphasize his points. "You're siding with her by legitimizing all this bullshit she's throwing on the table."

Bennett motions for Tuckerman to sit down again and the doctor slides back into his chair. The mediator leans forward to pull the doctor into engagement. He speaks calmly. "Ted, I can understand why you are frustrated. She seems to be contradicting herself. On one hand she agrees that her mother was obsessed with anxiety about her health. That admission was an important insight for her about you as her mother's physician. I also get the sense that something else might be going on with her. Any clues as to what that might be?"

"No clues. I'm not a mind reader." Tuckerman is fuming.

"She is grieving the loss of her mother, and she wants to blame it on someone," Bennett says. "You, Ted, are a safe pick. She is having a hard time accepting the loss, and she is putting all that energy into blaming you. Your statement that you too felt a sense of loss was heartfelt, and I could see that she heard you. She is going through a change, from seeing you as a murderer to someone who cared for and cared about her mother. That shift is not going to happen instantaneously. You might have to be a bit patient with her."

"It's hard being patient with someone who is so stubborn—and accusatory," Tuckerman says sharply.

"I understand. What's your choice?"

"You said it yourself, Bob. I can walk out of here whenever I want."

"What good would that do you at this point?" Bennett asks. "Wouldn't it just reinforce her impression of you?"

"Yeah, it probably would," the doctor replies.

Bennett stays with Tuckerman until he is calmer. Then he sends Tuckerman out to the waiting room and asks Long into the meeting room for her private session.

"Leslie, what are you feeling about where we are so far?" Bennett asks once she is settled in her place. It is obvious that she has been crying.

"I don't think Dr. Tuckerman gets it. He doesn't understand what I am feeling."

Bennett isn't sure that Long herself fully knows what she is feeling. "Leslie, what are you hoping to get out of this?"

"I went to a lawyer about this whole thing," Long replies. "He said maybe we could get some money for this. Insurance companies like to settle sometimes. But it wouldn't be for big bucks, nothing in the millions, because Mom was old and the medical facts weren't big-time wrong. Anyway, after I was done talking with the lawyer I realized that money is not what I am after. I want something more."

"What does 'more' mean to you?"

"I want to make sure this doesn't happen to anybody else," she says with conviction. "That's the main thing. That's why I made the formal complaint. So that he won't do this to somebody else."

"What could satisfy that?" Bennett asks.

"I heard that sometimes in these settlements, the doctor agrees to go to a medical education class about the subject. At least if he learned more about the warning signs for lung cancer, then he would know what to look for."

"That does not sound unreasonable to me," Bennett says.

"And one more thing, he should have to make a contribution to the American Cancer Society. That also will help make sure this is not repeated."

"And those two things would satisfy you?"

"Just one more thing," she says. "I need to know that he really is sorry. What happened will hurt us forever. I need to know that he understands that."

"When we come back together, may I present those three items to him?"

"Yes, I would like you to do that." Long is more composed than when she entered. Bennett feels that he has a good understanding of what will constitute an acceptable understanding for her.

Bennett brings Tuckerman back to the room and reopens the face-to-face dialogue. "My private sessions with both of you were very helpful. I have a better understanding now of what is going on for each of you, and thanks to your comments, there are some ideas for possible settlement."

"Ted, Leslie has mentioned three things that would make it easier for her to settle. The most important thing is assurance that this will not happen to another patient and family. She wants to know if you would be willing to take a medical education course on lung cancer?"

Tuckerman's defensiveness begins to relax. "No doctor can guarantee that every early cancer will be caught—even with all of the available tests. But I too want to make as certain as possible that this doesn't happen to another patient. I have to take medical education courses often, and if it will help settle this matter, I am happy to make one of them a course on the topic of lung cancer."

Bennett is encouraged and hopes that the next concession will come as easily. "The second is a little tougher," he says. "Leslie would like to see you make a contribution to the American Cancer Society. There is something significant about this request. The family members are not interested in getting any financial gain for themselves from what happened. They sincerely are more interested in making sure this does not occur for others."

"What level of a contribution are you talking about?" Tuckerman asks.

Long's reply is quick. "Three thousand dollars."

"Three thousand dollars? That's a lot of money," Tuckerman counters.

Bennett puts up both hands as if to call a time out. "Let's slow down for a moment. Can we first talk about the concept before we get to an exact dollar amount? Ted, in concept would you be willing to make a contribution?"

"Sure, in concept that would be fine. It just depends on how much."

"What would you propose?" Bennett asked.

"I think that one thousand dollars would be a fair amount."

Bennett turns to Long. "What do you think?"

"How about we split the difference?" she says. "Two thousand. It's a good cause."

Tuckerman sighs with resignation. "OK, if that's what it'll take to settle this thing, I'll make a two thousand dollar contribution."

"Finally," Bennett continues, "Leslie wants an apology."

Tuckerman looks directly at Long. "That's easy. Leslie, I don't know if you can imagine how hard it is for a doctor to lose a patient. I felt a tremendous sense of loss when your mother passed away. It's hard to accept this, but lung cancer is a terrible disease. There is a limit to what we doctors can do, and that is frustrating as hell for us. I wish I had caught your mother's condition earlier. Maybe if there had been a better prognosis she would have been more willing to try treatment. I was surprised and frustrated that she didn't want to attempt chemotherapy. It was her decision though, and we all had to respect it. Yes, Leslie, I feel terrible about what happened. I lost my father to cancer, so I have some feeling for how devastating it can be. I truly am sorry."

Bennett sees that Long is comforted by Tuckerman's sincerity. She waits a moment and says, "That helps. That helps a lot. I'm sorry about your father. I didn't know that he died of cancer."

Bennett has a sense of what Tuckerman is thinking. Bennett wants to raise it before Tuckerman fumbles over how to put it on the table.

"Leslie, given what Ted has agreed to and said, are you willing to settle and allow the complaint to be removed from the board's public files?"

Long hesitates and in that brief time Tuckerman again begins to escalate into angry frustration. He has a sudden impulse to push away from the table and run for the door. Who is she to determine such an important question for his medical career? Why is she hesitating? He's agreed to everything she asked for. The anxiety is driving him crazy. Bennett, seeing Tuckerman from the corner of his eye, senses his frustration.

"Leslie?" Bennett prods gently.

Long looks up from the table. "Yes, I'm satisfied. The case can be removed from the board's public files."

Tuckerman is overwhelmed with relief. He looks at Bennett and then to Long. "I'm glad we were able to settle this."

Bennett summarizes what they have agreed to, jots down the points, and has each sign the draft document. Later, the settlement is reported back to the board of medical registration. A letter of acknowledgment for the donation is sent by the charity to both Long and Tuckerman. Tuckerman takes the course on lung cancer within three months of the mediation, and then the case is removed from the board's public files.

The Mediator's Role

Fundamental to the process of mediation is the impartiality and perceived neutrality of the mediator (Moore, 1986). *Impartiality* refers to the mediator's thinking and attitude. *Neutrality* defines the relationship and interactions between the mediator and the disputants: the mediator is neutral when he or she is so perceived by the disputants. What is the significance of neutrality for the success of a mediation?

The mediator serves as a fulcrum, helping to balance, connect, and resolve differences between the disputants. By not leaning to one side or the other, the mediator establishes the importance of finding a settlement that fairly accounts for the legitimate needs and interests of all sides. If a proposed settlement unfairly favors one party, it will likely be rejected by the other. Because agreement itself is voluntary, such a rejection represents a breakdown of the mediation process. The mediator personifies the common ground toward which the parties are encouraged to advance.

The generative value of mediation is in the discovery of formerly obscured solutions that simultaneously satisfy the interests of both sides. As the parties develop trust in the evenhandedness and neutrality of the mediator, they are more likely to reveal their underlying concerns, and as they do so the mediator helps them derive and combine workable solutions. Finding those options and gaining that consensus is the key to encouraging the parties toward a settlement.

Of course maintaining an impartial perspective and perceived neutrality is a monumental challenge. At times the mediator does form an opinion about the people or issues involved in a case. However, if the mediation process is to succeed, the mediator must not reveal those biases in what is said or done during the mediation process. To undermine that nonpartisanship would be to damage the very legitimacy of the method. The ultimate test of neutrality, however, does not lie simply with what the mediator says or does. Rather, the most significant measures of neutrality are the perceptions and beliefs held by the parties.

How do their perceptions of neutrality affect the disputants? Parties involved in a dispute often fear that outsiders will align with their opponents, thereby weakening their own position. Similarly, a party's position is bolstered by the outsiders who endorse it: contenders crave allies. In a highly polarized dispute the mediator represents a unique value-added dimension of the process. It is the responsibility of the mediator to ensure that attempts by the opposing sides to gain favor with the mediator are not successful. If the mediator were to take sides, the parties would reinforce their positions, thereby reducing their willingness to offer concessions. The fairness of the process is not upheld when the mediator is biased.

The mediator's impartiality offers a unique perspective on the dispute. (For a useful discussion of perspective in the negotiation process, see Ury, 1991.) Invariably, by the time the parties call upon a neutral person for help in settling their differences, the conflict has become obstinately polarized. The mediator is able to offer a fresh perspective: a new set of questions to reframe the parties' differences, an opportunity to reflect on real choices and consequences, and new options that the parties have not previously considered. The mediator moves each party away from the conviction, or perhaps even obsession, that theirs is the correct resolution. In its place, the mediator offers original thinking and new options for considering the dispute. There is less emphasis on whether each perspective is right or wrong. Rather, the mediator opens alternative angles on the problems in order to generate multiple options and opportunities for resolution.

In mediation the parties craft the settlement with the help of the mediator. Their participation in the process is voluntary, as is their acceptance of the settlement. To maximize the chances of reaching resolution, the agreement must be mutually beneficial, producing a *gain-gain* outcome. In such a scenario the parties recognize that they achieve more by accepting the agreement than by continuing the dispute.

The Mediation Process

The word *process*, an overused word at times, is often applied in reference to mediation, negotiation, arbitration, and communication. In this instance, however, it is apt, and a mediation may have a good process, a bad process, an ironic process, no process, or periodically, far too much process. What is process?

If substance is the ends, then process is the means. It is not the decision; it is how the decision is reached. At times, process is formalized into an established sequence of steps, clear roles, definitive authority, and specific criteria for reaching decisions. The parties follow a predetermined sequence and script. This formal process typifies the bureaucratic steps of governmental and legal decision making. At other times, the assumed steps, roles, authority, or criteria do not work, or there is no foreordained method for reaching a decision, or the parties do not accept their part in the script. In these cases an alternative process must be developed and accepted if the parties are to reach their objectives.

A good process is not defined by a set formula. The most appropriate vehicle delivers parties efficiently and effectively to a mutually acceptable agreement. The right people are involved in the decision, the criteria are fair and sensible, the information used is valid and objective, and the outcome is reasonable and legitimate. Sometimes the process is established beforehand. Sometimes it evolves naturally between the parties. The key is whether it capably prompts decisions, actions, and outcomes.

A bad process excludes people who feel they should be a part of the decision, does not use objective information or criteria when they are available, or reaches an outcome that is infeasible or unlawful. A bad process is inefficient: it keeps people talking without advancing them toward a destination. The greatest process conflicts are between people who appreciate the conversation as an end in and of itself and those who see the talking as only a means to a tangible result. Conflicts on process also emerge between those who find the process of no value and want to dictate a solution and those who are thereby excluded from contributing to the ultimate decision.

An ironic process is that unfortunate predicament in which the parties actually agree on most substantive points and yet are unable to transcend their own obstinacy. An absence of process hides the presence of concurrence. Even when the parties agree on specific points, their polarization has them repudiating statements that ultimately are reasonable. Paradoxically, they are simply unable to get themselves unstuck. The 2010 health care reform debate in Congress was such a situation. There were many points of agreement between Democrats and Republicans yet it became impossible for either to agree on a bill that would attract bipartisan support, in part because each group had made public statements characterizing the other as an unreasonable, unreliable partner. Those legislators who did try to cross the aisle were threatened with retribution from the more extreme and vocal elements of their own party for "sleeping with the enemy." There was common ground, though it was littered with mines of bitterness that made meeting upon it impossible. The public process made private negotiation fruitless.

In order for the parties in a mediation to reach an agreement on the substance of their heated dispute, there must be some broad consensus on and acceptance of the means for getting there. This is often a stumbling block, because process itself may appear secondary to the substance of the conflict: everyone is so focused on the ends that little attention is placed on the means. Relationships, status, and recognition—all features of process—when not managed well can overwhelm the discussion of tangible outcomes and thereby can shelve the possibility of reaching a resolution.

In fact process may be central to the dispute. One party complains, "If you had asked my opinion in the first place, maybe we wouldn't have gotten to this impasse." Another retorts, "It is not my intention to talk endlessly. We have a job to get done here, and in the long run, that's all that counts."

Certainly, if the parties are overwhelmed by hostility on substantive matters, there will be little attentiveness left for focusing on process. That is where the contribution of mediation matters. The mediator structures and guides a procedure, first to prove that it is possible to get the parties talking, and then to turn their discussion into a constructive outcome: the resolution of their dispute based upon overlapping yet different objectives. It is this methodological balance of process toward outcome that is the essence of mediation.

In this way the mediator reframes the tenor of the disputants' negotiation. At the point when a mediator is brought into a conflict, the parties are most often locked into a positional, or distributional, negotiation posture. The mediator hopes to transform that posture into an interest-based, integrative process. The task is to assess whether an appropriate reframing is possible given the histories and attitudes of the disputants. If there is a reasonable chance that a settlement can be achieved, the mediator must construct a process to move the parties from confrontation toward cooperation and ultimately to resolution. As mediation is voluntary, at any point either of the parties or the mediator himself or herself can suspend or postpone the mediation. (For a discussion of ethical questions in dispute resolution, see Laue & Cormick, 1978; Cooks & Hale, 2007.)

The Mediation Sequence

There are seven steps in a formal mediation process, which correspond to the steps of the Walk in the Woods. These steps address (1) premediation determination of appropriateness, (2) premeeting investigation and party buy-in, (3) self-interests, (4) enlarged interests, (5) enlightened interests, (6) aligned interests, and (7) implementation. (See Chapter Seven for more detail on the Walk in the Woods method.)

1. *Premediation determination of appropriateness.* There are many avenues by which a dispute can reach mediation. At times one of the disputants brings an inquiry to the mediator. Often it is someone who knows or is associated with one of the disputants who suggests and contacts the mediator. At times the disputants request mediation together. The initial task of the mediator is to assess whether the matter is appropriate for mediation (see Potapchuk & Carlson, 1987). The mediator describes the process and then poses a critical question: "Are you interested in finding a settlement?" If the answer is yes from all parties, then the mediator has established the basis for continuing to the next step. If, however, every party or even just one of the parties prefers to pursue conquest over resolution, then the mediation effort most likely will be fruitless. An affirmative response here need not specify the conditions of the settlement. It needs merely to express a general desire to move beyond the dispute and a willingness to accept mediation as a reasonable process by which to attempt finding a resolution. It is a signal from each party to the other that there is a willingness to put aside the

weapons and negotiate a settlement. Having brought the parties to this point, the mediator informs each about the general approach and process of mediation.

2. *Premeeting investigation and party buy-in.* Having completed a cursory analysis of the issues and parties to the case, the mediator delves deeper into the dispute background, the parties' objectives, and the obstacles facing settlement. Although not every mediation case allows for a set of private mediator-disputant conversations before the parties formally reach the table, those that do provide many advantages for all involved. The parties are introduced to the process and the mediator, and the mediator is able to develop an understanding of the issues, of each party's perspective on the issues and perceptions of the other parties, and of the individuals involved. The mediator's most important tool throughout the mediation process is the good question. Even before bringing the parties together, the mediator uses his or her inquisitiveness to discern options and opportunities for settlement and encourage the parties themselves to see the dispute from multiple perspectives. In the course of this investigation, the parties develop trust in the mediator, usually owing to the mediator's good listening skills. By the end of this premeeting stage, the mediator has developed a strategy for building the mediation process, a portion of which is shared with the parties. The mediator plans the format for the meetings and establishes a timeline for moving forward. These proposals are shared with the parties for their approval, with the cautionary note that each should be reasonable about the expectations for the outcome: there can be no promises about what will or will not be achieved. The mediator has now gained support for the process and objectives of mediation.

3. *Self-interests.* There is often a good deal of tension between the disputants, and sometimes just being in the presence of one another will take them to the basement. In most cases the parties are well known to one another and are accustomed to the emotions of adversarial discourse. It is the inclusion of the neutral third party that makes their first joint meeting with the mediator different. The mediator uses this opportunity to create a clear change in tone from the parties' prior encounters. At the opening of the session the mediator sets the table by explaining the process, what each can expect, and what is expected from each of them. He directs the course of discussion, and ensures that everyone has a fair chance to express his or her interests and perspectives and to be heard. The mediator opens the forum with a brief discussion of mediation, the purpose of the meeting, and the processes that will be used in the hope of reaching a settlement. It is important that the mediator reminds all parties that everyone at the table has agreed that he or she is ready to find a settlement and that each has agreed to participate in this process in order to find it. Particularly during this initial session, it is not uncommon for the parties to vent their anger and frustration toward one another. Some

opportunity must be allowed for them to let off a measure of steam, though it is up to the mediator to decide when to move on toward the next steps in the process.

4. *Enlarged interests.* The mediator arranges the parties' issues into two broad categories: points of agreement and points of disagreement. The disputants are often surprised to discover that there are items on which they agree: they both want a settlement, they both have found the dispute to be painful, and they both hope that the settlement will be consonant with their values. Beyond these general points of agreement, the mediator may find specific points of agreement on substantive issues related to the conflict. Next the mediator points to matters of disagreement. These points are arrayed from the easiest to settle to the most difficult. This conversation can change the tone and tenor of the meeting, reframing the negotiation from a struggle between die-hard disputants to a pursuit of even greater common ground. It is hoped that the parties will recognize that their wide set of agreements could portend the discovery of other substantive agreements upon which a settlement eventually could be reached.

5. *Enlightened interests.* The mediation process helps the parties discover settlement options they could not find on their own. Often the mediator finds two incompatible proposals advanced by the disputants. The challenge is to generate a new set of choices that creatively combines the essential ingredients of each party's interests. The mediator helps to prompt this new set of options, some combination of which will be acceptable to all sides. To do this, the mediator uses brainstorming and laundry list techniques to bring his or her imagination to the process and likewise to spark the imaginations of the disputants to create plausible ideas not readily apparent to them before. Brainstorming asks the parties to quickly express a range of ideas without editing or comment: it is intended as an unobstructed, creative exercise. The laundry list exercise asks the parties to categorize the brainstorming ideas into lists, such as good options, bad options, feasible options, and unrealistic options. From this emerges appreciation for options that are *deal makers*, options that would be *deal breakers*, and a set of options in between that could be combined to motivate the parties toward resolution. During this process, some of each party's ideas and options rise to the fore and others fade. Attention focuses on a set of proposals that is agreeable to each party.

6. *Aligned interests.* By this point the mediator has built an incremental process that has the parties converging on a range of specific settlement options. These options outline a substantive exchange, the process by which the exchange will occur, and the protections to ensure its implementation. The mediator notes on paper the key points of agreement and requests buy-in from each of the parties. What is each party hoping to *get* from the agreement, and what is each party willing to *give* in order to make it happen? The mediator repeats each point so

that the parties can voice concerns, changes, and consent. Their acceptance is focused on the items listed on the mediator's notepad, which are being clearly heard and understood by both parties. It is at this point that the *fantasy moment* is likely to occur: The parties hear what they are getting and giving and compare this real outcome with their original fantasy solution of "I win, you lose." The difference between the actual settlement and the fantasy solution is disappointing, and the parties begin to retreat from the agreement. Bringing them back to the table tests the mediator's patience and skill. As one party gets cold feet, the other says, in effect, "You see, I told you he can't be trusted." The mediator must once again remind them of choices, consequences, and reasonable outcomes. By the end of this stage, the mediator has reiterated the agreement and encouraged final acceptance.

7. *Implementation.* Moving from resolution to actual consummation of the deal is a delicate stage in the mediation. The parties have progressed from their initial adversarial stance and anger to a feasible proposal that offers them some degree of satisfaction and closure. The mediator hopes for more than a mere handshake: the outcome must be one that will endure, an agreement with which the parties will abide. Therefore the agreement should include incentives and a means of enforcement to ensure that each party adheres to its provisions. Often there is limited trust between the parties, so such assurances help build mutual confidence in the agreement. At times it is wise to build in a formal implementation process, to be monitored and executed by an outsider. This outsider may be the mediator or, more likely, some other third party trusted by both sides.

The Mediator's Activities

The mediator engages in six streams of constant activity interwoven throughout the mediation process. (For further discussion of mediator actions and technique, see Honeyman, 1990; Honoroff, Matz, & O'Connor, 1990.) In each step the mediator simultaneously engages in investigation, empathy, neutrality, managing the interaction, inventiveness, and persuasion.

1. *Investigation.* The mediator is much like a detective, searching to understand the problem, its history, the people themselves, and the interests and objectives of each side. The mediation process is like piecing together a puzzle, exploring different shapes and trying various arrangements in search of the right fit. What might one side offer the other to spur settlement? Were there any key moments or points of misunderstanding that escalated the dispute? What are each party's interests, and how might they complement one another? Investigation requires a heavy measure of curiosity. In the course of this activity the mediator distinguishes

truth from exaggeration and falsehood. The better the mediator's insight and understanding, the better the likelihood of moving the parties toward a mutually acceptable agreement. Mediation requires a good deal of information gathering, and the mediator searches for and encourages the use of high-quality data: objective information that is verifiable and accepted by both sides.

2. *Empathy*. In order for the involved stakeholders to accept the process, they must build a trusting relationship with the mediator. That relationship is the antecedent to their developing a more trusting relationship with the other parties to the dispute. Key to this building process is confidence that their concerns are acknowledged and understood. The mediator employs active listening to offer tangible assurance, voicing and demonstrating his or her own concern for and understanding of the disputants' feelings and emotions. At moments when the parties are feeling overwhelmed by emotions that could derail the process, the empathic listening and assurance of the mediator can keep the negotiations on track. At the same time, the mediator needs to take care that empathy doesn't slide into overidentification or agreement with a party, which could compromise the mediator's perceived impartiality.

3. *Neutrality*. As discussed earlier, the parties bring an understandable suspicion of the mediator's neutrality into the mediation process. It is natural for them to test the mediator, closely watching what is said as well as what is implied by body language and voice intonation. The mediator is alert to these tests and slips of confidence in his or her neutrality. Similarly, the mediator is conscious of the fact that pure neutrality is a mix of myth and professional credo: all people, even mediators, bring their own biases and history into any dispute. Effective mediators are able to competently distinguish what they think from what they say and do. The proof is in the outcome.

4. *Managing the interaction*. The mediator is in charge of what occurs at the mediation table. He or she establishes the rules of interaction—one person speaks at a time, no one person dominates the discussion, everyone arrives at the session on time—and then enforces compliance by each of the parties. The key to this process is creating an equitable balance of time, concern, and attention. In so doing, the mediator fosters a reasonably level playing field, allowing the parties to accept that their interests are being fairly represented at the table. Even when the parties are engaging in constructive negotiation on their own, the mediator periodically interjects a comment into the discussion—perhaps to note progress, contribute an observation, or pose a question. Why? The mediator is aware that at any moment, friendly discourse can turn confrontational with one hostile comment. He or she wants to maintain a presence in order to protect the mediation from potentially stumbling down the slippery slope of positional comments and dissolution.

5. *Inventiveness*. Not only must the mediator help the parties develop resolution options that they had not previously considered. He or she must also fashion the process so that the parties feel they are part of the creative endeavor. The mediator wants the parties to own the discovery of ideas and solutions. Rather than merely announcing an option, the mediator may lead the parties through a series of questions so that they find solutions on their own. In so doing, the mediator not only takes the parties through a new line of thinking, he or she likewise learns a great deal about the background of the dispute and the possibilities for resolution. The mediator is attempting to build compatibility of ideas, proposals, and people against a background of significant discord. To do so requires an abundance of creative and imaginative thinking and maneuvers—and patience.

6. *Persuasion*. The mediator seeks to create movement toward agreement. To do so the mediator must convince the parties to recognize their predicament. In so doing they begin to change their attitudes about each other and the settlement proposals facing them. The parties, of course, ultimately shape their own choices. The mediator, by definition, is without authority to impose a resolution upon them. He or she encourages the parties to reframe their understanding of the problem and potential common-ground solutions. This is accomplished by clarifying the choices and the consequences that face the parties. There are costs to conflict, measured in wasted time, lost opportunities, and expended resources. The parties are encouraged to honestly weigh these costs against the benefits of settlement. It is this contrast that is the mediator's most effective tool of persuasion. In this process the mediator persuades by questioning rather than by prescribing. The temptation to advocate an obvious solution—apparent to the mediator and stubbornly refused by the disputants—is one that the mediator must constantly resist.

The Mediation Forums

In conducting the discussions between the parties, the mediator may employ a variety of meeting arrangements. The classic image is of the mediator sitting with the disputants evenly distributed at a round table. Indeed, the shape of the table, the closed-door atmosphere, the arrangement of the parties, and the placement of the mediator are all carefully orchestrated to illustrate and enhance the principles of mediation: neutrality, a level playing field, confidentiality, privacy, and voluntary participation.

As mentioned previously, in addition to meeting with all the disputants, the mediator may conduct private sessions with each of the parties. Before mediation begins the mediator often contacts each party to gather information necessary for assessing whether mediation is appropriate for the case. Also, during a joint mediation session the mediator or one of the parties may call for a private caucus. In most cases this is a meeting between the mediator and one of the parties. However, when there are two or more disputants on one side, they may want to hold a private caucus among themselves to assess what is happening and their next steps.

Mediators are often flexible with forms and formats in order to enhance the parties' inclination toward settlement. In most cases the mediator meets with the parties to work together face to face. However, in some cases it is prudent to avoid bringing the parties into the same room: their meeting would so inflame emotions that progress would become impossible. The mediation then becomes a process of shuttle diplomacy in which the mediator carries information and proposals back and forth between their private locations. In other cases the antecedent to an actual meeting is a long procedure that ignores substance in favor of process: the shape of the table, who will be there, the rules of order, and the manner for concluding a settlement. Progress on these logistical questions then prepares the parties for their meetings on more substantive matters. Whatever it takes, mediation itself is an adaptive process, molded to facilitate progress toward resolution.

Two years ago CEO Iris Inkwater had established a dispute resolution committee at Oppidania Medical Center to handle the range of issues not dealt with by existing hospital procedures. At that time the grievance process for employee complaints was tending to become adversarial, especially when it involved unionized staff. The bioethics committee was dealing well with difficult patient-related conflicts; however, this committee was sometimes approached to resolve other kinds of disagreements simply because no other mechanism existed to address them. Standard management procedures were handling most issues smoothly, except of course the most difficult. And more disputes than necessary were going to court, including malpractice, medical privileges, and even building contractor disputes.

The dispute resolution committee was designed to temper the adversarial nature of conflicts, with the hope of helping parties find mutually acceptable solutions. It is composed of seven members: a representative from the medical staff, a representative from the nursing staff, the chief operating officer, the hospital's general counsel, the social work director, a pastoral counselor, and a representative of the unionized staff.

The committee sees its role as providing a reasonable forum where people can talk out their differences. Such discussion ideally comes at a specific moment in the course of a conflict: at the crossroads between the vociferous venting of rage and the onset of full-scale war. The committee's work doesn't replace existing hospital governance procedures. Rather, it stands alongside them, clarifying the issues and often offering solutions that are much preferred to a reprimand, censure, or dismissal. The key to the process is the active participation of the disputants in expressing, understanding, exploring, and resolving the issues. The role of the committee members is to informally and at times proactively aid this process. Since its inception this committee has been used for physicians' privilege disputes, interstaff conflicts, and several management squabbles, to name just a few.

The committee is flexible in how it goes about its work. Each of its members has had training in dispute resolution. The group meets monthly, with special meetings called for specific problems. Its role is not to act as judge. Rather, its purpose is to facilitate and encourage the adoption of a negotiation process acceptable to both sides. At times members meet with disputants as informal mediators. At other times the committee recommends the parties to an outside, formal mediator or arbitrator. Finally, the committee serves a counseling function, hearing the particulars of a case and recommending a process for resolving the dispute (though not an outcome). The hospital finds that the very presence of such a committee facilitates earlier and more amicable settlements.

Any committee member may be approached about a dispute, and periodically every member has received calls about various issues. Because there has been so much general discussion in the hospital about the Harriford-Cummings case, the committee learned about that issue through the grapevine. It seems like a natural for the committee's dispute resolution process.

After a few calls among themselves, the members of the committee conclude that this issue is quickly growing out of proportion to the initial incident. It is bringing to the fore a number of underlying controversies just waiting to explode: gender conflict, nurse-physician antagonism, nurse practice divisions, physician practice apprehensions, and the way the hospital does or does not deal with these problems.

The committee decides to attempt to bring Cummings and Harriford together for mediation. The physician on the committee, Larry Lumberg, calls Chuck Cummings; Wendy Winchell, the nursing staff representative, calls Heather Harriford. After a volley of calls among all of them, it is determined that Lumberg and Winchell will meet with Harriford and Cummings to informally mediate a discussion. Both parties were reluctant to accept such a meeting at first. They each agreed after they had taken some time to consider both the offer and the realistic options facing them. They accepted that it would be better to try for a settlement than to allow the matter to escalate further.

The meeting is in one of the small hospital conference rooms not far from the cafeteria. Lumberg and Winchell get to the room well before Harriford and Cummings. They agree that it will be best for Winchell to open the session and introduce the process. Lumberg will discuss the possible outcomes that might emerge.

Cummings arrives first and slides into a chair at the far end of the table. A few moments later, Harriford quietly walks in and takes her seat. She has taken to wearing a loose jacket over her scrubs top since the incident and her hair is pulled back primly against her head. Winchell and Lumberg greet them both. Cummings and Harriford share only icy glances with each other.

Winchell opens the dialogue. "First, I want to thank you both for agreeing to meet with us today. As you know, Larry and I spoke with both of you, and you both agreed that it would be best to sit down and discuss this matter privately, together."

"As mediators, Larry and I hope to facilitate a discussion about what happened, what it meant for each of you, and how it might be resolved. Our purpose is not to judge whether one of you is right or wrong. It is up to you to assess what happened and how it might be resolved. Also, what goes on here will remain confidential. Larry and I will discuss your dispute only with each other, and we will report to the dispute resolution committee only whether or not your dispute was resolved, nothing more. The purpose of this confidentiality is to try to get us away from all the hype, rumors, and gossip that have spread around the hospital regarding this matter." At this point Winchell turns to Lumberg to continue the introduction.

"Whether you can come up with a mutually acceptable resolution is up to you," Lumberg begins. "One part of this process is going over what happened, to see if there are any misunderstandings. Another part is exploring what each of you needs in order to move beyond the problem, what you need for yourselves and what you need from each other. Our purpose here is not to smooth over matters that should be addressed. Rather, we hope to encourage an open discussion of issues that are of concern to both of you. Before we begin, do either of you have any questions?"

Cummings shakes his head silently. Harriford speaks slowly, "Let's say we can't reach anything through this process. Then what happens?"

"Then the complaint you filed will be reviewed through the normal administrative review procedure. The complaint will be assessed through the medical staff governance process. Your charges will be considered; though, as you know, you will not necessarily find that what they decide meets with your approval. The disposition of the complaint will be their decision, not yours, so you are no longer in the loop at that point. By contrast, if we can come up with something here, you are obviously a part of developing and accepting the solution." Harriford nods that she understands.

Winchell picks up the thread again. "We like to begin by getting a sense of what happened." She turns to Harriford. "Heather, you filed the complaint. Could you tell us what happened and what led you to take this action?"

Harriford goes through a very matter-of-fact description of the story, describing Mrs. Hayward's condition, her reaction to the morphine, and the touching and pressure she got from Cummings. ''It was inappropriate. It was terrible, and I felt violated. He was making an advance while I was trying to ensure that the patient would not get the wrong medication. There is no reason why I should have to put up with that. Actually, there is no reason why anyone here should have to put up with it. He and all his buddies who think this is cool deserve to learn a lesson. This is a hospital, not a bar. We all share responsibility for our patients, and it is not a responsibility that should be taken lightly.'' She stares straight at Cummings. ''This whole thing has been a nightmare for me. I did what I thought was right, and I am being punished for it. It's not fair, it's just not fair.''

Winchell pivots to Cummings. ''Chuck, what is your view of what happened?''

Cummings describes a busy and tense evening that had capped a twelve-hour shift. He says the tension was finally beginning to ease when he went into Mrs. Hayward's room. Her family was very upset, though they couldn't stop talking about how much they appreciated Heather. He explains that his intention was to pass along to Heather what they had said. He also wanted to relieve Mrs. Hayward's pain, because it was not only troubling to the patient, it also was very unnerving for the family to see her so uncomfortable. He says that he only wanted to do well by everyone.

He relates that he really didn't know about Mrs. Hayward's previous reaction to morphine. There had just been too much going on, and he hadn't had a chance to study her chart. He admits that he had been wrong, and he says he appreciates Heather's warning him about it.

''The more difficult issue for me,'' he continues, ''is the misunderstanding between Heather and myself. I just meant to be friendly, that's all. I didn't want her to feel uncomfortable about a come-on, or anything. It's not what I intended, and I am afraid that under the fatigue and stress I was feeling, I got carried away.''

Harriford jumps on this. ''Carried away? I would call that a bit more than carried away!''

Cummings pounces right back. ''Look, I didn't feel you up or anything. I was touching your shoulders. That's all that happened. I'm trying to be reasonable here, OK? If you want to rile things up, then this whole thing isn't going to work.''

Lumberg intercedes. ''Time out. Let's go back to the facts. Heather, what exactly did Chuck do that you found offensive?''

''Several things. He was rubbing my shoulders as if he were giving me a massage. He was playing with my bra straps. Then he blatantly stared down at my breasts. It was all very suggestive—all while he was ordering me to give the patient inappropriate medication.''

Lumberg waits for Harriford to finish. ''So, Heather, if I understand correctly, it was the combination of touching, staring, and making suggestive remarks in a context that was very inappropriate. Is that correct?'' Harriford nods.

Lumberg looks across the table at Cummings. "Is that what happened?"

"Yes, that's what happened," is Cummings's quick retort. "I think it's fair, though, to consider what didn't happen, especially given all the fuss being made over this. I did not fondle her, molest her, or touch what is not ordinarily considered OK to touch between people who know one another. We're talking shoulders here, nothing more."

"You're right, Chuck," Winchell says calmly. "There is a distinction. Nonetheless, even though it was just a shoulder, what makes the difference is how long you touch it, the movement you make while touching, and the context of that touching. Can you see that?"

This time his response is slower. "Yes, I can see that. I just think the punishment should fit the crime."

Harriford's reaction is lightning quick. "What punishment? You haven't been punished. What's happened to you anyway?"

Cummings looks straight at Harriford. "What are you talking about? A physician lives by his reputation. It is as essential as breathing. Whatever happened, and whatever might happen, this whole thing has put an indelible black mark on my reputation. You couldn't think of a worse punishment than that."

"Oh, give me a break." Harriford's voice drips with sarcasm. "What the hell is a reputation? And are you so dense that you didn't know about your reputation among the nursing staff long before the incident between us? Your reputation stinks, Cummings, and you might as well face up to it."

"I'm not talking about my personal reputation, which I can sense is what you are probably referring to. I'm talking about my professional reputation as a physician."

Winchell asks the next question. "Chuck, you are making a distinction. What's the difference?"

Cummings shifts his gaze to Winchell and leans back in his chair. His voice is calm. "One thing has to do with who I am as a person. Yeah, I've had a reputation since high school of being something of a lady's man. And Heather, you are not the first woman to tell me that I'm a bit too fast. What I'm talking about is my reputation as a doctor. That's what is at stake here for me."

Harriford leans forward, twitching with irritation. "How can you see those as separate? You *are* a doctor. That is the responsibility you took upon yourself. Every minute you are in this building, you are a doctor. You can't turn it on and off at your convenience, especially in the middle of talking about a sensitive patient care issue."

Cummings does not reply. Lumberg notices a change in his expression. He speaks into the silence. "Chuck, what's going on for you?"

Cummings hesitates, staring at the grain in the wood veneer of the conference table. "This whole thing is getting mixed up for me," he finally says, quietly. "It seems that we're talking about two separate things, and when they get mixed up is when it gets so complicated."

Harriford senses that he is genuinely struggling. She is feeling a speck of empathy for him. "Do you understand why this upset me so, why what you did was wrong?" she asks.

"I think so."

Winchell senses an opening. "Chuck, I have a feeling that Heather would find it helpful to hear why you think it was wrong."

He looks up and inhales deeply. When he speaks, he is crafting each word. "I think I crossed a boundary that is important to her, a boundary I may not have understood." He pauses.

Lumberg coaxes him. "What was that boundary, Chuck?"

"I think Heather felt I was making a sexual overture, and I felt I was just being friendly," he says sheepishly.

"Really, Chuck? Just being friendly?" Lumberg asks.

"Well, maybe more than being friendly. I guess it's important to me that women find me appealing, especially women I find attractive." He smiles wanly at Harriford. "I was sort of checking out whether there might be a spark there. You know, just being innocently flirtatious."

Harriford is listening intently and is focused on Cummings. "Maybe if the setting had been different, what you did could have been considered 'innocently flirtatious.' If we were at a party or at a dance and you did what you did, I would have turned around and gone for the punch—I mean the drinking kind—if I wasn't interested. Or if I was interested, I would have responded differently, and we might have danced. The problem is that our conversation about Mrs. Hayward was not at the prom. We were in the middle of a discussion about a patient, about giving her medication that would have been dangerous for her, and you started playing with my bra straps. You were taking advantage of your position of power as a physician to intimidate me. I can't accept that as simple flirtation."

Cummings again stares at the table, considering and clearly working with what Harriford is saying. Harriford's words hang resonantly in the air. Winchell and Lumberg look at both of them and then glance silently at each other, nodding slightly; they will let Heather and Chuck work through this next exchange on their own. They do not interrupt.

After a tense moment, Cummings looks up. His expression has turned from docile to hostile and his body seems to swell. "Fine. So you didn't like what I did. You told me that just when it happened. You could have left it at that and it would have been done with. But you couldn't do that. You had to turn this whole thing into a capital crime. You blew it out of proportion," he hisses

"You jerk. And I thought you were beginning to get it!" Harriford slaps her hand on the table.

Winchell leans into the table and with palms down presses the air to create some symbolic space. She knows they are about to go down the slippery slope. She knows it is important for Chuck to express honestly what is on his mind and that Heather's quick attack will cause him to recoil. Because he seems to have been working on understanding the issues, and because deep down he seems to be conflicted himself, she wants to keep him in the process. "One second, Heather. Chuck, what are you saying?"

Cummings takes a controlled breath. "All I'm saying is that this thing has grown so out of proportion that it's making me sick, OK? I don't think my whole career should be shot down because of this one complaint."

Lumberg picks up the discussion, asking calmly, "Who said your whole career is being shot down?"

"Well, it's obvious. Because of this complaint, I'm branded. You think that's fair?"

Lumberg intentionally does not answer his question directly. "Let me tell you what I see. Both of you have a line that can't be crossed, a line on a matter of great concern to you. Heather, for you the line is on someone making inappropriate sexual overtures at a time when there is a serious patient-care issue being discussed. To do that is unforgivable. Right?"

Harriford nods.

"And Chuck," Lumberg continues, "having someone threaten your career goes over your line. You feel that if someone has a problem with you, they should let you know about it, not file a public complaint. Does that capture your sentiment?"

"Precisely," he says firmly.

"So, given that, it's hard to respond to what Heather is saying?"

"Yeah, that could be."

Lumberg looks to Harriford. "Is there anything Chuck can do that would satisfy you and, at the same time, assure him that it will not ruin his career?"

There is nearly a minute of silence as Harriford contemplates the question. Her arms are crossed as she answers. "Yes, if he sincerely apologizes, and does something concrete, such as getting some sensitivity training, then I would be willing to drop my complaint. And he would have to convince me that it won't happen again."

"Chuck, is that something you could do?"

He is eager to put this behind him. "Yeah, I'll do anything," he replies almost nonchalantly.

Harriford is annoyed with his response. It was too quick. It sounded as if he was willing to say anything just to get her off his back. Then he could go back to his old ways. "No, it's not 'I'll do anything,'" she says. "I said I want sincerity, and I want to know what you'll do specifically."

Hearing her emphasis on the word *sincerity* triggers something for Cummings. He begins to realize that Harriford is looking for something deeper and that he will have to respond at her level—and really mean it—if there is going to be any movement. He understands that he will have to try harder. He looks directly into her eyes. "Heather, I am sorry for what I did. Truly sorry. I'm not sure what more to say."

Harriford lets the apology linger. She measures its tone and intent against the message she felt from his hands on the day of the incident. Finally, she is satisfied and replies, "Actually, there is something more to say. The Multicultural Institute is running a three-evening seminar on gender issues. Would you be willing to go?"

"What's involved?"

"Three, two-hour sessions. People speak on just the type of issues we've been talking about here. And there is discussion time after the sessions. Will you go?"

"Yeah, I am willing to go. Actually, I think it might help me out. Maybe that, plus I can tone down my libido some." He offers an apologetic smile. Harriford slowly nods back.

"If I do this, there is something I would like in return," Cummings says.

Winchell responds. "What do you want in return?"

"My apology, Heather, is genuine. If I take this class, and if I assure you that I truly have learned a lesson, will you drop the complaint?"

Harriford hesitates. "Yes, I will put the complaint on hold pending your completion of the class."

Lumberg summarizes what had been discussed during the session. Winchell makes crystal clear what has been agreed to by each of them. She asks Cummings to contact her after he's attended the class. She confirms that she will let Heather know that he has complied, and only then will the complaint be formally withdrawn.

That evening, Heather meets with Sally, one of her closest friends, to talk about the session over a salad and a glass of wine. Her friend asks if she feels that Cummings has gotten off easy. "On the one hand, yes," Heather says, "but any mark on his record would have been relatively insignificant in the long run. On the other hand, everybody knew about this and was talking about it. If I had pressed the complaint, there were no guarantees about the outcome except that there would have been blowback that would have worsened the relationships between the men and the women on staff as well as between doctors and nurses. He wouldn't have learned anything from it. It probably would've just ignited his anger without helping him get beyond it, and that anger would have been more of an obstacle to his changing than anything else. This way, I think the guy really learned something. He saw that what he did threatened something he deeply values: his professional reputation and his career. If I wasn't convinced of that—if I hadn't seen the change in him even in the course of that short meeting—I wouldn't have agreed. He realized something about himself and others that I think he will carry for the rest of his career. On the chance that he will learn a positive lesson, it is worth the risk of withdrawing the complaint."

"But did it give you the satisfaction you were looking for? You've been through hell with this," Sally says with a gentle squeeze of Heather's arm.

"You know, it did. It gave us the chance to deal with this as two mature adults. I felt like the hospital was taking me seriously and that Cummings really heard me. That means a lot."

Even as she hears herself saying the words, Heather Harriford wonders for a moment if she really has done the right thing. Then she realizes that both the process and the outcome have left her with a sense of calm that she hasn't felt in some time. She accepts that she didn't need to destroy Chuck Cummings with her anger or become vindictive in order to get an acceptable outcome. She thinks she has done something far more profound and is content with that.

Adapting ADR to Health Care

Ideally, differences and disagreements between people involved in the work of health care are resolved before they reach a point where mediation or arbitration is necessary. The premise of this book is to advance resolution of health care disagreements by combining prevention and cure. In this integrated model, interest-based negotiation resolves most matters and prevents their escalation into distracting and costly conflict; mediation and arbitration are used to resolve only those that have become a major burden and disruption. Disputes arising from routine decision making and staff interactions are then seen on a spectrum from low-level matters that can be resolved on the spot to full-scale conflagrations that can benefit from ADR. Disagreements are identified and resolved at the least adversarial and most constructive level possible: the earlier you incorporate constructive resolution, the less likely it is that disagreements will escalate. As with surgery, ADR should be avoided if less intrusive and less costly options are available. (For a discussion of dispute system design, see Ury, Brett, & Goldberg, 1988; Slaikeu, 1989.)

Nevertheless, when heated disputes do arise, an easily accessible and pragmatic mediation procedure is a useful and efficient way to bring parties to the negotiation table. These methods can be molded and tailored to fit the particulars of any case. Mediators who work with formal processes are settlement oriented, and they naturally adjust their methods to the situation at hand. Health care professionals can likewise adapt informal mediation methods to the unforeseen circumstances that regularly confront them in their practice. Perhaps the greatest attraction of mediation is the consistent inclusion of the relevant parties in the dispute resolution process. By definition, the parties have a voice in the final decision that is reached. The mediator upholds that perspective to ensure that it is reflected in the settlement.

Bioethical disputes offer an illustration (see Dubler & Nimmons, 1992). Bioethicists are caught in a professional dilemma. On the one hand they want to effectively help the parties reach a resolution. On the other hand they have a responsibility to uphold both the laws of their jurisdiction and general moral principles. What if the parties are considering options that would breach either the laws or the principles? Using these laws and principles as the boundaries of what is acceptable, the bioethicist guides the parties through the mediation process. As a result the parties are often able to find a number of options they hadn't previously considered, all falling within the range of what is legally and morally acceptable. Sometimes *when a decision is made* is at the crux of the issue, and a short delay facilitates agreement. Sometimes *who is involved in making the decision* is the primary point of contention—family members want to know that their concerns are heard. Sometimes the *criteria used to determine an action* are disputed: for example, the bioethicist can help to ensure that clinical measures are applied sensitively in assessing conditions and determining outcomes. The mediation process allows bioethicists to balance their organizational and societal roles while helping the participants to resolve the most wrenching dilemmas that one faces in life and in the work of health care. The process (mediation) and the outcome of their efforts are, taken together, termed *principled settlement*—a mutually acceptable and ethically responsible agreement that conforms to both legal requirements and moral principles.

Mediation certainly is not appropriate for the resolution of every dispute. When a fair determination has been made that a decision will be imposed upon one or all of the parties as a function of legal, moral, organizational, or clinical considerations, and when there is no room for negotiation, then mediation is improper. It is fraudulent to even suggest that there is room for discussion when a given decision is foreordained. Such is the case when someone has clearly violated the law.

In addition, a word of caution is appropriate here about using ADR procedures in health care: at times the process itself can become needlessly ritualized. Because the field of ADR has its origins in formal legal settings, the process can assume an aura of restrictive formality, despite its proponents' eschewing the use of procedural impediments. For the most part these protocols make perfect pragmatic sense. For example, in order to disclose his or her role and to offer protection from any subsequent legal ricochet (when a disputant takes legal action against the neutral mediator), third parties employ a formal, contractually specified process to inform and protect all parties to the dispute. Certainly during formal mediation these procedures are necessary and wise. However, as mediation methods are adapted to the unique and informal circumstances of health care disputes, these procedures too must be applied with flexibility.

Another important adaptation of ADR to health care concerns organizational or professional learning. Pure ADR is not always instructive or corrective in its orientation. Dispute resolvers measure their success on the basis of a concluded settlement. However, for those involved in the ongoing work of health care, conflicts and their resolution are also a vital source of invaluable information about measures that might improve the quality of patient care or of staff members' work lives. When the dispute or problem involves an error that reduces patient safety, one point of the settlement is typically the adoption of methods or mechanisms to eliminate the possibility that the same error will be committed with someone else. When former disputants resume a close working relationship or when someone must return to the circumstances that generated the dispute in the first place, the lessons learned must be incorporated into a reformed practice style and system design. When a practitioner returns to routine patient care following a malpractice case with one patient, when nurses resume collaborative work following a dispute with the medical staff, or when administrators reestablish business ties following a disputed billing issue with a vendor, what follows that resolution must be different from what happened before. It is essential to ask, How can we enhance the likelihood that the same dispute or problem will not be repeated? This question becomes a routine aspect of the settlement process, so that systemic learning amplifies the value of the settlement. In this way mediation can be helpful well beyond the culmination of a single dispute.

Finally, *alternative* in alternative dispute resolution, left over from the field's origins in labor relations and law, is somewhat of a misnomer in health care situations. Mediation and arbitration initially were promoted by reformers as an alternative to litigation or other escalation. However, with the growing recognition and acceptance of mediation and arbitration, litigation itself is becoming the last-resort alternative, used only after all else has been tried and has failed. Wishing to change the term and preserve the catchy three letters that have become a trademark for the field, some practitioners therefore have renamed the process *appropriate dispute resolution*.

Conclusion

Mediation and arbitration are adaptive processes. They have been used to advance resolution of a wide range of complex issues. (For a critical overview of the applications of mediation, see Kressel, Pruitt, & Associates, 1989.) In each of these applications, ADR has been formed and reformed to fit the circumstances of its new arena. Its entry into the health care field is a relatively recent phenomenon. It is a two-way learning opportunity. Health care has much to learn from dispute resolution, just as the dispute resolution field has much to learn from health care about unique decision-making criteria, conflicts, and implications. In this way, new concepts, techniques, and methods are emerging as the processes of dispute resolution adapt to the requirements of the health care field.

CHAPTER 10

META-LEADERSHIP

THERE ARE leaders whose scope of thinking, influence, and accomplishment extend far beyond their formal or expected bounds of authority. These *meta-leaders* generate widespread and cohesive action and impact that expands their domain of influence and leverage. Derived through observation and analysis of leaders in high-stakes, high-pressure circumstances such as crisis response, the five dimensions of meta-leadership practice and analysis serve as an organizing framework for understanding the foci needed to effectively build influence in the complex domain of health care. These dimensions are (1) the *person of the leader* and his or her self-awareness and problem assessment; (2) *the situation*, problem, change, or crisis that compels action or response; (3) *leading down* to one's organizational base and operating in one's designated purview of authority; (4) *leading up* to bosses or those to whom one is accountable; and (5) *leading across* to other entities and organizations beyond one's immediate scope of authority to build system connectivity (Marcus, Dorn, & Henderson, 2006). Meta-leadership is particularly valuable when addressing health care challenges that require different departments, organizations and entities to be brought together to achieve a common purpose.

What is the difference between leadership and meta-leadership? *Leadership* most commonly refers to the acts taken within a leader's recognized or expected span of authority in his or her formal role (dimension three of meta-leadership). *Meta-leadership* takes a broader view. For example, the chief executive officer of a hospital is expected to demonstrate leadership in the way the organization is operated, setting the vision and the strategic direction of the enterprise, and in achieving its performance objectives. That same CEO is practicing

The meta-leadership framework and practice method were collaboratively developed by the authors of this book, along with Isaac Ashkenazi, MD, MSc, MPA, MNS, former surgeon general of the Home Front Command of the Israel Defense Forces; and Joseph M. Henderson, MPA, of the U.S. Centers for Disease Control and Prevention.

meta-leadership when he or she, for example, creates a regional initiative to combat adult-onset diabetes by engaging other health care organizations, area universities, and the media, along with businesses and nonprofit community groups. What could be accomplished by these organizations acting together to address this critical health problem would be far more than each entity could achieve in isolation. Thus the meta-leader demonstrates effectiveness with constituencies beyond those that would traditionally be described as his or her *direct followers*. Able to identify the gaps between what could or must be done and the will and capacity to do it, meta-leaders coalesce knowledge, organizational workings, and context to achieve an otherwise unachievable cohesion of effort (Kotter, 1999). They navigate multiple environments and constraints in order to achieve an overarching objective.

Meta-leadership combines two aspects of the leadership equation to create a broad platform of influence. The first aspect is traditional hierarchical leadership, a leader's primary source of recognition and authority (Jaques, Clement, Rigby, & Jacobs, 1985). The second aspect is akin to social movement leadership (Barker, Johnson, & Lavalette, 2001), what religious leaders, political figures, and humanitarian advocates exercise to inspire and engage people when they do not have the power of a paycheck, promotion, or sanction to persuade them to be followers. It is that blend of commitment to a purpose, charisma, the talent to motivate, and appreciation of the fine art of timing that is at the heart of the informal side of meta-leaders' influence and performance. Although the exercise of formal leadership incorporates a measure of these qualities, those who practice meta-leadership do more as they influence and rally others—without direct authority to command participation—to a shared, broader purpose.

Although one can be hired to the role of leader, one must earn the mantle of a meta-leader. It cannot be bestowed simply by formal sanction. To be sure, there are many who occupy positions of formal authority who may think themselves leaders when in fact their influence is marginal and they are leaders in name only. Not all CEOs, clinical chiefs, or community activists have a wide impact or play large roles in the environments in which they operate; those who do have discovered the potential of meta-leadership.

Why is meta-leadership important in health care systems? Compared to traditional manufacturing organizations or service companies, which have a relatively clear-cut order for developing strategy, making decisions, and measuring success, health care organizations and the health care system are exceptionally complex. There is no one really in charge of the system: different people and entities have oversight and authority over various portions. Within a hospital, managers control administrative variables; however clinical decision making—a critical component of the financial health of an institution—remains, as it should, with clinicians. If patient care is to progress smoothly, these different departments and administrative sections must carefully coordinate their interdependent transactions and their interactions with third parties such as testing laboratories and insurance companies. If a hospital is to meet its patient outcome, productivity, and fiscal objectives, different departments and professionals must leverage and link with the capacities and activities of one another. And if overall health policy objectives are to be achieved, insurers, governmental agencies, businesses, and health care providers must synchronize their work in order to maximize the efficiencies and effectiveness of the system.

Absent overarching authority, how are system components synchronized to get the work accomplished in a cost-effective, high-quality, and value-motivated way? When it applies to the complexities of many departments, organizations, professionals, and systems effectively interfacing with one another, the answer often lies with capable meta-leadership.

To successfully exert meta-leadership in health care, you must exercise leadership across a network of entities both within and outside your organization. For example, in a large medical center, flat and matrixed structures have increased the complexity of accountability, control, and exercise of power and influence. A premium is placed on nonhierarchical leadership (Meisel & Fearon, 1999). For the first time in the United States, four generations are working at the same time, each with different expectations and norms for leader and follower behavior and motivation (Hackman & Johnson, 2004): the medical and nursing school graduates who are in their twenties differ greatly from their counterparts who are in their sixties and seventies. Confronted with this, leaders cannot afford to lead in traditional ways. The transformation of the traditional organization requires the transformation of the traditional leader (Ashkenas, Ulrich, Jick, & Kerr, 2002).

In this environment, authority and accountability structures have become more reciprocal and relational (Wagner, 2008) and health care leaders find themselves challenged to use influence as much or more than formal levers of control. Organizational boundaries function as semipermeable membranes rather than hard walls: there is active involvement with other internal and external entities in the health care value chain—from independent primary care and specialist practices to hospitals, clinics, labs, insurance companies, and more. These mazelike networks of business and clinical enterprises are often complex, and when there are problems, they can become emotional and chaotic (Green, 2007).

The complications of providing direction in such an environment are often obscured by the focus of traditional theories that view leadership as a top-down, leader-subordinate construct, typical of hierarchical organizations (see, for example, Weber, 1905; Lewin, Lippitt, & White, 1939; Likert, 1967; Tannenbaum & Schmidt, 1973; Burns, 1978; Bass, 1985). The conventional boss-employee relationship, for one, has been formalized through clear roles, authority structure, rules, job descriptions, and responsibilities that prescribe performance and productivity expectations (Fernandez, 1991). Many relationships critical to leadership success are not so structured. Organizations that employ matrixed structures build cross-functional relationships but generally within the single entity (Thomas & D'Annunzio, 2005).

Customary leadership approaches also do not fully capture what occurs when leaders must catalyze action well above and beyond their formal lines of decision making and control, as is common in health care. Meta-leadership addresses these leadership challenges that cross interorganizational as well as intraorganizational boundaries. The most effective strategy for leadership in these circumstances is unified action incorporating a wide scope of stakeholders in pursuit of a common goal—what we call *connectivity*. To achieve this, leaders must exert meta-leadership by simultaneously leading *down* to the people who are accountable to them (as is traditionally expected of leaders), *up* to influence the people or organizations to which they are accountable, and *across* to activate peer groups and others with whom they have no formal hierarchical relationship. These activities are parts of an integrated whole, what we earlier in this book referred to as *whole image negotiation*. Meta-leadership embodies this overarching approach to problem solving (Marcus et al., 2006). The concept and practice integrate a wide body of leadership scholarship and map critical interdependencies. Here we apply these theories and concepts to the complexities of health care delivery, management, and administration.

The Meta-Leadership Model: Origins and Extensions

The meta-leadership model was born from observing and analyzing the actions of leaders in the aftermath of the terrorist attacks of September 11, 2001. Along with Isaac Ashkenazi, we were asked by U.S. Centers for Disease Control and Prevention (CDC) to study and assess leaders preparing for and responding to unprecedented events facing the nation. Our contact at the CDC, Joseph

Henderson, joined the research effort. Our research took us up close to leaders during major events in this country and abroad. We were, for example, on the front lines observing the leaders who responded in 2005 to Hurricanes Katrina and Rita in the Gulf Coast. More recently, members of the team were able to observe the aftermath of the 2010 earthquake in Haiti and the 2010 Deepwater Horizon oil spill response. We discovered that these crisis situations brought already complex leadership challenges into much higher relief. We were able to develop a profile that distinguished effective leaders from those who were less so. Beyond simply a descriptive model, we hoped to extend what we learned to a normative framework: a set of practice guidelines and a curriculum that leaders could learn and apply to their work in complex, crisis scenarios.

Although the leaders we observed were for the most part working in public agencies, these were large, complex organizations with thousands of employees, hierarchical management structures, multiple stakeholders, and exposure to fierce public scrutiny. We found these large public sector agencies ideal for the investigation of leaders and development of the meta-leadership strategy, as these organizations exhibit many of the characteristics of traditional bureaucratic settings such as are often found in health care. There is the need to develop influence well beyond one's authority, there are the complexities of overlapping jurisdictions as well as gaps in authority, there is significant value in building connectivity of effort, and the work must be accomplished with intense public exposure combined with expectations of perfection. Meta-leadership has its greatest impact in situations with high stakes and a high number of stakeholders—scenarios typical of health care and ones that can be ripe with potential conflict.

The prefix *meta* is taken from ancient Greek and refers to that which is transcending or extending above and beyond. Consider, for example, the term *meta-research*, which refers to research that systematically identifies cross-cutting themes found in many different studies, or *meta-analysis*, which refers to a process of combining and synthesizing findings about a range of questions in search of overarching thinking and conclusions, or even the term *metamorphosis*. Similarly, as a meta-leader, not only must you catalyze change, viewing evolution as an active rather than a passive process. You must also build and maintain a capacity for intentional direction, remaining proactive amid circumstances that could otherwise be overwhelming. Meta-leadership as a framework connects what have otherwise been disparate areas of thinking about leadership into a cohesive, interdependent model to help you do this.

With the continuing unfolding of health care reform high on the state and media agendas, the state governor has appointed his talented lieutenant governor, Sarah Smith, to lead and assist efforts to translate cutting-edge policy into everyday practice. She has the knowledge, capabilities, and intuition of someone who knows and practices meta-leadership, a necessary set of tools given the importance and volatility of the issues and decisions that lie ahead. And given that the governor has privately decided that he will not run for another term, this will be an opportunity for Smith to showcase talents that may position her for a run for the top office. His charge to her was clear: "Bring this state together on health care and make us the best in the country."

Smith is a quick study and she soon impresses health experts, the state legislature, and the general public with her insightful understanding of health care, health policy, and the political process. She is a good connector—of people to ideas and ideals and of problems to better understanding and solutions. By design, the approach to the whole process of reform implementation has been framed as open and inclusive. A number of health care summits are being held around the state. Smith participates enthusiastically in these open forums, which include testimony from consumers, health providers, the business community, and political leaders. The topic and the format have caught the attention of the press, in part because health care is such a hot issue and in part because of the lieutenant governor's compelling personality and flair. She truly is leading.

Before the health summit in the City of Oppidania is even announced, Dr. Larry Lumberg, medical director of the emergency department at Oppidania Medical Center, has been asked to participate. Lumberg is outspoken and politically active on community health issues. He is pleased to have been invited, and he happily accepted the offer.

On the day of the summit, an animated crowd streams past a row of television remote broadcast vans and into the civic center. Lumberg strides through the throng thinking how fortunate he is to be at this point in his career now, when the system is in the midst of such important change and the public is paying attention. It is a rare opportunity to help shape what he believes will be a new era for the health system and for health care. Sure, many of his colleagues looked upon the process with disdain, worried about the independence, earnings, and status they might lose. He just doesn't see it that way. He sees a better, more responsive system truly dealing with the health disparities in the community.

Rows of seats fan back from a stage with a square table at which fifteen chairs are set. The room is brightly lit to accommodate the bank of television cameras perched on a platform at the back of the room. Lumberg finds his seat at the table, off to the right of the lieutenant governor.

Smith opens the forum with an articulate and inspiring assessment of the need to move forward with health care reform and the tremendous opportunity that faces the state. She speaks in terms of people's well-being and the interests of the business community and even mentions her family's experience with the system. The reaction of the crowd indicates that she is hitting the right notes. Lumberg is impressed with the breadth of her knowledge and the spontaneity of her remarks. When Smith finishes, each of the other individuals at the table makes brief opening remarks. First on the agenda are the laypeople, consumers who for the most part have been denied care because of insurance or administrative obstacles. Then come the providers. The moderator turns to Lumberg and says, "Dr. Lumberg, you work in a hospital emergency department here in Oppidania. What do you think needs to be changed or improved?"

Lumberg remembers the admonition from the organizers to be brief and to the point. "Yes, thank you. I direct the emergency department at Oppidania Medical Center. Within one mile of our building are the affluent neighborhoods of Oppidania Heights in one direction and the low-income areas of the Crestview housing projects in the other. When people come to our door for emergency care, they are each treated equally, no matter their socioeconomic status. Health and health care are the great levelers in our society. And in the emergency room, we see it all."

He leans into the microphone, warming to his task. "In moments of frustration in the ER, there is a phrase often heard behind the desk or in the lounge among the nurses and doctors: 'Another preventable!' That phrase refers to another victim of violence, to a pregnant crack cocaine user in crisis, to a person critically injured in a vehicular accident because he wasn't wearing a seat belt, to a casualty of domestic abuse, and to a heart attack victim whose poor health habits made the tragedy almost inevitable. We know that the hospital will somehow get paid for its work with these people, either through Medicaid, private insurers, or through the state's universal coverage plan. Nonetheless, we should all like to see fewer of these preventables in our ER and more of that money going to help keep these people safe and healthy. This is a human catastrophe that is afflicting our society, and it can't be fixed by our ERs and hospitals alone. Health reform is not simply about a new insurance scheme. It is about reforming what we do as a society to keep ourselves healthy. And if you take it from a mere business perspective then, as some people have commented, for making a small investment in keeping our community well, you get a generous return on investment in the form of a productive, healthy population and you spend less money on preventables—avoiding the human heartbreak that accompanies every case."

"I have another point. We must remember that hospitals are businesses too. They have payrolls to meet, bills to pay, and investments in maintenance and new equipment to make. Just as we cannot treat people if we do not receive compensation to cover our costs, we cannot work with the community around us if that work is not supported. We have begun a number of programs already, with modest state support and in conjunction with several foundations that encourage community groups. These programs have been welcomed in Oppidania, and we are seeing very positive results. If they were expanded, I know that we would see far fewer preventables in our ER—and that makes both health sense and business sense."

"Here is an example. Our cardiology and nutrition departments are currently being reimbursed by several HMOs for running health promotion workshops for their subscribers. Yes, it is hard to pinpoint exact savings or positive outcomes from prevention programs. Some people who avail themselves of them might not have gotten sick anyway. That is true. But in general, the programs do improve the overall health quality of life of these people, and I believe that is a worthy outcome in and of itself. These programs require a copayment on a sliding scale, so their overall expense is modest compared to their overall benefit."

"To conclude, Mrs. Smith, I do hope that plans for changing the system include not only shifts in the structure of health insurance but also the shifts we need in our health care priorities, spending, and objectives. In our society I believe we value life and a high quality of life. There is a price on that value, a reasonable one when compared to the real costs of illness and unnecessary death. There is much that we as health professionals can offer to keep this state healthier. I do hope that you and the governor and other major players who affect health policy and practice will help to lead us in a positive shift in what we do and how we go about doing it."

Lumberg's thoughtful and passionate remarks captivate the room. The moderator is taken off guard, and he turns to the lieutenant governor. "What do you think, Lieutenant Governor Smith?"

"First, Dr. Lumberg," says Smith, "thank you for those moving and important comments. I do agree with you. If we merely change *how* we finance health care, without also changing *what* we finance, we will have accomplished little. This is perhaps the most perplexing piece of this complex puzzle, because it is the most intangible. We have concrete numbers to calculate what needs to be changed in the insurance realm. What you describe is what we need to be attending to, and it is difficult because there we enter the unknown. What will it cost? What will it accomplish? How do we go about doing it wisely and efficiently? These health summits will continue prodding us to ask these important questions and to continue searching for the answers, no matter how elusive. I commit to you that we will find a way, and once we do, we will open those doors, carefully evaluate what's working and not, and then put the attention and the money where it will make a difference. And you in the health system must be part of that process, though you must understand that the money cannot chase after interesting ideas. We will look for results and impact and then make the case based on the data. This is a historic moment for our health care system, and we would be cheating ourselves and our constituents if we did not take up this challenge to re-create the system so that we can intentionally promote health and avoid—by design—what you and your colleagues aptly call *preventables*."

Dr. Lumberg and Mrs. Smith exchange gestures of gratitude, and the summit moves on to the next speaker.

Five Dimensions of Meta-Leadership

The meta-leadership model and its five dimensions serve as an organizing framework for the many factors that you as a leader must account for when working in a complex enterprise that is intensely knowledge and specialty driven. Just as when driving a car, you must be simultaneously attentive to what is ahead, behind, on the gauges, and around the corner. So too must you pay wide attention to a flexible set of personal, social and organizational considerations. Meta-leadership is a framework for keeping focused when there is so much with which to be concerned.

By design, meta-leadership speaks to the complexities of generating a unity of action when many different people, organizational units, and even competing priorities are focused on a broadly adopted strategy, plan, or mission (Marcus et al., 2006). The model generates a series of questions that bring to light and then engage the variety of interests and considerations that must be connected to align a wide scope of stakeholders. In concept it is a question of how to best align the plan of action with the problem or opportunity: What personal and contextual factors affect what meta-leaders see, perceive, decide, and ultimately act on? (Northouse, 2004). In practice it is a puzzle of optimally creating organizational connectivity: Who are the many stakeholders who must be influenced, and how can they best be leveraged to catalyze forward progress? What other entities should be engaged to create a greater probability of success? Anticipating resistance and push-back to new ideas, working relationships, and other change, what are the likely sources of conflict and what preemptive actions can be taken, or systems created, to mitigate them? The Walk in the Woods and other conflict resolution practices discussed in prior chapters are tools for the meta-leader.

These broad themes translate into the five dimensions of meta-leadership practice. Dimensions one and two, the leader's self-awareness and having an accurate perception of the situation, are foundational conditions: optimal action is not possible without them. Dimensions three, four, and five are the foci of organizational and interpersonal action: leading down, or leading in one's designated purview of authority; leading up, or leading those to whom one is accountable; and leading across, or leading connectivity across various entities. Deploying meta-leadership requires using all five dimensions, variably leveraging each aspect of thinking and practice as called for by circumstances, and always having these different yet complementary perspectives in hand. Meta-leadership concept and practice are distinctive owing to their intent to draw these many elements into a unified framework.

Dimension One: The Person of the Meta-Leader

Meta-leadership begins with you. You must know yourself: your likes and dislikes, your strengths and weaknesses, your ambitions and your fears. If you do not know yourself and if you are not comfortable with who you are, it is less likely that you will be able to know and make others comfortable. If you are angry at your core, you will be an angry leader. If you are at peace with yourself, it is more likely that you will be at peace with others. With a measure of self-awareness and self-control, you can be intentional about the role model you present and the impact you have upon others.

Meta-leadership practice requires a high degree of emotional intelligence (Burns, 1978; Goleman, 1996). Although smart people have a high intelligence quotient, truly successful people possess a depth of emotional intelligence. The attributes of emotional intelligence are (1) *self-awareness*: knowing yourself, the experiences that color your perceptions, your hopes, passions, and even demons; (2) *self-regulation*: having the capacity to control your desires, your moods, your look, and your interactions with others; (3) *motivation*: being motivated yourself and being able to motivate and move other people; (4) *empathy*: having the capacity to understand other people for their distinct experiences, needs, and interests; and (5) *social skills*: feeling comfortable in being with other people and having a talent for making others comfortable in your presence. Self-awareness, in particular, has been shown to correlate with leadership effectiveness (Tekleab, Sims, Yun, Tesluk, & Cox, 2008). People who demonstrate emotional intelligence possess an understanding of the impact that their personality, experience, culture, emotional expression, and character have on themselves and others: this is the internal *you* of the meta-leadership construct (Kirkpatrick & Locke, 1991; Trompenaars, 1994). Self-discipline, drive, understanding, and capacity to form meaningful and satisfying relationships are critical to crossing the usual divides and boundaries of organizational, professional, and cultural associations (Goleman, 2001).

Whenever you operate outside your formal and comfortable purview or across clearly drawn boundaries, risk for you and for those with whom you work is increased. You may not know the qualities and characteristics of those with whom you are dealing, just as they don't know yours. Thus meta-leaders must also understand how to build, manage, and maintain trusting relationships. This is especially important in circumstances in which decisions and actions must be taken without complete information or certainty, as when leading through a volatile health crisis, such as a pandemic, or launching a joint business venture. It is to be expected that when people are evaluating whether or not to trust others, they will weigh factors related to the decision maker and the situation (Hurley, 2006). You must understand this dynamic and the appropriate actions to take in order to achieve the greatest commitment from a wide scope of stakeholders; integrity is a must—it is the glue that binds the interests of the stakeholders. Organizational cohesion in high-stress situations has been found to be lacking where trust-based relationships are absent (Kolditz, 2007). In practice, when you present a model of composure, balance, and appropriate perspective, your followers are both calmed and persuaded to subtly follow and mimic your behavior.

Other important qualities of the meta-leader are curiosity, courage, and imagination: these attributes make it possible to take a large, complex problem and filter it through a wide range of possible solutions (Giuliani, 2002). By applying abundant curiosity you can imagine that which has not otherwise been discovered (Sternberg, 2006, 2007). An aptitude for seeing the bigger picture is particularly important in fast-changing, emotionally charged circumstances, especially when an organization faces a crisis situation: an adverse outcome that results in the death of a patient, a financial crisis, or a volatile and unforgiving marketplace. Any of these and more can send the enterprise into crisis mode. The meta-leadership framework can help you maintain perspective, ready to take appropriate action.

Our discussion in Chapter Two about situations that can send people to their emotional basements is at the core of practice for this first dimension of meta-leadership. Being able to rise out of the basement when all around you are heading downward and then being able to lead others toward more productive thinking and activity is an essential behavioral aspect of dimension one of meta-leadership.

Dimension Two: The Situation

The task of diagnosing and eventually communicating the operational context—what is happening—is among the most difficult yet most critical tasks for a leader. Finding the most appropriate solution to a problem depends first on precisely determining the nature of the problem (Bransford & Stein, 1993; Pretz, Naples, & Sternberg, 2003). This involves not simply observing surface phenomena but also "tuning into the organizational frequency to understand what is going on beneath the surface" (Goffee & Jones, 2006). It requires you to form a "picture of the situation," and that understanding frames for you what has transpired and what more you need to know.

Because there is often a gap between objective reality and subjective assessment, getting an accurate, focused picture is a job in and of itself (see, for example, Hazleton, Cupach, & Canary, 1987). This is why the emotional intelligence of dimension one is so important in achieving effective *situational awareness*, the combination of dimensions one and two. This gap between objective and subjective is further magnified when many different stakeholders are involved, when a great deal of information is required to diagnose the problem, when the stakes and emotions are high, or when the analysis and action are time constrained. You must grasp, work with, and narrow the likely reality-belief gap, aided by good questions, the collection of necessary information, new facts that become apparent as the situation evolves, and the perspective of hindsight. Complex circumstances—the very scenarios typical of large health care organizations—demand capacities and skills for strategic situational awareness (see, for example, O'Brien & O'Hare, 2007), resulting in an evidence-based, clear, and actionable description of what is occurring. It is the tireless pursuit of situational awareness that leads you to the most appropriate response.

Especially in times of stress, there can be difficulties in information flow between organizational units, competition among hierarchies, and priorities that are in conflict. You can be caught in the cross fire. In a high-stakes situation the many stakeholders involved naturally have individual perspectives, analyses, and interpretations of the *objective problem* that accord with their distinct interests, concerns, and purposes (Australian Public Service Commission, 2007). You must understand that each stakeholder uses a distinct *frame*, built of personal values, experience, objectives, and priorities, that filters what is seen and how risk is perceived. These frames, or guiding operational assumptions, are difficult to discern, appear complete though rarely are, and are resistant to adjustment (Clyman, 2003).

In keeping with the lesson of the cone in the cube illustration presented in Chapter One, you must seek and encourage observations that integrate different perspectives. Are there ways in which differences might complement rather than contradict one another? Might divergent perspectives be integrated into a cohesive, new proposition that adds value for the relevant stakeholders? A meta-leadership perspective drives you to close the gaps by encouraging connectivity and identifying leverage points that could transform discord into opportunity. Applying the mediation methods discussed earlier in the book, you should be less interested in judging who is "right" or "wrong" and more interested in fostering a common-ground understanding of the situation in pursuit of common-ground solutions. With a cohesive image of the problem, it is likely that a wider variety of stakeholders than before will be motivated to contribute to achieving a solution. This is what meta-leadership requires; interest-based negotiation and conflict resolution provide tools to aid and abet its practice.

The process of developing situational awareness is an iterative progression of divergence—through both internal and external debate over what is happening—and convergence—through intermittent points of agreement or understanding (Roberto, 2005). Herein one finds both the tension and the paradox of dimension two. In a complex situation, a quick assessment that is close to the mark and moves the process forward can be better than a slow though more accurate one that comes too late to make a difference. Time is a critical factor in situational awareness and meta-leadership. Before a fast-moving, high-stakes situation erupts, time is your ally: the more time you have to lay the groundwork and prepare the better. However, once a crisis hits, time is your enemy: the longer you take to develop your picture of the event and take action, the worse the consequences. Think of the *crash cart* found in a cardiac care unit. A great deal of time is taken to decide exactly what should be on it and where it should be placed. People are trained to know precisely where each item is located and exactly what they should do in the event that a patient goes into cardiac arrest. This extensive preparation allows all members of the team to work seamlessly, almost without words, to treat the patient as quickly as possible. In this moment every second counts, so the initial response is intricately choreographed; no one has to ask, "What should I do?" Whether it is a matter of a high-stakes financial dilemma facing your hospital, a personnel issue that is plaguing your department, or a life-or-death clinical decision on your service, the longer you take to develop situational awareness and to implement a plan of action, the less control you will have of the consequences and implications. The meta-leader understands that even though success and failure may be measured differently by different stakeholders (Daly & Watkins, 2006). A leader must make decisions and must take action, especially in a crisis situation. Each action helps to close the gap and further clarifies the multiple dimensions.

What happens in the absence of meta-leadership? Pragmatic situational awareness and problem assessment suffer when the leader is distracted or simply misconstrues what is occurring; the lingering gap between perception and reality has its dangers (Mullin, 2002; O'Brien & O'Hare, 2007). There are numerous reasons why this happens and why it happens often. It can be a function of a parochial point of view: the leader experiences a strong case of denial prompted by a multitude of personal or professional explanations, seeing the expected or the desired information and overlooking information that does not correspond. It can arise from a lack of the experience necessary to identify and understand what is happening. Some leaders demand to have all the information before making a decision and in the process cause a delay that exacerbates the original problem. At other times leaders encounter an overload of information that is difficult if not impossible to decipher because it does not distinguish between important facts and unimportant facts; it's just a mass of indiscriminate data (O'Reilly, 1980). Functionally, these conditions describe the leader who is in the basement, blind and impotent, or as often happens, who is solving what he or she sees as the convenient or soluble problem rather than the one that is really at hand. When this happens the leader magnifies the extent or implications of the problem by preventing effective corrective action. Myths, like mold after a flood, appear and thrive.

Meta-leadership practice requires the perspective and measured patience to work with ambiguity. When the situation is clear and every action has a certain and predictable cause and effect, the skills of the meta-leader will likely not be called into action. However, complex, multi-tiered relationships, high-consequence organizational predicaments, and difficult interpersonal conflicts do not come with obvious computations of what is right and what is wrong. Individuals faced with these ordeals are not equally able to establish a calculated assessment and then rise to the challenge—and these are among the strategic and analytical capacities uniquely associated with meta-leadership.

When Manuel Mendez was appointed city health commissioner last year, the media were abuzz with profiles of the new mayoral appointee. He did not fit the mold of previous commissioners. He was not a physician: he had a public health degree and served as director of a community health center. He was young, a member of a minority group, and energetic. He came into the position with a reputation as a "weaver." After taking a seminar on meta-leadership, he commented, "That's sort of what I've been doing all along. Now I have a name and a discipline for it."

Mendez is an activist. He organized the neighborhood surrounding the health center, putting together an economic revitalization program to help local businesses, an antigang coalition to combat violence, and a support group for mothers to ease their access to public services and provide nutritional and child-rearing instruction. He had instilled a fresh pride in Oppidania's City North neighborhood. Though he has received countless honors and awards in his community, he was not known citywide until he assumed the commissioner position.

When he took the helm of the Oppidania Health Commission, Mendez decided to study the job for six months before he became the public policy activist he had always aspired to be. He confided to one of his aides, "For six months I'll manage the department. After that I'll begin to lead it; actually, in my newfound description, I'll *meta-lead* it.'' He used the first half year to learn the agency's policies, to meet the people inside and outside the other organizations integral to its mission, and to develop trusting relationships. He believed that keeping his head down and attending to the business of the agency would earn him the credibility he would need as a policy advocate.

Now nine months into his appointment, Mendez is well liked. He has the magnetic capacity to get people excited about conceiving a new vision for health and health care in Oppidania. After much study, consultation, and assessment, he decides on a banner under which the department will direct its work: *community health*. He knows that this move is not without political risk. Are transients and homeless people included or excluded? How about undocumented immigrants? Nontraditional families? Not everyone is comfortable with programs that give even an implied endorsement of gay, lesbian, and transgender households. Does the community end at the city line?

Mendez decides to define *community* as the sense of belonging that is vital for every human being. Although people may belong to different types of clusters, it is through belonging that people meet their vital needs, in particular those needs that are critical to keeping them healthy and well. Of course homeless people are included, he says. ''If they don't have their own sense of belonging to someone, then it is our responsibility as a community to give them that sense of dignity and respect.'' At the press conference announcing the new program, he makes it clear that he is not proposing the answers. Rather, the city's community health project is about posing the questions and helping the families, the health system, and individuals themselves find the solutions together. Mendez gets the mayor enthusiastically behind the initiative. The mayor proclaims that he will ensure that every department in city hall will cooperate to make this program a success.

Mendez pulls together a representative group of fifteen of Oppidania's civic movers-and-shakers to guide the program. He draws on his network throughout Oppidania and so, far from being the usual collection of the well heeled and well connected, the group reflects the diversity of the community, the institutions that serve the community, and the work that needs to be done. Mendez asks the CEO of Urbania Medical Center to sit on the steering committee. Mendez knows him well, because Urbania is located adjacent to the City North area and the two had often collaborated. A representative from Oppidania Medical Center is also needed, and Mendez asks the hospital's medical director, Dr. Fred Fisher, to join the project. Although it takes some time and some prodding, Fisher finally agrees.

On the day of the first meeting, Fred Fisher steps into his outer office pulling on his coat. ''I'm off to this 'community health meeting' that the health commissioner has put together,'' he tells his administrative assistant. ''I have no idea what he wants *me* there for. Maybe he just wants a doctor in the room to make up for his own lack of credentials. Hopefully, I'll be back soon," he grumbles, as much to himself as to her as he heads into the corridor.

Fisher has never had much patience for committees. He can think of a hundred better uses for his time. He remembers his military days: declare an objective and go get the job done. None of this bureaucratic baloney. However, Iris Inkwater is his commander now and she told him at their last meeting that it would be an embarrassment for the hospital if he said no or sent a junior staff member in his place. He remembers her exact words: "Urbania is on this committee so we have to be too. Especially now, with the public turmoil over the Community Health Plan's deal with Urbania."

He hears his name called and turns to see Inkwater scurrying after him. "I'm glad I caught you, Fred. Let me ride down in the elevator with you and review what we need from this meeting."

"I'm thinking of taking the stairs, Iris," he replies with resignation.

She scoffs at that and takes his arm to guide him into the open elevator cab. On the descent to the parking garage she reminds him of the many community projects the hospital has initiated. She also reminds him that it is the city that issues zoning variances—an absolute must if that doctors' office building idea is to ever to become a reality. He nods blankly after each point she makes, his eyes fixed on the floor indicator above the door.

"This hospital needs to be seen endorsing and actively supporting the mayor's new pet project," she says as the door opens. "So don't just sit there like a lump." She gives him a gentle prod and a wink.

"I've got it, Iris. No need to worry." Fisher wants to encourage good things for the hospital and certainly knows that he has to get on board with all this new thinking. So after Inkwater's pep talk he heads off to the meeting feeling less antipathy but more ambivalence. And Fred Fisher doesn't like ambivalence.

Dimension Three: Leading Down

Although the bulk of the leadership literature focuses on leading within one's immediate base of operations, dimension three of meta-leadership emphasizes aspects of that practice that complement the other dimensions. Individuals who rise to effectively practice meta-leadership—whether they are hospital CEOs, clinical department chiefs, or heads of public health agencies—generally have their own organizational base of operations within which followers see them as in charge (Phillips & Loy, 2003). Although not all leaders practice meta-leadership, all meta-leaders operate from the base of influence and capacity derived from successful leadership of their own organization or frame of reference.

In that entity, the leader carries formal authority, has subordinates and resources at his or her disposal, and functions within a set of rules and roles that define expectations and requirements. Those subordinates expect adherence to allegiances and loyalties, trusting that the leader will advocate on behalf of their best interests (Heifetz, 1994). In bureaucratic terms, these accomplishments are often measured in expanding resources, authority, or autonomy for the unit and its members. In many bureaucratic settings, departments and divisions compete among one another, and followers expect their leaders to triumph on their behalf (Lee & Dale, 1998).

The support of your constituents is essential to achieving influence within the larger health care system and beyond. Understanding how you are perceived (dimension one), demonstrating an ability to diagnose and explain the context in which the group is operating (dimension two), and having a productive relationship with your boss (dimension four) are all critical to garnering that support. The size of your follower base as well as the regard in which the followers hold you are clear signals that can be read by other constituencies.

When you practice meta-leadership, you are a leader of leaders. It is your responsibility to advocate leadership development broadly through the system, though first at home among your immediate constituents. Leadership, after all, does not reside with one person. In robust organizations it is embedded among many people and at multiple levels of the hierarchy (Northouse, 2004). Effective leadership is a continuous learning process. Your meta-leadership will be enhanced when you drive this leadership learning curve, encouraging those who work under your supervision by building, marshalling, and communicating a vision and a message that is crafted, executed, assessed, and persistently adjusted and improved as contingencies require (Senge, 1994). In this way you foster meta-followership within your base; your subordinates become proactive thinkers and doers who are able to greatly expand and inspire the impact which they together seek to achieve. Accomplishing this requires a sense of leadership confidence and security, so that you see strong, smart, capable followers not as a threat but rather as a vital asset (Sternberg, 2007). Seek followers strong enough to challenge you on occasion (Goffee & Jones, 2006). It is your devotion and commitment to your followers that generates the same loyalty from them to you. If you are to achieve extraordinary results you will need subordinates who do not follow you because of a pay-based transactional relationship but rather because they believe in what you stand for and are striving to accomplish. If you are to effectively practice meta-leadership, you must seek people who U.S. Coast Guard Commandant (ret.) Thad Allen described to us as "dogs that hunt"—individuals who are proactive problem solvers. empowered people who share the passion, commitment, instinct, and capacity to get things done.

Guiding and directing behavior from atop the hierarchy, you must recognize that a collaborative, attuned strategy among the senior leaders sets the tone and tenor for the organization. To be sure, problems, differences, and conflicts are likely to emerge among people in charge. The question is whether those differences are readily resolved or, conversely, played out as policy and procedural contests that put lower-ranking personnel at cross-purposes. Operations on the front lines are directly affected by both collaboration and conflict at the highest levels. Whether the state of affairs at the highest levels of the organization is collaboration or conflict, it sets a tone throughout the operation. You must understand this *shadow effect* (Marcus, 1983) and proactively ensure that it is a positive force, enhancing moral and shared purpose throughout the organization.

What if you have not effectively engaged the commitment of your direct followers? It will be awkward and difficult for you to establish credibility in the wider health system if that same quality is not first established in your home base of operations (Romzek, 1990). Your followers serve as ambassadors of your meta-leadership, amplifying your efforts and attitudes as they create their own linkages among counterparts in other departments and organizations. Without their support, it will be difficult to leverage influence and activity beyond the scope of your immediate authority. And of course much of leadership is modeling—displaying thinking, behavior, and action that others not only follow, they mimic. Both strengths and weaknesses are imitated (Hermalin, 1998). A leader's closest colleagues and constituents know him best and often are the arbiters of that leader's climb or fall.

The unity of purpose and reliability of achievement that meta-leadership inspires and coalesces within your direct domain of responsibility form your foundation for work beyond the immediate confines of your official authority and power. The strength or weakness of confidence, direction, and dependability fostered within is what will be communicated to the larger system of influence and action. Those same factors can impress or intimidate your boss, a critical factor for the fourth dimension of meta-leadership.

Dimension Four: Leading Up

With rare exceptions, people who work in organizations have a boss. The chief executive officer of a hospital reports to the board of directors; below the CEO are a series of senior managers who report to him or her and who in turn serve as bosses to their staff. Embedded in the culture of this country—founded through a rebellion against a monarchy—is a reluctance to invest too much power or authority in any one person, to avoid its being exercised for abusive or inappropriate purposes. As a result our culture has in both its public and private sectors a complex system of checks, balances, and oversights that limit the autonomy and autocracy of any one individual. We have bosses but we also have power-limiting laws, rules, and safeguards (Haynes, 1959).

Dimension four—being able to effectively influence those to whom you are accountable—is an important element of exercising wider leadership within a system. Followership, like leadership, is a matter of both rank and behavior (Kellerman, 2008). You will likely not start at the top of the hierarchy. However, by carefully cultivating and managing a productive relationship with your boss, you may be able to leverage extensive influence within the larger system, enjoying a *halo effect* generated by your relationship with your boss. Bosses come to depend on subordinates who have gained their confidence (Kellerman, 2008).

In health care organizations, subject-matter experts—such as chiefs of clinical departments—often report to managers who are responsible for strategic organizational policy direction and decision making. Although a subordinate may or may not know more than her boss, she will often have a perspective on the work at hand that the boss does not. Because they are in closer proximity to that work, subordinates can have a better sense of both real problems on the ground and solutions to address them. This perspective and functional interdependence can be a valuable asset to the boss, because it generates vertical connectivity: the strategic thinking at high levels is in sync with what occurs at the front lines, and problems at the front lines may signal the need to reconsider strategic direction. Much, though, depends on how the information is delivered to the boss and how it is received.

How is this leading up accomplished? Those proficient at meta-leadership are great subordinates: dependable, honest, reliable, and loyal. They validate the power and authority equation, respecting and serving the objectives and proclivities of those in charge. When you do this, you can craft vertical connectivity and stimulate bidirectional feedback. Your influence is built by informing and educating your boss. Bosses vary in style and temperament of course, and you must appreciate that like any other relationship, this one must be carefully and strategically managed (Marcus et al., 2006). When your leading up works well, the boss appreciates your prioritization and management of problems and decisions: he or she is able to focus on the truly important questions and not waste valuable time on distractions. In shaping that focus, you should intentionally and transparently communicate information and a variety of reasonable options in order to contribute to strategic assessment and solution building. The great subordinate manages assumptions, does not promise what cannot be delivered, and ensures that the boss is never surprised. This last point is a sensitive matter. Although bad news and valid criticism are hard to deliver, you must practice telling *truth to power*: anticipating and managing the dangers and distractions of explosive problems. In the best of circumstances, compliments balance criticisms, and both are equally welcomed when honest and deserved (Kotter, 1999).

Sometimes, Iris Inkwater finds she needs to sit alone and think. As much as she appreciates the great people around her, there are times that the greatest clarity comes from solitary reflection. She plops down on the couch in her office, flips off her shoes, and rests her feet on a low glass table. She has her "green book," a journal that she uses for capturing her thoughts and working through vexing challenges. A freshly brewed cup of coffee in her hand, she is ready to think.

"So it was a good retreat," she muses. "Better than expected. The ratio of good talk to hot air was favorable. I performed pretty well. Actually, not bad. Not one faux pas the whole day. The facilitators did their job with aplomb. The participation was robust. Now, what do I do with it? Even better, what would a meta-leader do with it?" She writes that question at the top of the page.

"OK, so there are five dimensions to meta-leadership," she thinks. "A tool box. Like a carpenter's. Focus. So how am I going to reframe this place?" She jots down keywords and phrases as she thinks.

"Dimension one—the person of the meta-leader. That's me and that's also every other person here whom I expect to be on board. We're going to be in the basement—a lot. Every time we see the news there will be another basement dive. Every time we get a new set of financials—to the basement. So I'm going to need to engage my emotional intelligence for the road ahead. Self-awareness: got that. Self-regulation: Mom called that 'poise.' I've got that. Empathy: got to work on that. There will be rough times here, and I need to show people that I care, in their own terms. Motivation: I have to be energized and I have to get other people energized. That I can do; I rally people well. Social skills: I am better at that with people like me than with foreigners, like doctors. When they get arrogant I go to the basement. They live in the basement, which sort of makes sense given what they do with their patients. Doctors, OK, I have to work on the doctors. If they are not with me this whole thing won't work."

"Dimension two—the situation. This is a lousy situation. I hate feeling out of control. Everybody hates feeling out of control. It's a bummer. We are out of control. Anxiety can take over. Back to dimension one. Ouch. So what do we do? First, we have to be objective. We have to see the numbers for what they are. We are going to have to take some of the emotion out of our analysis because it clouds people's capacity to get a good hold on the situation. We have to be more data and dollars driven. Ask tough questions—and then more tough questions. Soften the tone by being curious. We can be in control of our analytical excellence. We can't afford to miscalculate the market, policy trends, demographics, and technology advances. Technology. Why can't they just leave us alone for a few years with all their new machines and software so we can pay off what we've already bought? Oh well, the situation is what it is and we can't wish it away. We just have to drive hard to make sure we are always as accurate as possible in our reading of what's happening. We have to continually gather information and not let lack of some details prevent us from taking action."

"Dimension three—leading my troops. We have many good people here. Unfortunately, not all of them are as productive as we need. We are going to have to make some tough cuts. I will have to make sure that the people we keep on board don't feel vulnerable. I need to support them and let them know that I hear them. They need to know that I will create the conditions that will make them a success. There are a lot of people here who believe in me even after all that we've gone through in recent years. They need to see that I believe in them. I also have to get a hold on the internal fighting that goes on. It can't be tolerated anymore. We are not going to be competitive in the outside market if we are eating each other up inside here. I'll need to invest in training to make sure people have the tools they need to get the job done. They'll appreciate that and it will make them better at what they do. I love feeling that people are loyal to me though I am going to have to earn that by showing them that I am loyal to them. I can do that."

"Dimension four—leading up. Oh, the board of directors: quite a cast of characters. Some of them are great. Thank goodness for Arlan. There are some old-timers too. I always get the feeling that they view all this turmoil in the health market as my fault. As if they were thinking, 'Health care was great before you came along and now look at the mess you've created.' Well, that sage advice I got years ago about educating your board members in order to engage your board members—it's never been truer than now. They have to feel involved without feeling hassled about the details of running this place. I mean, they have to own this bigger problem and the solution because, if they do, my life will be a lot easier. There is no slam dunk, 100 percent solution that is going to make all our troubles go away, and if the board starts mulling over firing me, then my credibility is gone and everything is shot. So I need to be paying attention to that part of my job more than ever before."

"Dimension five—leading across. Connectivity. I'll need it in many ways. First, I need internal connectivity. Meta-leadership has got to be the way we run this place on the inside. Not just talk the talk—walk the talk. We've got to have our internal leaders living and breathing a culture of working together like never before, forging internal linkages, leveraging one another's efforts across departments. If we can build that cohesion internally, the other stuff will come in line. Then I need to think about the outside too. I need a higher profile. I've got to spend a bit more time with folk on the outside, including those political folk—more lunches. *Relationships, relationships, relationships* has to be my new mantra. I need to know what they are thinking and then maybe I can influence some of it as well. Maybe I should do more speaking at Chamber of Commerce meetings and other venues. I need to be a presence in the community. We ought to be better at reaching out to the media. They should be on our side, understanding what we are up against. And then of course there are the naysayers, our resident community of complainers, always ready to give the press a good quote. Maybe this is time to read a line from the book of strange bedfellows. Maybe I need to be more proactive about building alliances, even with our detractors. That would be a good idea. I should remember that old saying, 'Keep your friends close and your enemies closer.' Finally, CHP and Urbania. Ouch, I didn't see that coming. Maybe I need to reframe that whole set of questions. Maybe there are options that none of us have yet considered, options that would shift the whole story. All that stuff at the retreat about new thinking. We have to use our imaginations."

And with that, Inkwater summarizes her notes into a to-do list. She slides her shoes back on her feet and moves back to her desk. She has a new sense of mission in her head and some concrete steps to take. Time to get to work.

There is another important aspect to the fine art of leading up. What if the boss engages in immoral, illicit, or dangerous activity with the expectation that followers will accept what he does without questioning? Herein lies a moral responsibility for followers. Just as the checks-and-balances system works from boss to subordinate, so too must it at times function from subordinate to boss (Kellerman, 2008). Being a good subordinate does not imply passive compliance with inappropriate, unlawful, destructive behavior: it is not blind loyalty. It also at times requires the subordinate to draw the line, bypass immediate bosses, and lead up to bosses above them, or at the extreme, to demonstrate the courage to resign.

It would be difficult if not impossible to practice meta-leadership without the concurrence and support of your boss. Because one function of the boss is to rein in and curb abuses of power, a boss with an overly active subordinate may not only stop the subordinate's activities, he or she may find them threatening to the point of dismissal. An unsympathetic boss could limit the would-be meta-leader's access to outside people. Obstacles and barriers could be erected and worthwhile ideas and proposals could be disparaged.

Conversely, with the boss on your side, you may be able to fashion wide influence throughout the system by virtue of the support and opportunities your boss is able to open to you. This brings up the larger and very sensitive question of who gets the credit and reward. There are some bosses—often those high on the self-confidence continuum—who welcome and encourage a subordinate with valuable ideas and strategies and who will endorse that person's larger presence in the system of influence and impact. That independence and those accomplishments are viewed by such a boss as a testament to your talents and motivations as well as his or her own. Other bosses—obviously those far less secure with their role and presence—prefer to claim sole credit for those ideas and strategies, in order to enhance their own recognition and status on the larger scene. As appropriate to the situation, you may very well conclude that it's best to allow the boss to take the recognition if it advances larger purposes. In other words, you can at times generate significant though quiet influence through the domino effect: having other people join in carrying the ideas and intended impact forward. Most important, you must recognize that you can guide the direction of an organization or system from numerous vantage points, and they are all worth exploring.

Dimension Five: Leading Across the System

When you are building a wide sphere of influence, your vertical, or up and down, linkages need to be complemented by horizontal linkages. By leveraging adjacent centers of expertise and capacity, including resources and assets outside your own organization, you will be able to engage a spectrum of departments and other organizations that can be recruited to your extended network (Ashkenas et al., 2002). This is the added value of meta-leadership: it unlocks the ability to generate a linked, multidimensional thread of interests and involvement among entities that look at a problem from very different yet complementary vantage points. By combining and leveraging these entities' assets and efforts, you can envision and activate more than any one entity can see or do on its own. The connectivity that results may be limited to proximate departments or organizations or may extend more broadly to incorporate constituencies, such as patient groups, that exist beyond the traditional professional and organizational bounds.

Why is this both important and difficult? Often, wide social problems and questions—such as how to improve the health and well-being of a community—demand the engagement of an extensive set of organizations or constituencies. These varied groups will not, on their own, recognize the lines of influence and capacity that they could generate together. In fact they might very well see themselves as being in competition with one another: if credit or benefit falls to one entity more than to another, noble purposes may be undermined by those who ask what's in it for me? For example, early versions of the health care reform legislation passed in 2010 were criticized because a number of senators agreed to support them only after securing sweetheart deals that benefited their individual states. It was only public exposure and the resulting pressure that caused the Senate to remove these provisions from the final legislation. This barrier to collaboration is especially likely to arise when collaboration requires sharing proprietary knowledge or technologies, opening systems or processes, or contributing valuable assets, such as a brand name or staff resources, that are viewed as a source of competitive advantage. You can exert meta-leadership to focus the attention of a wide set of constituencies on the shared purposes of a shared mission while at the same time tempering those forces of suspicion and jealousy that constrain the achievement of those purposes (Marcus et al., 2006).

How is this accomplished? Aligning disparate yet complementary cognitive spheres into a unified plan of action requires that you first be keen to identify and understand the intrinsic interests and motives that each organization or constituency has in generating a connectivity of thinking and action. Each entity must be recognized for its unique profile of needs, experiences, and contributions to the shared enterprise. Although it is common for any set of people to focus on their differences and conflicts, you must turn their attention to their points of agreement: shared values, aspirations, objectives, and circumstances. Following the example of step 2 of the Walk in the Woods, in which self-interests are expanded to discover agreed-upon enlarged interests, turn *what's in it for me* into *what's in it for us*. With a new appreciation for their points of commonality, stakeholders will be able to creatively envisage what they could accomplish if they were to join forces, building new equations and strategies centering on common ground and achievement. Actions speak louder than words, and early triumphs are a critical factor in demonstrating the value added of working together.

Your first meta-leadership challenge is defining what working together looks like, along with its benefits, and why it is urgent to act now (Kotter, 1996). To be effective as a meta-leader you must influence and engage the many different entities that are to be linked into the envisioned shared enterprise. The people representing each entity must be moved by the powerful advantages of acting in concert and by the enlarged possibilities generated by working together. The compelling message, if effective, influences, perhaps inspires, and certainly engages the many different people that are to be linked into the shared effort. The purpose of the effort must appeal to *logos, ethos,* and *pathos*—to the reasoning and logic, to the character and credibility, and to emotions, motivations, and convictions of those who will be involved. People must be convincingly moved by the powerful advantages of a wider purview for a problem of mutual concern and by the possibilities generated by working together to solve it.

Likewise they must be assured that individual stakeholders will "stay in their lanes," avoiding any tendency to veer into another's areas of responsibility or authority, a move that would raise competitive ire and ruin opportunities for collaboration. In pragmatic terms, each stakeholder must accept three discrete propositions: (1) its own distinctness: what it does exclusively or least differently in relation to other stakeholders; (2) others' distinctness: what it doesn't do and someone else does do; and (3) collaborative possibility: what all stakeholders might be able to do together to address system gaps—critical tasks or topics not belonging to any one entity—and objectives that no one entity can achieve independently. This role clarity reduces both collisions among those involved and chasms where no one is involved. Once established, clear role delineation translates into less attention devoted to competitive forays and more energy directed at what can be done together (Hughes, Ginnett, & Curphy, 2006). The possibilities are expanded, and with that, so too is the capacity to satisfy more appetites.

Push-back and resistance are to be expected in fashioning this new alignment of strategy and action. There are many hurdles to overcome. Chief among them is egocentric opposition from potential collaborators, which may take the form of a *silo mentality* or a *turf battle* (Hughes et al., 2006). Bureaucratic organizations characteristically reward internally focused leaders who simply build the budget, authority, and autonomy of their own endeavors (Thompson, 1965). The potential for creating cross-cutting benefit is curtailed when different areas, or silos, that could be working together see themselves merely as competitors (Schuman, 2006). Building collaboration does not require—as is often heard—tearing down the silos. In fact silos have important functions. Training, practice, and professional advancement occur and new knowledge and skills develop in the concentrated environment of the silo. There is so much to know and to do that no one person or group of people can do it all. Strong silos not only foster proficiency in complex work environments; they also offer a modicum of familiarity and comfort that can be reassuring, especially during periods of high stress or crisis. Connecting and empowering silos is a far more encouraging way to characterize what the meta-leader hopes to accomplish in shaping constructive flows of information and lines of coordinated activity.

The introduction of collaboration, however, may require some traditionally antagonistic constituencies to turn away from well-entrenched attitudes about and behaviors toward one another. When such conflict is anticipated and planned for, it is far less likely to undermine the shared purposes (Yukl, 2002). You should expect such conflict and respond to it by crafting an alternate reward structure that acknowledges and encourages work that builds shared solutions. This reward structure should reflect and amplify the central message or theme of your meta-leadership work and should speak to what can be accomplished if these traditional rivalries and conflicts can be replaced by the advantages of the shared enterprise.

Cohesion of action will not begin in the moment a critical decision is made: it must be embedded into the thinking and activity of organizations and people before they must collaborate during a critical situation. This is a purpose and mission you can undertake as part of your meta-leadership. It is akin to carefully crafting interlocking gears so that when it is time to move, the cogs will link in a way that ensures movement and not stasis. To put it another way, creating cross-system connectivity requires strategic and methodical design and construction so that both the process and the outcome of the effort attest to the value and benefits of striving toward common purposes. As stakeholders experience the demonstrable advantages of leveraging the expertise and capacity of others, and as they recognize the added influence gained when their contributions are likewise leveraged by others, impact and collaborative value both rise. And with that initial success, you must recognize that to keep the connected effort on track, it must be carefully monitored and adjusted so it perseveres beyond the expected bumps and challenges and remains current with new developments.

Connectivity: The Work of Meta-Leadership

As should now be apparent, the critical work and distinctive benefit of meta-leadership is in forging a strategic connectivity for coordinated effort among stakeholders, reaching past the usual bounds of isolated organizational thinking and operating. This connectivity needs to be carefully orchestrated among the distinct groups that are involved in an endeavor and that must be intentionally assembled, shaped, and linked. In such a connected enterprise, each individual and organizational unit, whether part of your group's organizational chart or of your extended network, is aware of his, her, or its particular role in any ongoing whole image negotiation. There are a number of critical questions: How do we define success and encourage it across the organizational spectrum? What are the critical dependencies? How will information, resources, and assets flow? How will interests and incentives be optimally aligned to achieve mutually beneficial solutions? How will rewards be distributed? It is up to the meta-leader to compose a compelling, integrated picture and message, engage each actor, and chart the impact they will together achieve (Dorn, Savoia, Testa, Stoto, & Marcus, 2007).

Connectivity is fundamentally a very human process: people sharing a common and compelling purpose that blends their organizational allegiances with their commitment to a purpose that can be achieved only when different groups of people are working together. Igniting this process requires a strategic view of who needs to be involved and what will motivate their participation. People moved by your vision and message are inspired and empowered to reach out beyond the confines of their particular roles. They create linkages with others that enable a potential that would not otherwise be present. When they then embed those connections in their institutions, the connections can remain active beyond the tenure of the individuals initially involved. These people-to-people and organization-to-organization linkages overcome the barriers and gaps imposed by strict silo thinking. Whereas organizational structures can mold and confine the behavior of people in roles and procedures, people—when intentionally connected—can find ways to combine their efforts to achieve an impact that they all value and could not accomplish individually. This does not necessarily imply that rules are broken. It is more that rules may be seen as levers to make positive things happen. This process describes the difference between succumbing to obstacles and seeking out opportunities.

When connectivity is achieved, individuals and the entities in which they work are better able to leverage one another. They can do more because they have a wider scope of resources at their disposal. Information is more readily available, expertise is more widely accessible, and tangible assets are more generously shared. Competition as a primary motivator is reduced because success is less about prevailing in a turf battle and more about achieving the overriding goals of the shared enterprise (Dorn, Savoia, Testa, Stoto, & Marcus, 2007).

As we have tracked adoption of meta-leadership across complex public and private organizational systems and networks, we have found three important advantages. Meta-leadership encourages (1) thinking in terms of intentional networking and cohesion beyond formal organizational boundaries (and developing a vocabulary that fosters such thinking), in order to connect the purposes and work of different stakeholders; (2) adopting a purposeful strategy of action designed to advance coordinated planning and activity; and (3) supporting a compelling mission, one that can be a rallying cry for both leaders and followers—inspiring, guiding, and instructing, and ultimately setting a higher standard and expectation for performance and impact. Meta-leadership as a practice framework is outcome driven, building a broad connectivity of effort and thereby enabling a wider scope of achievement.

Organizational forms evolve to better meet the needs of the marketplace, the community, or a wide social purpose—so too must leadership styles and methods. For the first three-quarters of the twentieth century, command-and-control models dominated both management and leadership in Western countries, in part because many individuals in the managerial class shared the experience of military service. It was a familiar model with centuries-old roots. With the growth of information technology, industry restructuring, and globalization, however, health care organizations have become flatter, work has become more team centered, and multiple organizations have been linked in new and novel value chains.

The command-and-control model does not function well in the current environment when used alone. Relationships today are highly collaborative, are often guided by general principles as much as contractual requirements, and require commitment to an enlarged set of self-interests. The meta-leadership model and framework are well suited to the work of health care, as much of that work is built on trust and influence more than formal authority. Additionally, even formal leadership within large organizations has become more distributed as layers of management are shed, self-organizing teams are formed, and employees are challenged to find new solutions and provide checks and balances rather than simply executing orders.

As he crowds into an elevator with the masses of people going to various city offices in the civic center, Fred Fisher looks at his watch. "With any luck I'll be back in my office in two hours," he thinks. He presses the button for the top floor where the commissioner's conference room is located. At each stop along the way, more parents with crying babies, shuffling seniors, and other form-carrying citizens, dreading inevitable lines, exit the cab, until it is finally quiet for the last leg of the ascent. Once on the top floor Fisher pauses briefly at the hand sanitizer dispenser and rubs some of the gel vigorously into his palms, steeling himself for the meeting.

Fisher has not met Mendez in person but has seen him on TV and spoken with him on the phone. He expects more grandstanding than action. "Medicine would be better off without meddling politicians," he thinks.

Fisher announces himself to the assistant in the outer office and sits down to peruse a dated magazine. Within moments Mendez strides energetically out of his inner sanctum and both shakes Fisher's hand and grasps his elbow. "Dr. Fisher, I am delighted that you are able to join us! Let's go meet the others." As they walk together to the conference room it is evident that Mendez has done his homework. He remarks that he has a cousin who attended Fisher's medical school alma mater and asks a question about a journal article that Fisher had coauthored the previous year. Fisher notices that Mendez gives an engaging greeting to each person attending the gathering.

Arriving at the seat marked with his name placard, Fisher unbuttons his tweed jacket. Sitting next to him is a young woman adorned in vibrant jewelry and wearing blue jeans. "Had I known this was going to be a cookout," he thinks, "I would have come more appropriately dressed." The woman is talking animatedly with someone on her other side, and he has a chance to check out the others sitting around the conference table. He looks for a familiar face and seeing none, glances again at his watch.

He is trying to look absorbed in the information packet at his place when his neighbor turns around unexpectedly and places her hand out to shake his. "Dr. Fisher, my name is Melinda Martin. It is a pleasure to finally meet you. I've really been looking forward to this."

"Well, it's a pleasure to meet you, Ms. Martin."

"My mother, Pam Martin, has been a patient of yours for years," Martin continues. "She talks about you all the time. She says she owes her life to you. I'll tell you a secret. She's a very spiritual woman. She says a prayer for you every morning."

She is smiling ear to ear, and Fisher finds it infectious. "Well, that's wonderful to hear, Melinda. Your mother is a wonderful woman, one of my favorite patients. Please send her my regards. Tell me, what are you doing on this committee?"

"I direct the Harborside Youth Action League: H-Y-A-L, or as we say, 'Hi y'all.' I've been there about five years. Our center is in a rough part of town, and we have a lot of programs that are really making a difference in the community. Teenage pregnancy, HIV/AIDS education, violence—you name it, we have a project going." Though Martin had once stood up without an ounce of fear to a kid who brought a handgun into the center, she is nervous talking to Dr. Fisher. She continues, "Our staff motto is 'We work *with* the kids.' The kids are involved in everything. We do a lot of leadership development, and the kids are responding. Believe it or not, we even have a college prep club. My kid brother is in it. He says he wants to get into med school and be a doctor just like you. So there you go, Dr. Fisher!"

"Well, that's wonderful. It sounds like you are doing splendid work. Where do you get the money to keep the league going?"

"We scrounge. I get a little money for one project over here, a little money for another project over there. The city gave us the building, though we had to put together the money to rehab it. Money is my big headache. The tragedy is that the kids and my staff have loads of great ideas they would like to get off the ground. I want to bring in a grief counselor who is an expert in helping kids get through tough times when they lose someone, especially if it was through violence. I want to start a photography workshop. I've got room for a nurse or doctor to sit in the center for a few hours a week—the kids asked for it. Great ideas, and without moolah, they're just great ideas."

Mendez takes his place at the head of the table and calls the meeting to order. He personally introduces each person at the table, describing each person's purpose on the committee. Fisher is touched by Mendez's comments, though he is wary of the commissioner's hope for the medical community's support and involvement in the community health initiative. Support is easy, but what would involvement mean? OMC's plate is already full. What more can it do? If Mendez wants money, Fisher would be happy to write him out a personal check for $100 right on the spot. Maybe that can be his exit ticket he thinks, with a slight smile.

As the meeting unfolds it becomes more intriguing and involving than Fisher ever imagined it would be. There are some captivating ideas, and Fisher surprises himself by jumping into the discussion. Placing nursing students and medical residents into the community is listed as one of the community health program's action plans. The King Foundation is offering financing for community-based medical education. Fisher is particularly attracted to this idea. He thinks it will be great to move some residency training into the community, especially into a place like HYAL. With the hospital census down, there have been comments about the residents' not being busy enough. It would be a good idea to expose them to health care experiences outside the hospital. The nursing school dean is also interested in the proposal. Nursing students could do some clinical work and also help with health education. He will talk it up at the next medical school department meeting.

Fisher is also captivated by the notion of a health profession internship for neighborhood kids. For his own children and those of his friends, the thought of a medical career is not unusual because they see their parents or friends' parents in these roles. Harborside kids' experience of people working in a health care setting is probably limited to technicians and food service workers. Yet if they were to enter the medical professional field, their background and experience could make them enormously helpful in community public health. He promises to discuss the idea with Iris Inkwater. He likes the thought of bringing something tangible back to her so she'll quit nagging him about community involvement, and he is genuinely enthusiastic about the idea.

After the meeting, Fisher rides down in the elevator with Melinda Martin. Before they part company, he again asks her to send his regards to her mother.

Settling into his car for the ride back to the medical center, he realizes something changed for him during that meeting. He isn't sure exactly what it is.

Conclusion

In the complex web that is health care, extraordinary individuals emerge. These people are able to create greater value by balancing and leveraging the expectations, needs, resources, and contributions of all of the stakeholders in the extended enterprise. Through their strength of character and keen analytical skills, along with their ability to lead, influence, follow, and engage others, they are able to forge both impact and collaboration that would otherwise not have been achieved.

These meta-leaders—who as a type certainly predate this model that seeks to describe them—deserve further attention and regard so that their important work and their example can be better appreciated and supported and so that their strategies can be adopted and replicated by others.

This chapter has described a framework that can help you find your path to be one of these extraordinary individuals. The practice of meta-leadership enables you to galvanize others through your capacity to articulate and achieve extended vertical and horizontal linkages, appealing to more than just personal gain or parochial organizational interests in order to achieve important outcomes representing shared interests. Through meta-leadership you can convincingly define a higher purpose—making the case that by acting above, beyond, and across the confines of their own organizational entities, individuals and groups will accomplish more and function with less friction. Over time, the work in which each is involved will be far more rewarding.

PART FOUR

EVOLVING HEALTH CARE PRACTICE

CHAPTER 11

DESIGNING A MORE COHESIVE, BETTER-LINKED HEALTH SYSTEM

July 30, 1965, and March 23, 2010, were two landmark dates for health care in the United States, separated by forty-five years. On the first date, President Lyndon Johnson signed the Social Security Act of 1965, an amendment to existing Social Security legislation that established the Medicare program and marked the beginning of an entitlement to government-funded health service for millions of elderly and disabled people. On the second date, President Barack Obama signed the Patient Protection and Affordable Care Act, marking the beginning of a series of changes in access to health insurance along with changes in financing, health services, health profession education, and public health initiatives intended to unfold over the decade to follow. In retrospect the extraordinary innovations launched by the 1965 law are relatively clear. As of this writing, what the 2010 law will mean and how exactly it will unfold are still unknown.

It is evident though that there will be a decade or more of significant redesign of the U.S. health system, a period begging for effective negotiation, renegotiation, and meta-leadership so that this redesign will—it is hoped—result in an infrastructure that better meets the needs and the spending tolerance of the American public.

Unless otherwise noted, quotations and summaries of comments from Donald Berwick, Mary Bylone, Christopher Crow, Eddie Erlandson, George Halvorson, Richard Iseke, Mitchell Rabkin, Scott Ransom, and Andy M. Wiesenthal are taken from interviews conducted by the authors in 2009 and 2010.

Systems Thinking, Acting, and Results

In the United States, the manner in which health care is provided is euphemistically called a *system*. The debate about whether it is or is not hinges on how well the different pieces are believed to be connected. Those who would argue that it is not a system point to the independent and disconnected management of services, the fiercely entrepreneurial development of devices and pharmaceuticals, and the divide between those who pay for and those who receive care. To the extent that the pieces making up health care operate independently of one another, health care as we know it is not a system but rather a disjointed set of services, payers, populations, patients, and professionals. The more disconnected the people, organizations, and money are, the less likely the country will be to achieve the quality, access, and health improvements envisioned and the opportunities presented by the 2010 health reform bill and other initiatives. For each modification to leverage a larger transformation—and significant transformation is exactly what is envisioned and required—the components of health care must be linked in such a way that one motion can purposefully and intentionally cause another. One cannot activate a true transformation if all of the pieces are not carefully and deliberately considered, including their interactions and interdependencies.

For health care to meet both the challenges and the aspirations of a new era—producing a nation that is healthier, that enjoys high-quality health care services when needed, and that does all this at a balanced cost—what we call the health care system must operate more fully as a truly integrated endeavor. To clarify what this might look like in practical terms, this chapter presents the experiences and observations of health care leaders whose thinking about what has been and what might be can inform our vision for the future of health care in this country.

Donald M. Berwick is a professor at the Harvard School of Public Health (HSPH), president and CEO of the Institute for Healthcare Improvement, and a longtime advocate for integrating systems thinking into health care. He was named in July 2010 by President Obama to lead the federal Center for Medicare and Medicaid Services. In October 2009, he delivered the Dr. Herbert Sherman Memorial Lecture at the HSPH, beginning his talk by quoting a passage from an article he had written in 1991. It powerfully articulates the interdependencies in health care and the consequences that vary with the ability to master these interdependencies. It is just as relevant now as it was when it was first written.

> Kim, aged 3 years, lies asleep, waiting for a miracle. Outside her room, the nurses on the night shift pad softly through the half-lighted corridors, stopping to count breaths, take pulses, or check intravenous pumps. In the morning,

> Kim will have her heart fixed. She will be medicated and wheeled into the operating suite. Machines will take on the functions of her body: breathing and circulating blood. The surgeons will place a small patch over a hole within her heart, closing off a shunt between her ventricles that would, if left open, slowly kill her.
>
> Kim will be fine if the decision to operate on her was correct; if the surgeon is competent; if that competent surgeon happens to be trained to deal with the particular anatomic wrinkle that is hidden inside Kim's heart; if the blood bank cross-matched her blood accurately and delivered it to the right place; if the blood gas analysis machine works properly and on time; if the suture does not snap; if the plastic tubing of the heart-lung machine does not suddenly spring loose; if the recovery room nurses know that she is allergic to penicillin; if the "oxygen" and "nitrogen" lines in the anesthesia machine have not been reversed by mistake; if the sterilizer temperature gauge is calibrated so that the instruments are in fact sterile; if the pharmacy does not mix up two labels; and if when the surgeon says urgently, "Clamp, right now," there is a clamp on the tray.
>
> If all goes well, if ten thousand "ifs" go well, then Kim may sing her grandchildren to sleep some day. If not, she will be dead by noon tomorrow [Berwick, 1991].

What does it take to achieve this extraordinarily intricate connectivity of thinking and action? In Berwick's words, "Optimizing parts is not a path to system excellence." A major source of medical errors, for example, is mistakes made during handoffs between shifts, between departments, and between institutions.

Being intentional and deliberate about these handoffs and other linkages demands a template for thinking about health and health care that is different from what currently prevails. It also requires a concomitant set of shared frames to guide everyday work. The specific linkages, or points of interaction, are matters of everyday negotiation, and the template of thinking that can successfully guide this negotiation is a theme for compelling meta-leadership.

These points of interaction are also rife with potential conflict and demand effective conflict resolution. Scott Ransom, a physician and the president of the University of North Texas Health Science Center in Fort Worth, notes that systems are often made up of parts that were once independent. Although bringing them together into an integrated system can make logical sense, the people associated with these formerly independent units may retain diverse, passionately held viewpoints on numerous issues of control, authority, and responsibility.

Iris Inkwater has always liked the number seven: there are seven days in a week; seven is more than five and clearly nowhere near ten; and an odd number is convenient for breaking a tie. She wants to continue to build the momentum that resulted from the successful retreat, and she has decided to form a ''kitchen cabinet'' to help her do it. Thinking about who would be the right six people to join with her, she decides to call on Arlan Abbington, Fred Fisher, Janice Johnson, Perry Pudolski, Rajeev Rao, and Larry Lumberg. Though Lumberg's official rank as medical director of the emergency department is not as high up the leadership ladder as the others' titles, he has a good read on the medical center and people respect his opinion. Whatever comes next, Lumberg will have to be behind it.

Early in the morning on the following Tuesday, Inkwater has them all sitting at a table in her office. She's ready to get to work. There is a large whiteboard affixed to the wall on the far side of her office. It is shiny clean except for the words ''The New Oppidania Medical Center'' printed in bold letters at the top. Inkwater opens the meeting by pointing to these words: ''What is this?'' she asks. The group members sit in silence, both pondering the question and trying to figure out what to say. No one is quite sure of her intention, and everyone wants to avoid saying something silly.

Dr. Fred Fisher, Oppidania's medical director, finally gives in to his impatience. ''I'm not sure what you are asking, Iris. Perhaps I am speaking for my silent colleagues as well. I mean, we have a set of values and principles that have guided us and made us the respected institution that we are today. There is a lot of noise in the health care world right now. I am not sure that we want to be distracted by it and abandon all that we have accomplished. Yes, there are things we can no doubt adjust to get us more in line with reimbursement incentives. But I don't know that the community wants a *new* Oppidania. They count on us to deliver on our tradition and reputation for excellence. What are you driving at?''

Inkwater grips her pen and tells herself not to respond. It will be better today to listen, to see how others will reply. Though disappointed, she is not particularly surprised by Fisher's words. She knows that he represents the sentiments of many, and she has to learn how to handle and lead through those apprehensions.

Lumberg speaks up: ''Fred, I'm not sure I agree with you. I think Iris is trying to challenge us here. Without getting caught up in words, I think we have to transition from an accidental attitude to an intentional design for how we run this hospital. We simply have not been careful about aligning what we do here to ensure that we get both the most efficiency and the most effectiveness from our workflow. Everyone does 'their thing' and passively assumes that it somehow lines up with what everyone else is doing. When it works, that's terrific. When it doesn't, no one really bears the responsibility. It is the patient or the budget that suffers. If we took the notion of intentional design really seriously, it would be a new phenomenon for us. That said, we should not underestimate how hard it will be to make the change. Yet given all that is going on in health care today—the insurance market, the demographics, the new technologies—I don't really think we have a choice."

Janice Johnson, the VP for nursing, has been taking careful notes. Now she looks up. "Larry, I think you're right about the importance of being intentional though you're missing something important. We have been intentional though you may have not noticed all the intentionality that is already in place. While you doctors are doing your thing, we nurses maintain a steady framework in the background that keeps everything in place and moving along, straight from admission to discharge. We can't afford to be accidental. There is too much to do and too few people to do it. We always have to pay attention to what we are doing and figuring out how to do it better."

"So this is perhaps the first hurdle to overcome," CFO Rajeev Rao interjects. "If, Janice, you see a systematic framework and, Larry, you don't, then that's where some work needs to be done. I think parts of our organization are intentionally designed and parts are not. We can't afford that. It's not good for our patients, it's not good for our bottom line, and it detracts from our strength in the marketplace."

Board chair Arlan Abbington sees an opening and enters the conversation. "Let's look at what's happened in other industries. Maybe there will be lessons for health care. The airline industry went through cataclysmic change. The old-time and respected legacy airlines were stuck in their comfortable ways and could not or would not adjust. New and aggressively opportunistic players came into the market. These new airlines had lower operating costs and offered lower fares; they were more customer oriented, more nimble. The old-timers are still around but they have great financial difficulties. The same thing happened with the automobile industry. Foreign manufacturers had a better read on the market and produced what people would buy. American carmakers lagged behind and saw their market share deteriorate. I think Iris is right. Health care is at one of those major inflection points, and we have to be thinking in new terms or else we'll be left behind. What's going on in our insurance market here is a wake-up call, and we ignore it at our peril."

COO Perry Pudolski has been sitting quietly, sipping coffee, and following the conversation. Finally, he joins in. "Arlan, you miss something in your analogy. Yes, the airlines that nudged themselves into the travel market were in fact new. They appear to be nimble because they were able to start from scratch. They had new planes that were cheaper to run, no pension or other long-standing obligations to their workforces, and they reset service expectations downward. You'd be hard pressed to find anyone who finds flying enjoyable any more. The same could be said for some of the foreign automakers. Because they have lower legacy costs, they've been able to more quickly adapt. We have been around here for a long time and have ingrained ways of doing things. Iris, I think you're right," he says, turning to her, "it would be a great luxury to be, as you say, *new*. That would make things a lot easier. In fact though, I think we're going to face many of the same obstacles as those legacy airlines and domestic automakers." His voice rises in intensity. "We have a ton of tradition mixed with bad habits and, excuse me, privileged attitudes among some here. It would take a veritable revolution to clean our house of all that."

Pudolski has a way of speaking his mind without considering how that bluntness might offend others.

Fred Fisher is blunt in his own right and refuses to let this sit. "First, we are not an airline and we don't produce cars. We are a medical care system. Sick and dying people come here for a cure. And we do a darn good job of getting that for them. That is the reason people fly us and drive us. It's not for the peanuts and not the miles per gallon. If we somehow lose that central precept, then we'll be in real trouble." He taps his forefinger forcefully against the conference table. "I am all for finding ways to do better caring and curing. I am just afraid that the solution is going to be given over to some management efficiency consultant who doesn't understand medicine and who is going to pare us down and ruin the very things that make us great. I've seen it happen in other places, and it's demoralizing and detrimental to the purposes of an institution like ours. I think we have to be extraordinarily careful."

Lumberg feels that the conversation is getting off track. "I think we're missing the point. Look, I see this institution from a very telling perch, the emergency department. If we were a fine-tuned organization, it would be clearly evident in the way patients moved through the ED and into receptive departments upstairs. It's not evident because our process simply does not work that well. We are like a big, cumbersome machine in which the gears don't line up. Getting things done is more difficult, more time consuming, and takes more work than it should. There are inefficiencies and missed calls when it comes to patient care—and those must be remedied. I appreciate your point, Arlan, about the airline and car industries. I think, though, we're going to have to carve our own unique path to figuring out how to survive and then thrive in a new health care market. And I don't believe we're going to get there by congratulating ourselves or debating who has got it right and who hasn't. It's going to take an intentional process if we are going to achieve an intentional outcome. Janice, believe me, I know what you are doing in nursing to cover our backs. If there is glue holding this place together, it is and has been nursing, and we have to better link your sensibilities to ours as physicians. Where I do agree with you, Arlan, is that if we don't do this, we could very well find ourselves irrelevant. I don't want to see the Oppidania Medical Center on a list with TWA and Pan Am of once-great brand names. Other health care organizations are going to rise to the challenge. We are seeing consolidations, integrations, downsizings, and retoolings—and also collapses—all across the country. We can't pretend we have some sort of immunity. If we really believe that we have something special here, the test of that belief will be whether we can corral ourselves and work together to meet the challenge of taking what we have to the next level."

Inkwater has been intently absorbing all of these perspectives. Now she takes a deep breath and speaks, choosing her words carefully. "Believe it or not, I'm happy to hear such spirited discussion. I brought you together this morning because I believe that together you represent some of the key thinking in this medical center. I also thought that if it turned out that we had instant consensus, it would mean only that we weren't thinking hard enough. It is not that one of you is right and the others are wrong. Fred, what you say is true. We are a great organization and we have to figure out how to retain that. However, the world around us is changing. Janice, we are doing many things right, and we can learn from how we do them and also learn how we can do them better. Arlan, you speak to my deepest fears—that we will fall victim to our own rigidity. Rajeev, we do need therefore to do a lot of rethinking. Perry, I sympathize with what you say. It would be easier to start from scratch, but we don't have that luxury. So, Larry, what you see from your perch, and your willingness to articulate that, says a lot. We have to find a way to make this work. We have to be leaders and even meta-leaders to recalibrate this organization in a health care market that is moving a million miles an hour. And what you said is true, Larry: we have to build a process well matched with what we hope to achieve."

Inkwater glances up to the whiteboard and continues. "The word *new* was chosen to be provocative. We should not miss the fact that we have incorporated many changes here in the past decade. The hospitalist program started as a small experiment and now has grown significantly. It has had a positive impact on our metrics for length of stay, patient satisfaction, and quality of care. We have been working with our medical practices to make accountable care the normal course of business. I have no doubt that we are flexible and opportunistic enough to try adding new elements that will continue our pace of constructive and valuable change. At this point though, I think we need more than that."

She stands and walks to the whiteboard. "By *new* I mean a new organizing concept. Let's start with the patient experience. Let's say we organize ourselves around the patient rather than organizing ourselves around our departments, our professions, or our areas of expertise. That was the lesson, Arlan, that I took from all those successful insurgents in other industries. They asked themselves, 'What problem is the customer trying to solve, and how can we help her solve it?' Our problem though as a health care business—and we are a business among many other things—is that we have many customers and they all have very different expectations. The patient obviously is a customer. Private insurers are customers, and they also have customers in the form of companies who expect the insurers to manage their health care costs. And the government is a customer, with the power of both the dollar and the ability to regulate. I think the picture we stare at is so complex and so chaotic that we could just give up, we could make small adjustments, and then we could go back to our comfort zone, fighting to keep doing what we have been doing because it offers some degree of gratification."

"However, I think that we have the smarts here at OMC to get beyond that complexity. What I am suggesting is using the patient experience as our true north, as a guiding star that informs how we organize and deal with each other, with payers, and with all of our other stakeholders. I think that we will mold something that is, yes, *new* and different. I can't tell you exactly what it will look like, but we need an organizing principle that links what our patients want, what our payers demand, and where new technology and changing demographics are taking us. I think we'll find a new logic and a whole set of exciting opportunities. I believe in us; I think we can do it, though we are going to have to think, operate, and then commit to new ways. And that is what I mean by *The New Oppidania Medical Center*."

Everyone around the table stares at her, frozen in inspired silence. Finally, Fisher speaks up: "Iris, I am not sure I understand everything you said, but your passion is palpable. I will say though that what you said intrigued me, like a puzzle that I want to figure out and solve. As a clinician I'm attracted to the idea of using the patient experience as the 'true north,' as you put it, that can guide the entire organization." There are smiles and nods of agreement around the table, and the meeting ends with an agreement to convene again in a week. The group breaks up noisily, with conversations about the patient experience continuing as people disperse.

Physician Mitchell Rabkin led Beth Israel Hospital (now Beth Israel Deaconess Medical Center) in Boston for three decades as it grew from a community institution to a leading medical center. During his years in this prominent health care leadership position, he found a common theme in efforts to reform and improve the system: "Most of what we hear deals with symptoms. We have to ask: what is the pathology underlying those symptoms?" What if we were to think of the system itself as a patient? What pathology must we deal with in order to create a health system that delivers cost-effective, timely, high-quality, and satisfying health care?

Eddie Erlandson, a former vascular surgeon and chief of staff at St. Joseph Mercy Hospital in Ann Arbor, Michigan, and coauthor of *Alpha Male Syndrome* (Ludeman & Erlandson, 2006), put the issue of reform to us as a simple question: "Health care has not improved nearly as dramatically as our knowledge about medicine and the body or our technical capacity to diagnose and treat. Why?"

The U.S. health system has evolved through a muddled series of events rather than a linear or cohesive process: entitlement programs and legislation emerge from the politics of health care, market forces shape the business of health care, and research and technology drive actual medical practice toward protocol-based medicine. The development of research methodologies and the improvement of practice capacity have progressed far more methodically than have the politics, the business, or the shifting population trends that also affect health care. It is this disequilibrium that has produced the extraordinary incongruities in our health care infrastructure and that health reform efforts hope to overcome. For example, even though expensive treatment regimens have the potential to transform previously terminal conditions—such as lung cancer—into chronic illnesses, more than forty million people across the country have been excluded from these advances because they lacked health insurance and could not easily gain access to affordable care (Newport & Mendes, 2009). Furthermore we have yet to distinguish those whose quality of life can benefit from medical intervention from those whose condition is so dire that only palliative care is warranted. When the pieces do not logically fit together, incongruities persist.

Models for Systems Thinking and Organization

How does one incorporate systems thinking and operations into different types of health service settings? To encourage the sort of creative thinking that is at the heart of whole image negotiation, later in this chapter we profile two health providers who have devised very different models for building their systems. Their differences and the ways they have adapted illustrate the range of options available to the processes of true health reform. One, the Kaiser Permanente Health Care System, serves more than eight million members across nine states and the District of Columbia. The other, Legacy Medical Village in Plano, Texas, serves a few thousand patients in the suburbs north of Dallas. One employs more than 14,000 physicians; the other fewer than 10 in its core practice. Although these two systems are at opposite ends of a spectrum in scale, they share a vision and passion for redefining health care and they are both masters of health care delivery integration.

In the rest of this section, we set the scene for these examples with a brief review of the concepts and practice of integration and systems thinking.

From a design perspective, integration is conceptually straightforward: fashion individual components to fit together as perfectly as possible, and minimize friction to optimize desired outcomes. If you were to go about the task of creating and building a picture puzzle, you would first sketch or select a picture and then cut the individual pieces from it, so that these parts interlock and the original image reappears when they are assembled. One aspect of this process is having a clear initial image: What is it that your health system hopes to achieve? Is it health promotion, disease treatment, care delivery, or some combination of these or other services? What is your marketplace demanding? If that image is not clear, the pieces of your puzzle will not fit together. There will be a lot of friction and conflict.

One branch of *systems thinking* emerged from the field of engineering (Bertalanffy, 1968). Take, for example, a machine found in many hospitals and clinics, the magnetic resonance imaging (MRI) machine. The engineers who design this complex piece of equipment employ a systems approach to devise and build a machine that produces high-quality images while being easy to operate, reliable, comfortable, and affordable. Each of the components is carefully chosen and crafted—from the magnets to the display screens to the padding on the bed on which the patient rests—with careful attention to how they will work with one another and how the operation of each affects the overall end result. Linked to the engineers are the marketers who have assessed what purchasers are shopping for, because customers vary and having the best MRI but no customers willing to purchase it does not serve the purposes of the manufacturer. One portion of the market may be looking for affordability, another for patient comfort, and yet a third for its compactness. Each of these is a valid consideration, and it will be to the engineers to determine how many different objectives can be incorporated into a design. Once chosen, the objectives will be prioritized, and those priorities will inform a multitude of decisions in design, purchasing, manufacturing, marketing, and distribution. When all these elements from design through distribution are well linked, what emerges off the assembly line is a marketable product.

One might disagree with the notion of importing systems thinking into the lexicon of health care practices. It is after all a method that appears at first to be more about engineering and manufacturing than it is about the humane provision of care. A systems appreciation (Deming, 1986) of the provision of care, however, is simply an understanding of all of the interacting processes and entities that add something to or take something from that which we call health care. Indeed W. Edwards Deming, known most widely as an authority on quality improvement, held that "all people are different" but that "the performance of anyone is governed largely by the system that he works in" (Deming, 2000). Deming's work has been applied to health care by Donald Berwick and others.

The push-back against systems thinking has come from those who see medicine more as art than as a mechanistic set of steps. They are concerned that imposing this line of thought will discourage the creative exploration and inspired discovery that yielded medicine's most important breakthroughs. Furthermore, they fear that this method serves only to dehumanize the people working in and receiving health care. Health care, it is argued, is not manufacturing. A hospital is not an assembly line. Doctors are not robots. Patients are not products: every individual is unique. We're talking about people, not widgets!

This is all true. However, revisiting Kim's story, related earlier in this chapter, it is evident that many parts of the care process should not vary from patient to patient: the degree of sterilization of the instruments, the gas that comes out of the valves marked "oxygen" and "nitrogen," the cross-matching of blood—variance in any of these will increase the likelihood of a bad outcome for this young girl or any other patient. The question is how do you maintain this uniformity while also maintaining flexibility in those services that are best when customized to the unique circumstances of an individual patient?

Process, or routine, is not necessarily the enemy. Although some regard processes as a source of rigidity—the cause of hardening of the organizational arteries—they are essential to any organization (Stene, 1940; March & Simon, 1958; Cyert & March, 1963; Thompson, 1965; Nelson & Winter, 1982, cited in Feldman & Pentland, 2003); moreover, they can also be a source of flexibility and change simply through their ongoing performance (Feldman & Pentland, 2003).

Systems Thinking and Variations

Systems experience two kinds of variation: intentional and unintentional. In health care, *intentional variation* is a response to the uniqueness of each human body and medical condition. For example, Kim's heart may have some distinctive characteristic that prompts the surgeon to vary her procedure, applying careful assessment and purposeful action. This is an explainable and defensible variation that prevents a disadvantageous outcome. Other surgeons with similar training and expertise would be expected to take a similar action. This sort of variation is good and is to be encouraged. A system should be designed not only to allow intentional variation but also to endeavor to provide each participant with the right information at the right time and place so that correct decisions are reached.

There are two types of *unintentional variation*: common cause and special cause (Deming, 1986). *Common cause variation* includes the variations that occur naturally because people, unlike machines, can rarely do the same thing exactly the same way twice, no matter how hard they try. Common cause variations are typically acceptable and tolerated because their size, scale, and frequency are not disruptive or significantly consequential. For example, if you go out for your daily run and follow the same route at your typical pace, you will find that the time it takes to complete the run is approximately, but not precisely, the same each day. If in a week our surgeon performs another operation like the one she is performing on Kim, the incision may be a millimeter longer or shorter than Kim's incision and the procedure may take ten minutes more or seven minutes less, but the range of variation is predictable over a large number of such surgeries and constrained within a range deemed acceptable.

Common cause variation extends beyond the acceptable when there are dire consequences or disruptions resulting from the deviation. A one millimeter variation in the incision might not affect the outcome whereas a five millimeter variation might have fatal impact. A few extra minutes on one procedure is likely offset by another completed more quickly than planned so that the scheduling of surgery suites is not disrupted. A forty-five minute delay, however, can put the whole schedule in disarray. When no mechanisms are in place to anticipate and manage unacceptable common cause variations, conflict, disruption, and deterioration in the quality of care are likely outcomes. The control, discipline, and predictability necessary for smooth operation evaporate, and a sense of uncomfortable chaos overtakes those affected.

In *special case variation* the differences between one instance and another may be explained by knowable or predictable information. Let's go back to your run. Though you may run five miles every day, your time will vary based on whether you take the flat or the hilly route. If we know which loop you've chosen, we can predict the time of your return with relative accuracy; if we do not, we are much less likely to estimate your arrival correctly. Special case variation is acceptable when it does not create concomitant problems or unacceptable consequences. If taking the hilly route makes you late for a meeting that results in the loss of a major contract, then that is not good. Your colleagues will be angered and baffled by your irresponsible behavior.

Unexplained variations in care and outcomes were tolerated in health care for many years. The patient safety and error reduction movement, in the name of saving lives and improving outcomes, has championed the obliteration of these sorts of variations from the landscape. Among our medical colleagues at

HSPH, Luciane Leape has led the cause of error reduction and Atul Gawande has demonstrated the improved outcomes that emerge from the simple use of checklists in the surgical suite (Gawande, 2010). With fewer mistakes and forgotten steps—in other words, less special case variation—there is significant improvement in the quality of care.

The objective of systems thinking in health care is to reduce variation as much as possible, especially when it places patients' lives in danger. The goal is predictable, intentional, and deliberate uniformity in matters where variation has negative consequences. This ambition requires data-driven decision making, so that variations can be systematically observed and tracked and corrections made where necessary.

Those working in health care rarely disagree about the need to have tests run according to an exacting protocol. There is much more resistance to having direct patient care made more systematic, especially among those who consider their work an art as much as it is a science. Be they doctors, nurses, or administrators, these "poets of health care" see complete freedom of action as critical to their ability to perform at their peak. They see their ability to improvise and make judgment calls as part of the genius that they bring to the table. They bristle at the thought of becoming *robo-docs* focused on controlling variation. Unfortunately, improvisation when it is not really needed tends to increase mistakes and to make outcomes less predictable for patients, life more difficult for colleagues, and costs higher for everyone. Standardizing protocols and establishing norms for common cause variations also makes it easier to spot special cause aberrations so that the proper focus and resources can be dedicated to rectifying them.

Because health care has been a system more in name than in operation, differentiating between common cause and special cause variations has been difficult to document and rectify. The belief that the best outcomes for patients will arise from the good intentions of the various players is based more on hope than design. Thanks to the dogged efforts of Donald Berwick and others, systems thinking is becoming more accepted and common in health care. Along with this, more intentional system design is being recognized for the improved outcomes it can achieve on many fronts of health care (McLaughlin & Leatherman, 2003; Contandriopoulos, Denis, Touati, & Rodriguez, 2003). This means the health care that will dominate the scene a decade after the Patient Protection and Affordable Care Act of 2010 was signed will be significantly from what preceded it. Those who craft health care legislation, those who pay the bills, and those who get the care will expect more, and they will get it by recognizing and rewarding those who provide it.

VP

Rumors. David Dickenson hates rumors. Dickenson is vice president of human resources at OMC. He has been here, moving up the ranks, for twenty years. It's the last twelve months, though, that have given him gray hairs.

Dickenson is well liked and well respected at the hospital. His style is open, responsive, and helpful. Many on the hospital's management team regularly call on him to be a sounding board for human resource problems in their departments. He is solution oriented. In fact he believes that most problems have the solution built into them. He asks questions—good questions. He offers perspective. He rarely gives outright advice. He prefers, when he is able, to help people discover a solution on their own.

This morning his e-mails are piling up at an unusually busy pace and ten voice-mail messages await from people who want more than an e-mail exchange. Each message has the same theme: employees are hearing rumors about everything from the imminent closure of the hospital to a consolidation with another institution that could cut jobs in half. There is even a rumor that Inkwater herself has been fired. The problem with a good rumor, of course, is that there is usually an ounce of truth in it. There have been daily articles in the newspapers about turmoil in the city's health care organizations, with OMC prominently featured. From the Community Health Plan contract surprise to the budget problems that were already in play, any rumor is easily ignited and spread. What can be done about it?

Dickenson decides to call Iris Inkwater before anyone else. It is a difficult, though constructive discussion. Inkwater is not surprised about the proliferation of rumors. She and Dickenson agree chances are good that the media will continue pushing on the issue—they are selling papers and building their ratings by hyping the issue and not much can be done to stop that feeding frenzy. They also agree, however, that it is time to be proactive internally. Inkwater is convinced that an e-mail should go out from her to the employees by the end of the day. Dickenson offers to prepare a draft but Inkwater wants to write this one herself: "This has to sound like it comes directly from me, David. Unfiltered. If it comes across as too scripted, it will be worse than saying nothing at all."

"Just remember that there can be policy and legal implications," he cautions. "Will you show it to me before you hit 'send'?"

"Sure," she replies. Her mind is already ruminating on the message. She knows she has to convey that she understands the situation from her perspective and also that she grasps the perspective of all the people who are affected. She begins to sketch an outline: (1) this is what is happening, what we know and what we are doing about it; (2) this is what we don't know and what we are doing to explore options and learn more; (3) this is what you should do as an employee of OMC. She wants to be empathetic but realistic: employees need to know that layoffs are a very real possibility and that in areas where layoffs are needed people will be given financial and career support for the transition. With these thoughts as a guide, the actual e-mail flows smoothly. ''And once this is out,'' she thinks, ''I have to start walking the halls myself. People have to see me and be able to ask me questions.''

Dickenson returns to his growing pile of messages. The one from Evelyn Edelman looks most urgent, so he calls her first. Edelman is the director of the dietary department, with overall responsibilities for both the clinical and the nutritional services operations. She asks for a quick meeting, and a half an hour later she is sitting in Dickenson's office. Dickenson notes the bags under his colleague's eyes.

''David, it's awful what's happening,'' she says with a weary sigh. ''I'm afraid I may have a mini-revolt on my hands. The food service employees' morale is very low. Many are earning minimum wage or a bit more and the loss of their jobs would be catastrophic. The old-timers who have been around a long time feel confident they'll keep their jobs, and the younger workers resent that they may be the ones who take the hit. The supervisors are having a really tough time keeping operations on track. And of course, for the patients, we know that their experience with their food and the person who delivers it makes a difference to their overall experience in this hospital. It is something they can understand and evaluate, and it becomes a surrogate measure for whether we are providing good care. Believe me, that lesson was drilled into me a long time ago. And after all, the patients are seeing the same stories on TV and in the newspapers as our employees are.''

She goes on for more than five minutes, recounting stories and problems, before pausing to gauge Dickenson's reaction. Dickenson sits quietly, knowing that the most productive thing he can let her do is vent. Tension has taken its toll and Edelman needs a release. He also understands that she'll be in a better place to solve her problem once the frustration is off her chest. Edelman concludes with a question: ''What should I do?''

Dickenson shares Inkwater's plan for an organization-wide e-mail and more or less what that message will and will not say. ''What impact do you think that will have?'' he asks.

''That will solve one piece of the problem,'' she replies. ''If there is a downsizing, the severance pay and outplacement service will probably offer some relief for those people facing layoffs. For those staying, the anxiety will continue unless there is an absolute assurance that there won't be more layoffs to follow. I'm not sure what I should do.''

''What do you think would be helpful for people facing a job crisis in their lives?'' Dickenson guesses that Edelman also has some nervousness about her own job. After all, laying off minimum-wage employees will have far less financial impact than eliminating more senior positions.

"Well, it probably would be helpful to talk it out with someone," she says. "I imagine it is difficult for people to bring news of possible layoffs home because it will unsettle their families. Perhaps we can give them a chance to vent some of their feelings in the relatively safe haven of the workplace. If we combine that with whatever information Iris feels she can share, that might help things out. I know just talking with you about this has sure calmed me down."

Dickenson smiles and gently shakes his head. He wants to let the benefits of Edelman's sense of release settle in. After a moment, he speaks quietly. "Evelyn, I've been in this hospital for almost a generation now. I've watched it go through some pretty tough times. Sometimes they were other people's problems, like the restaurant fire twelve years ago that stretched this place to the max for five days straight. Sometimes they were our own problems, like that budget scandal that hit the hospital just after I started working here. To be sure, this period is a really rough one. Yet there is a healthy resilience to this place. I think it is because we all believe in what we're doing—and I know that commitment extends to the people who deliver the food trays. Somehow, I trust we'll survive this one too. Probably we'll look a bit different afterward, perhaps smaller than we were in the past. I think we'll make it, though. Of course," he leans forward, "if we don't believe we can make it, we certainly won't."

Edelman reflects for a moment, then she too finally smiles. "David, once again you've been a real help. Thanks for your ear." Edelman returns to her office, ready to do for someone else what Dickenson has just done for her.

Design and Operation of Integrated Health Systems

As of fall 2009, only about 5 percent of heath care services in the United States were being delivered through a fully integrated system like Kaiser Permanente or Intermountain Health System, according to Harvard Business School professor Clayton Christensen (Blagg, 2009). The evolution of the U.S. health care system will no doubt cause that number to steadily grow. In this section we consider two organizations that use integration and system design as the keystones of their practice and delivery of care: one is a *vertical* system in which system elements are integrated from top to bottom to provide accountability throughout, and one is a *horizontal* system in which independent though linked side-by-side organizations are integrated to provide coordination and continuity of care.

The Kaiser Permanente Health Care System (KP), based in Oakland, California, operates 35 hospitals and more than 400 medical office buildings in which each year more than 36 million doctor visits occur, more than 500,000 surgeries are performed, and more than 129 million prescriptions are filled (Kaiser Permanente, 2009). Organizationally, KP is a partnership between the nonprofit Kaiser side—which operates the insurance business and runs the hospitals and the clinics—and the Permanente Medical Group side, to which KP doctors belong. KP is recognized as an example of a rare type of organization in U.S. health care, the large, vertically integrated health care system: everyone from the chief surgeon to the maintenance worker is an employee; its pharmacies and labs are in-house operations; it is the insurer and the caregiver. If you are a KP customer, every facet of your health care falls under one umbrella.

Organizations such as Kaiser Permanente were once known as HMOs—health maintenance organizations. That designation fell out of fashion when it became synonymous with miserlike attention to costs at the expense of quality patient care: the effort to better manage care became so financially driven that its potential health advantages were lost to the drive to lower costs. Despite being a former HMO, Kaiser has received numerous accolades. For example, according to the J. D. Power and Associates 2008 National Health Insurance Plan Study, it had the "highest member satisfaction among commercial health plans in California," and *U.S. News & World Report* has ranked Kaiser Permanente of Northern California as the top commercial plan in that state and among the top fifty plans in the country (Kaiser Permanente, 2009).

Vertical integration, and the near-total control that comes with it, allows Kaiser Permanente to analyze outcomes, costs, and other variables based on an end-to-end, data-driven view of the efforts of thousands of clinicians and administrators and on the experiences of millions of patients. It enables KP to deploy standardized treatment protocols and best practices for everything from medical procedures to information management across the entire system. Oncology offers a good example.

"Thanks to the work of Dr. Sydney Farber (founder of the Children's Cancer Research Foundation, which later became the Dana-Farber Cancer Institute, and the 'father of the modern era of chemotherapy' (Miller, 2006)), pediatric oncologists have been using common protocols for the treatment of childhood leukemia for 60 years," according to Andy M. Wiesenthal, associate executive director for Clinical Information Support at the Permanente Federation. "Every doctor has been able to learn from every case and the survival rate is now 95%+ as a result." Conversely, in adult oncology the protocols vary hospital by hospital and even doctor by doctor across the country. However, at Kaiser Permanente, standard, evidence-based protocols are used for the 350 top malignancies. Imagine the insights that could be gleaned from the data if all treatment of all adult cancers across the country started with the same set of default protocols?

Think of the effect this could have on increasing the overall survival rate and the dissemination of best practices.

Another advantage that KP clinicians have is an advanced electronic record system. This information technology platform allows the consistent collection of data and a continuous feedback loop that encourages ongoing improvement and refinement of KP's system. Doctors and nurses are able to get the information they need when and where they need it. So too are patients: they have access to their laboratory test results, for example, at the same time as their clinicians have access.

Providing information to patients as quickly as it goes to their caregivers is an example of transparency. So too is sharing performance data among the medical staff. Transparency increases the pace of change. "Change comes to health care when patients refuse to accept suboptimal outcomes," Kaiser Permanente CEO George Halvorson told us. With more traditional component-based health care systems, it is not only patients who may not have all of the data available to optimize their decisions. "Many doctors (nationally) don't get the data," Halvorson continued. "The outliers don't know that they are outliers." At Kaiser Permanente one of the goals is to keep everyone in the appropriate loops through extensive data availability and transparency.

Halvorson also noted that about 80 percent of the chronic care costs in the U.S. health care system are driven by six conditions, with comorbidities, and that chronic care is "entirely a team sport." This is an area where he sees the Kaiser Permanente model of integration as a decisive advantage in the market and a harbinger for the future of the U.S. system as a whole. KP is able to build tools, structures, and incentives for collaboration that may be missing in a less integrated system. The doctor isn't competing against the hospital or specialty care facility, and the payer and provider are aligned.

Having everyone on your payroll—the vertical integration model—removes an important source of conflict. According to Mary Bylone, assistant vice president of patient care services at the William W. Backus Hospital in Connecticut, a community hospital must maintain its financial health, just like any other business. And yet the physicians who order tests or admit patients have little stake in or control over whether the hospital is reimbursed for those services. Although doctors expect hospital-provided state-of-the-art equipment and facilities, as do patients, it is the hospital that must finance their acquisition and upkeep. Without integration, there is no direct relationship between the commitment to the investment and the gains or losses that derive from it.

Integration also reduces the conflicts over how to "divide the pie" said Richard Iseke, chief medical officer of Winchester Hospital in Massachusetts. He noted that when doctors have a financial interest in nonintegrated, for-profit facilities that compete with the community hospital where they have privileges, things can "get complicated." These practices may "cherry pick" profitable procedures to the lower-cost comfort of their offices, leaving the more expensive and less well reimbursed procedures to the local hospital. Without a mix of procedures that can balance overall costs and reimbursements, hospitals are left in precarious financial health while their doctors reap the benefits. Conflicts grow as the hospital resents the physician practices and the physicians resist efforts to constrain their business undertakings.

Vertical integration is not the only alternative for health care providers. Legacy Medical Village in Plano, Texas, is an example of horizontal integration. The village is made up of independent yet interconnected and colocated practices that range from the core primary care practice to practices in sports medicine, cardiology, ophthalmology, pain management, and other specialties. The village also has a full imaging center. The practices share interoperable patient record systems that make it easier to share information. It also allows them to cross-refer patients when appropriate. For example, a patient arriving at the primary care office with complaints of a respiratory problem might be reminded upon check-in that she is also due for her annual mammogram, and the appointment can be made right from the primary care office, with the service delivered down the hall.

Christopher Crow, a cofounder of the village and a primary care physician, explained to us that his patients are looking for "access, communication, and convenience" and that his team designed the village to provide just that.

"The specialists to whom I refer patients are key to my reputation," said Crow. "Colocating with them helps me both have a closer relationship with them and have deeper insight into their interactions with my patients. If my patients aren't happy with the specialists I send them to, they won't be happy with me."

The connections between the village practices are deeper than simply sharing a physical location. The doctors in the primary care practice choose the specialists they invite to the village based on "a shared philosophy of continuous, coordinated care and evidence-based medicine." The practices all agree to use interoperable health information technology.

The village has found that its systems-based approach has helped it to lower administrative costs significantly, meet or exceed many national quality standards, and increase income for its physicians. It reports some of the highest compliance rates in the country for preventative measures such as mammograms and colonoscopies, in part, Crow says, because the village makes it easy and convenient for patients to comply.

The attraction for physicians is a triad of interests: professional, financial, and personal. Professionally, they can be confident that they are delivering the best

As a rule, Dr. Nick Norton does not like committee meetings. He defines a committee as a body that can take a five-minute decision and turn it into a five-hour conversation. Despite that, he knows that every so often he has to do his duty. When he was asked to join the OMC patient safety committee, he had an unusual twinge of ambiguity about the assignment. On one hand, how could anyone be against patient safety? It's good for the customers, good for the hospital, and it's the best way to keep pesky lawyers out of your hair. On the other hand, the patient safety crowd has a lot of wide-eyed do-gooders who have a penchant to think that adding more time and bother to the workload improves patient safety. As far as he's concerned, if patient safety can be improved without too much interference in his work, he is all for it.

The agenda for today's meeting has him peeved. The topic is surgeon checklists, forcing surgeons to go through a mechanical ritual before starting to operate. He has read about this practice in one of his journals and has had a fascinating discussion with a neighbor who is a pilot and who described the checklist routine that goes on in the cockpit before a plane takes off. He knows there has even been a widely read article on medical checklists in a well-regarded general interest magazine. He can understand why a neophyte surgeon might find it useful. Not for him though; it would be a waste of time.

The patient safety committee is chaired by Dr. Beatrice Benson, from the emergency department, and includes, among others, Dr. Ken Kavanaugh, chief of the ICU; Stuart Schilling, the bioethicist; and Dr. Rusty Rice, who is chief of OMC's hospitalist department. Norton is the most senior surgeon on the committee and feels responsible for holding the line if committee members get too close to his turf. When the committee had previously become involved in developing protocols for the operating rooms, he had been able to keep its attention away from fiddling with the surgeons. He prided himself on this small victory for the "home team."

Benson expects push-back from Norton and has planned to open the meeting with a solid, open-and-shut case validated by indisputable evidence. "I hope you've all had a chance to read the articles I distributed in advance of this meeting," she begins. "A considerable body of research on surgical checklists has been amassed, and the results are impressive. Errors have been significantly reduced, and there are considerable savings associated with better outcomes and reduced avoidable care. With this evidence, it's hard to imagine why we wouldn't want to require their adoption here."

Norton is caught a bit off guard. He had only had time to scan the articles that Benson had shared. He is ready to make the case for the value of each minute in the OR and the costs associated with delaying the start of surgery to accomplish a required ritual. Even two minutes more, multiplied by the number of procedures performed each year, times the cost per minute of a busy room would make an impressive case. He realizes that his efficiency argument suddenly seems weak in light of Benson's opening. Not to be deterred, he gives it a try anyway.

"Beatrice, you have to look at this from many angles," he says. "We have been working really hard over the past two years to improve the efficiencies of the operating rooms. We have had some significant success. Speeding things up by as little as an average of five minutes helps the bottom line to the tune of thousands and thousands of dollars over the course of a year. What you are proposing flies in the face of those two years of progress. Our surgeons, particularly the more experienced ones, have honed their skills and have personal techniques for focusing their attention. An artificial program like a standardized checklist will only slow them down and, frankly, break their rhythm."

Benson has heard variations of the "doctor as artist" argument against any kind of standardization for years and has taken preemptive strategic action. Prior to the meeting she asked Rusty Rice to be prepared to respond if Norton goes on the offensive. Rice has been a force for improved patient safety in the hospital for years and his credibility derives from his systematic tracking of outcomes, errors, readmissions, and patient satisfaction. He has been counting everything in sight ever since completing his master of public health degree. With his wry sense of humor, Rice is often heard joking about his cosmic philosophy: if something can't be measured, it probably doesn't exist.

"Nick, you are dead on right," Rice now says. "You multiply the minutes, procedures, and dollars, and you get an impressive number. But that isn't the only relevant number. The question is how does your number compare with another impressive number: the minutes it takes to fix an avoidable error, times the number of times avoidable errors that occur here per year, times the cost of the OR? And you know that when an error pushes you into crisis mode, the cost per minute jumps because more people and resources are needed. Add to that the added costs of postoperative care, the legal costs, and the time everyone has to put into documenting and reconstructing what happened. And with all that, we're still just talking dollars. Insurers compare our metrics to those of other institutions, and we're not far from consumers being able to do the same. That creates a multiplier effect that costs us business."

"Wait a minute, Rusty," Norton protests. "We're damn fine surgeons. Our error rates are not out of whack."

"The only defensible error rate is zero, Nick. That research Beatrice shared with us shows that checklists reduce errors even by experienced surgeons. That alone should be enough reason to adopt them. I know this too well. My dad suffered as a result of an error, and it was hell for him and all of us for three painful months until he pulled out, and he'll never fully recover." Rice's face was flushed with intensity. "But since you want to talk dollars and cents, I've looked at what implementing surgical checklists would add to our expenses. It is a fraction of the downside costs of avoidable errors. I'll be happy to show you the numbers. And of course I haven't even tried to put a monetary value on patient satisfaction and or on the human toll that an avoidable error can have for a patient and her family."

Ken Kavanaugh jumps in to steer the conversation to less emotional ground: "I think we should also consider that checklists can be a useful training tool for our residents." He goes on to explain that medical students and residents are coming into OMC with a new attitude toward what they are doing, what they need to memorize, and how they access and use information technology. "What we used to commit to memory they believe they can access via a handheld or computer far more reliably and efficiently," Kavanaugh says. "This is particularly true given the pace at which new knowledge and information is being introduced. They think and act differently from those of us who have been around for a long time. And the generations after them are going to be even more tethered to their information systems. I know. I watch my kids on their computers and wonder what medicine will be like by the time they may be deciding to go into the profession." Turning to Norton, Kavanaugh continues, "Nick, it comes as no surprise to hear that you are ambivalent about going through a checklist before each procedure. When you and I were in medical school, doing something that basic would have been considered a weakness. It is different today, and we need role models among our senior folk who are willing to embrace where the future is going, as hard as that may be."

Norton wonders if Benson orchestrated this ambush. He wishes he had a gavel and could make a motion: all in favor of adjourning this meeting and forgetting the conversation that just happened say "aye." He feels attacked and humiliated—and he doesn't like it. It takes him a minute to climb out of the basement and recover. What can he say?

As Benson watches his discomfort, she wonders if they have piled too heavily on him.

"Look," Norton says, "I want to make it clear that there is no one in the surgical department who is not 100 percent in favor of taking steps to improve our outcomes. On the whole we have done a good job of building patient safety mechanisms into the OR and we are proud of what we have accomplished. I think we have to be very careful every time we add something to our protocols because it is much easier to add something than to take it away. I will commit to sitting down with Rusty to go through the numbers and, from there, will look into presenting this to the surgical department. I can't take it further than that today."

Norton feels a bit relieved. Benson is satisfied and thanks Norton. Rice agrees to meet with Norton to discuss the numbers. Benson moves the meeting on to other points of business. Stuart Schilling has said nothing during the checklist debate, though he is now thinking, "One step at a time this place is going to become a safer place to be a patient."

possible standard of care: "We are committed to establishing best practices and spreading them as quickly as possible," says Crow. Financially, five of the seven doctors in the primary care practice are in the ninetieth percentile or higher for pay relative to their peers. And finally, personally, they "have a life," said Crow. "We've achieved efficiencies that give them back time."

This sort of horizontal integration is not without its challenges. First, an *anchor tenant* is required to get things started. In the case of Legacy Medical Village, Crow's practice—Village Health Partners—was both the philosophical and the financial engine behind the enterprise. The practice is larger than most private practices, with about ten principals rather than the two to three that are typical nationally. The extra resources and patient base of a practice that size have allowed Crow and his colleagues to build an attractive institutional support structure, with a top-notch chief information officer, chief financial officer, and staff who provide traditional business functions. With that in place, the founders were able to attract quality specialists to the village, professionals who would complement their work and attract the patient volume necessary to fund infrastructure costs.

Crow feels that his primary care–centered model is sure to spread. "Payment systems are going to need to change, but primary care isn't going away," he said. "Care coordination is a softer skill but it is essential for higher quality and lower costs."

Standardization will be an inevitable part of integration as quality imperatives demand that physicians adopt and adhere to established best practices of care. Market imperatives will do the same, as physicians are persuaded to balance high quality with cost efficiency. "'Variance equals cost' is one of my favorite phrases," says Crow.

The continued pressure on the health care system to increase quality and decrease costs will inevitably encourage the emergence of better-connected and better-integrated linkages. Market pressures will demand this, technological innovations will make it easier, and a more informed patient population with better knowledge and higher expectations will seek it out. Although they are an important development, we do not suggest that integrated systems will solve all the problems found in the organizations that preceded them. Whether vertical or horizontal, these systems are subject to conflict: clashing egos, budget battles, and the other foibles of all large-scale organizations. They present many opportunities for employing the Walk in the Woods, mediation, and meta-leadership to anticipate, manage, and resolve these differences. And because integration removes many institutional road blocks to collaboration while at the same time rewarding collaborative successes, intentional connectivity is likely to become more prevalent across the health care landscape.

A New Era of Integration

In the late 1990s, systemwide efforts to spur health reform sparked new forms of integration and collaboration—including mergers and consolidations among large medical centers, the purchase and joining of medical practices, and the development of national chains to provide allied health services. Those moves coincided with related efforts to improve the quality and speed of care. Similarly, this next round of health system change seems certain to spawn new models for integrating services and care. For example, the adoption of a more universally implemented electronic medical record (EMR), an innovation that has lagged in the United States, could very well draw and encourage new lines and forms of integration, especially as patients themselves become more actively vested in the EMR's transparency and transportability.

As integrated systems become more common, they will reshape the roles of each participant. The most significant change will be for physicians. Accustomed to autonomous control as part of a small practice, the physician in a vertically integrated system will be an employee subject to policies, procedures, and decision-making hierarchies not fully of her own design or choosing. By contrast, in a horizontally integrated system, the physician will need to be as much savvy businessperson as medical expert, because new entrepreneurial models are making the economics of medicine more complex and therefore more demanding of the physician's time and attention.

Herein rests the paradox of integration. On one hand the deliberate linkages that constitute the infrastructure of integration offer encouraging opportunities for beneficial collaboration among different professionals, organizations, and clinical services. On the other hand the many advantages of independent operation—in the comfort of one's familiar sphere of work—are surrendered. Standard procedures and business operations impose constraints and conditions and frustrate time-honored expectations. Clinicians can already be heard to complain that integration and its fixed rules violate the professional independence, autonomy, and art of their work. Rather than disregarding these complaints, leaders should view them as offering chances to engage and translate frustrations into meaningful opportunities that do not disrupt the overall objectives of the enterprise.

How can this be accomplished?

For a system to succeed, those involved must behave in accordance with the overall game plan. Behaviors can be identified and incentives offered to encourage the specific cooperation and compliance that are keys to the success of the design. Often those in charge expect that people will simply go along; they fail to recognize that those affected must make accommodations—sometimes with difficulty—in ways that might not be apparent.

Good behavior deserves to be rewarded. This insight should guide the change strategy. If you are leading the charge, the five dimensions of meta-leadership can serve you well: understand what motivates you and others and strive to keep everyone out of the basement; integration is a fluid process, so ensure that you are mindful of the situation and circumstances as they evolve; be attentive to your supervisees so that your commitment to them is mirrored in their commitment and support for you; your bosses may not appreciate the complexities of an integration process, so position yourself as both subordinate and teacher for them; bringing together disparate organizational cultures and ways of doing business can be tricky and it demands robust and resilient leadership: be deliberate in all your actions.

Change—no matter how confident or well intentioned—provokes push-back and resistance. Do not ignore this behavior. Resistance should be anticipated and planned for and not simply with strategies and mechanisms to quell it. Change should be understood for what it means for those expected to make it happen. Their concerns should be heard, their suggestions considered, and appropriate accommodations made. Buy-in is a valuable asset to any change endeavor. Buy-in is not automatic. It is earned. You attain it as a function of a process that engages those whose cooperation is required. The Walk in the Woods is one tool for actively involving stakeholders and achieving their buy-in.

Once in place, any change or integration will suffer problems, setbacks, and disappointments. No major shift is as good in its implementation as it was in its planning or on paper. Those responsible for managing and implementing changes and integration should have appropriate opportunities to monitor and assess progress. These assessments provide the best chance for the continuous quality improvement necessary to ensure that systems designed to improve the efficiency and effectiveness of the workload are in fact doing that. And when conflicts emerge—and they will—there should be standing dispute resolution committees and procedures already in place. When access to a conflict resolution mechanism is easy, they will be used early, before a standoff significantly disrupts the morale and the productivity of the very people you count on.

Helping people to work better together is a difficult undertaking. It is often not given its proper attention. A well-designed system remedies that. Deliberate procedures can eliminate many sources of conflict, though it should not quell opportunities to constructively and meaningfully express differences when they contribute to decision quality (Gero, 1985). You can negotiate accepted *rules of engagement* between stakeholders. You can establish shared priorities and benchmarks for mutual benefit. And among the complex issues to be addressed, there is none more sensitive than the issue of money. As Richard Iseke reminded us, "Every change that affects the payment stream threatens someone and can be a source of conflict."

Conclusion

It is not uncommon to focus abundant attention on the ostensible markers of integration and in doing so to lose track of the complex people dimensions. Yet it is the people dimensions that are your most important success factors in any integration process.

Yes, gleaming new signage declaring a consolidation attracts attention. So too do new contracts, new machines, and new wires linking buildings and computers. Those markers, however, are not the predictors of a flourishing combination of people and processes that formerly worked in independent fields of activity.

The most telling markers are the high morale and satisfaction of those involved and their capacity to reap increased effectiveness and new efficiency from a better operating system. That result emerges from a deep appreciation for and attention to those people dimensions.

Those responsible for making systems work and work well will find that the process of constructing integration reaps both triumphs and disasters. If it is to succeed, motivations must be intentionally aligned in the direction of mutual success and reward. Though difficult, this is possible and is eminently negotiable.

When personal and professional motives are aligned with a shared drive to save lives, to improve the quality of life, and to advance the health of populations, compelling advancements can be accomplished. When people believe in you as a leader, it is astounding what you can accomplish. The key is in understanding where you are going and which people you need on board to help you get there. Recruit those people to the cause, and you can make a real difference.

One common thread and driver for more integrated health systems is technology. This is the topic of the next chapter, which also addresses this question: How do you marry the people dimensions of your system with the technological dimensions that can enhance your total system operation?

CHAPTER 12

EVOLVING WITH TECHNOLOGY

THE EVOLVING accomplishments of technology have for centuries defined health care. Humans long ago discovered that instruments of manipulation and chemical compounds could be used for curative purposes. They sought ways to record and communicate what they were able to accomplish. With time these tools and formulations became increasingly sophisticated. They framed what healing purposes could and could not be accomplished and explained the factors that promoted or detracted from good health.

That same progression of scientific and technical evolution continues today, as research, information technology, nanotechnology, and robotics expand what we know and what we can do. Clinicians are able to delve into the smallest reaches of human anatomy and manipulate tissue with increasing dexterity and precision. Epidemiologists probe with growing certainty the far reaches of the environment and most intimate reaches of human behavior to understand causal factors associated with health promotion and disease prevention. What we know and our ability to assimilate and communicate that knowledge grows exponentially each decade.

These new capabilities redefine what can be accomplished on behalf of health and well-being and the venues through which it can be done. As technology evolves, so too must everything that surrounds and supports it: organizational structures, professional curricula, insurance financing, and the people involved and affected. And insofar as there is a correlation between the phenomenon of change and the presence of conflict, the advent of the newest technological

Unless otherwise noted, quotations and summaries of comments from Mary Bylone, Kimberly Costa, Christopher Crow, Martha Crowninshield, O'Brien, Richard Donahue, Cindy Ehnes, Eddie Erlandson, John Halamka, George Halvorson, Richard Iseke, Paul Levy, Gordon Moore, Scott Ransom, Pamela Wible, and Andy M. Wiesenthal are taken from interviews conducted by the authors in 2009 and 2010.

advances and opportunities are accompanied by measures of friction. This conflict has been ever present—even in the days of using leaches and bloodletting to relieve illness—as existing technologies and methods are defended by their practitioners and challenged by mavericks and innovators.

Evolving Technology and Emerging Conflict

The invention and introduction of a new technology has implications for many people. Simply put, for some people the new technology brings exciting new opportunities and benefits, and for others it carries downsides such as losses and inconveniences and with them come anxieties about what this new technology could mean. This distinction is the fundamental source of technology-driven conflict. There are enthusiastic and creative idealists on one side of the table and concerned and proficient defenders of the status quo on the other. Negotiating a resolution requires finding some balance and common ground between the two. Zealous defenders can raise an impervious wall in order to stop change, and idealist innovators can provoke many unintended consequences in their drive to move change forward. And the parties on each side like to portray themselves as the "good guys" at the table.

How is this conflict manifested? One effect of new technology is to afford medical professionals greater independence from once-necessary hospitalization of their patients. For example, conflict emerges as new technologies allow procedures that once required in-patient care to be performed in a doctor's office. In other cases, the doctor and patient do not need to be in the same facility: a patient who might once have required an open prostatectomy can now have one performed robotically by a physician hundreds or thousands of miles away. The same is true when new pharmaceuticals render older treatments obsolete, such as circulating tumor cell blood tests that may one day replace biopsies, and when testing that had once been performed by a physician is automated so that it can be administered by a nurse or even the patient herself.

There are those who argue that relocating care or allowing others to perform newly routine procedures is an infringement on quality of care. The central issue often veiled in the background in these conflicts is the matter of compensation. Advances in technology shift who does what, and that changes who gets paid for what. Scott Ransom, president of the University of North Texas Health Science Center in Fort Worth, provides an example. If technology facilitates the migration of high-reimbursement procedures to specialty hospitals and clinics, that migration can starve the general hospital that continues to support the community by providing a full range of services. That shift can spell *fight!*—sending those in the hospital's administration straight to the basement.

One often cited advantage of new technology is its capacity to reduce expensive personnel costs by turning routine tasks into efficient, machine-run operations. In the field of banking, for example, automated teller machines, or ATMs, have replaced some bank workers. Although some may lament the loss of the interpersonal banter that came with a cash withdrawal, few saw this personal touch as essential to the provision of banking services, and many more found the added convenience was far more important than chitchat.

The degree to which this dehumanizing aspect of technology is useful in health care is still being debated. There are those who argue that bedside and clinic-based conversations and banter with patients are essential to the diagnostic and curative process, providing the clinician with necessary physical and psychosocial information and the patient with the confidence that comes with being carefully attended. In this perspective, new technologies are seen as reducing the human touch that defines the most personal and intimate aspects of health care service. This loss becomes a source of conflict. It is believed that a robot, machine, or computer cannot replace the warmth or comfort of another person. Machines also cannot discern the subtle nuances of human behavior that yield valuable clinical insights. Conversely, proponents of new technologies that allow clinical care to be delivered in new and varied settings note the many advantages. These include the greater independence offered by technologies that allow people to remain on their own at home rather than being institutionalized or to have medical procedures done on an out-patient basis rather than being hospitalized. These changes of course also offer bounteous savings to the health system. New machines, it is argued, are allowing fewer people to accomplish more work, integrate more information in a quicker fashion, commit fewer errors, and thereby better serve patients. Despite the arguments for improved care on both sides of the table, one can often find the contours of this conflict along the lines of who benefits and who loses financially.

Costs are a critical factor in an environment in which expectations for service and outcomes are rising and pressures to constrain the budget are growing. As in many lines of business, new technologies are pursued and championed for their efficiencies and cost-saving potential. Cost saving capitalizes on the mandate to accomplish more while spending less. Conflict arises though when more money for one clinician means less for another or when clinicians are altogether removed from the mix. This is the point when the human touch conflict can arise from the ledgers of cost-savings proposals. For example, as the process of collecting a patient's medical history occurs more often through an interface between patient and computer screen than between patient and clinician, the loss will be significant for those who transition through this change, and it will ultimately raise questions regarding quality of care and outcomes. Furthermore, as highly specialized procedures become more routine through the application of technology, the demand for care by previously busy specialists will decline, a matter that predictably will ignite significant angst and conflict.

Remuneration is a potent source of conflict. New technology-enabled diagnostics and procedures that offer significantly improved results may fetch higher rates of reimbursement. Patients may demand them as news about the advantages and benefits spreads across the Internet. Advocates of evidence-based care will clamor for technologies that feed their databases with information on what works and what doesn't. Payers, however, will want to discourage the ballooning demand for these new technologies and procedures except where there is a clear and compelling benefit. Clinicians and their employers will feel market pressure to deliver cutting-edge care and to keep their expensive machines active and generating revenue. They will also succumb to the temptation to hone and practice their skills using the latest methods. The line of motivation between what is financially beneficial for the provider and her facility and what is essential for patient care can quickly become fuzzy. This has been a well-documented phenomenon: for example, one classic study demonstrated that an X-ray machine located in a doctor's office correlates with increased utilization (Childs & Hunter, 1972).

The conflict surrounding technology revolves around many themes. Money is one: who pays, who benefits, and who loses. Control is another: who controls information, the patients, and the revenue stream. Control is at times managed by sustaining the mystery of health care, designating only particular people as having the expertise or skill to know or do something. Knowledge and skill are power levers in health care, and their legitimacy and importance can be sources of conflict as the answers to the question of who really has the know-how become more diffuse. These answers often translate into matters of ownership and territorial domain. For example, there is significant conflict about which specialty "owns" the vascular tree and the treatments and technologies to diagnose and provide care to it: cardiologists, cardiac surgeons, vascular surgeons, radiologists? And although people rush to get on board with a technology when it offers obvious upsides, they also stampede to distance themselves from anticipated downsides when a technology fails, becomes a source of liability, or does not deliver.

Technology-based conflict occurs on three primary planes. The first is enterprise-wide conflict regarding the wholesale adoption of new technology, such as the electronic medical record. Enterprise-wide change is national in scope and comprehensive, involving all aspects of the health endeavor. The second is system-based conflict, such as adoption of a new technology that involves many different departments and professionals within a large organization. The third is more individually based conflict that occurs within a much narrower field of people and organizations and concerns specific business- or treatment-related questions and negotiations. Though these three planes of technology-based conflict are closely related, they differ in their stakeholders; the scope and scale of the motivations that frame the frictions; and the strategies, methods, and venues used in resolving the conflicts. One of the stumbling blocks slowing the adoption of new technologies has been the difficulty of negotiating their introduction and teasing apart the sources of agreement and disagreement for each plane. Each of these three planes is individually discussed in the sections that follow.

Enterprise-Wide Technology: Conflict and Negotiation

There is no better example of the problems and conflicts of adopting new technology than the saga of the electronic medical record (EMR) in the United States. Although electronic recording and tracking of information is a routine matter in most businesses—such as overnight shipping, to mention just one example—it remained a mystery to health care organizations for a puzzlingly long time in this country. At the point when many countries in Western Europe had 100 percent penetration of EMRs, the United States had only a 17 percent adoption rate in physicians' offices (Burt & Hing, 2005), and a large portion of that was accounted for by the country's two largest health care systems, the Veterans Health Administration (VHA) health care networks and the Kaiser Permanente Health Care System. One 2005 study suggested that under current circumstances, EMRs would not reach maximum market share in small practice settings until 2024 (Ford, Menachemi, & Phillips, 2006). Although circumstances are constantly changing and government requirements and incentives may finally accelerate the adoption of this particular technology, it is useful to understand why this process has persisted so long and has been so tenaciously slow and painful, given that the same negotiation barriers and conflicts could stall national adoption of other important technological and health-promoting advances.

The electronic medical record is a unique example of an advanced technology that can have ramifications across the entire system. It set out to replace a technology that at one time was itself novel and interesting—pen and paper. There was a mountain of resistance against changing that simple though cumbersome record-keeping and communication system. However, the conflict between advocates and opponents was hard to locate because it did not center on one pressure point or decision-making venue. The battle, though palpable, was largely a clash of trends, fears, and sentiments. It was not a pointed difference of opinion among stakeholders who could easily assemble themselves about a table to negotiate and then settle their differences. Why was the conflict so thorny? And why in spite of the many benefits that could derive from its resolution did the standoff persevere for so long?

To place the conflicts surrounding adoption of the electronic medical record into proper focus, consider first how the collected set of obstacles is likely to be understood by a single physician with a private practice, the simplest unit of analysis. This lone physician plays two primary roles: clinician and small business owner. Both roles impose powerful pressures on the doctor. The clinician wants to provide quality care to his patients in a way that is both professionally and intellectually satisfying. The business owner has to be concerned about a wide set of managerial matters for which he has little training. To ensure an adequate patient volume that will generate the necessary revenue, the practice must be marketed, efficient and effective in its care of patients, and connected to other practices and organizations that can provide additional services or referrals.

When the matter of the electronic medical record comes before this doctor, it is the business owner as well as the clinician who must go through the difficult adoption considerations. An EMR is a costly investment in, first, capital and, second, time to learn the new system. There are no revenues to offset these costs. In the days of strong resistance, insurance did not reimburse for the purchase of the equipment and software necessary to launch an electronic medical record. In addition, the business owner has a number of vendors to choose from—what if he chooses the wrong one and it does not conform to systems adopted by others in the market? Finally, this doctor, like many others, may reason that he is comfortable with the system in place and has already invested a great deal in making it work. Why change it? He can see no major incentives or motives to do so. When these individual reservations are combined on a massive national scale, moving from an admirable idea to actual implementation is a slow and cumbersome process. Any small carrots that might encourage the change have looked insignificant compared to the arguments of the widespread wave of resistance. Narrowly conceived, no logic about the advantages of an electronic medical system could overcome the immediate downsides seen by the single physician in private practice. The notion of "build it and they will come" has simply had no traction among the many entrepreneurs who populate the medical delivery system in communities across the country.

Resistance to a massive investment by a single practitioner with a modest revenue stream can be understood, but what about large health systems and medical centers? Although there were some early adopters, on the whole even those who could bankroll the hardware and software that are central to the adoption of new information technology have been resistant. The opposition manifests itself on a number of substantive issues. First has been the internal battle previously mentioned with physicians reluctant to take the time and to invest the energy to learn how to use a new system. The EMR has been seen more as a distraction from their core clinical responsibilities than as a new tool they could master and use to their advantage. Second, there were concerns about the early software and hardware necessary to launch a new electronic medical record: what if the wrong vendor were chosen and the system had flaws? Or what if other providers were to select a different system and that other system became the industry standard? A tremendous amount of capital and clinical time would have been invested in a program that could require change down the road. Few leaders were willing to take the responsibility when that difficult set of decisions had to be made and many deferred to the point that these collected reservations became a national trend.

What early advocates of the EMR did not recognize as they sought to introduce a national system is that orchestrating an enterprise-wide evolution of the health care system requires multiple and simultaneous transformations. Focusing only on specific questions and stumbling blocks regarding costs, vendors, software systems, privacy concerns, or clinician opposition cannot break the logjam. Gaining the momentum for enterprise-wide adoption will take something more.

On the enterprise-wide level, introducing a new technology is an exercise in leading—actually meta-leading—change. One must not only generate interest in the technology and its advantages but also address questions of culture, process, and system alignment. EMR adoption must be tied to other innovations and developments, such as *pay for performance*, or P4P, which reimburses clinicians and hospitals for compliance with quality and outcome standards; the emerging reimbursement arrangements that require an EMR as part of the method for tracking charges and paying bills (Burt & Hing, 2005, found that 73 percent of physician offices were using information technology for billing patients); consumer-friendly report cards that reach the Internet and inform the marketplace of the qualifications and practice records of clinicians; and the existence of a new crop of medical students and residents who are more digitally oriented than their older colleagues and whose experience in VHA medical center residency programs has made them proficient with the EMR and expectant that their next employer will have this technology as well. Quality, reimbursement, the market, and education together make up the package necessary for generating enterprise-wide change. Attempting to fix one piece of the system—without adjusting the motives, inducements, dynamics, and linkages of the overall enterprise—is unlikely to succeed in achieving enterprise-wide acceptance of a new technology or other innovation. It is like trying to change one gear in a gearbox without adjusting the other gears: without somehow changing all the workings, the desired motion will not be generated. (This same lesson holds true for other enterprise-wide change campaigns, including efforts to address significant public health problems such as childhood obesity and tobacco control.)

An enterprise-wide application such as the electronic medical record will change the way that many people go about their work. This must be accounted for. Some will embrace it enthusiastically. Some will doubt that the benefits outweigh the costs. Others will resist adopting new processes or sharing information. Still others will resent the time that it takes to get the data into the system even though they see the value in what they get out of it. Nurses may be eager to learn how to operate a new heart monitor, and doctors may line up to try the latest gadget applicable to their specialty. However, these same people will be reluctant to try a new method of data entry unless it makes their lives easier and less complicated. Analyzing and developing methods for linking the advantages of a innovation to the ways people do their work on an enterprise level is an essential part of conceiving and implementing enterprise-wide change, from the micro level up to the macro level and then back down to the micro level. It is an exercise in meta-leadership.

Those who advocate broad change must also take into account the fundamental concerns shared across the enterprise, even though this step might, at first blush, counter the notion of linking one element of change to overall system change. In keeping with the practices of whole image negotiation, leaders must consider enterprise-wide fears and concerns when promoting an enterprise-wide change. As the EMR collects and collates data in ways that make them accessible and easy to analyze by a broad range of entities, caregivers may fear the implications of exposure of what they do and their success in doing it. Caregivers may be unable to see the benefits of collected and coordinated information and may see only the exposure of any inadequacies in their care as well as failures to treat according to accepted protocols. This will tend to frighten caregivers because once data are collected and exchanged they become a powerful tool for determining whether care has been "good" or "bad." This determination can then be linked to reimbursement and malpractice issues. How does one both create linkages and allay the fears about those linkages at one and the same time?

John Halamka is chairman of the Healthcare Information Technology Standards Panel at the American National Standards Institute. He is also a member of the Health IT Standards Committee, a federal advisory body to the Department of Health and Human Services that is charged with making recommendations to the National Coordinator for Health IT on standards, implementation specifications, and certification criteria for the electronic exchange and use of health information. He brings rubber-meets-the-road experience to this topic, as he serves as chief information officer for Harvard Medical School and for

Beth Israel Deaconess Medical Center, among other roles. A physician himself, he has had extensive experience persuading health care professionals to adopt new technologies. "Almost everyone sees the benefit of automating medication management: writing and refilling prescriptions electronically, checking drug interactions and the like," he told us. "Most see the benefit in managing laboratory test results, particularly when automated exception reports can save them the time of looking at 100 'normal' results reports just to find the one or two that really need their attention. Beyond that, there is resistance because it is always going to take more time to enter data into a system than to scribble a note." That sentiment was echoed by others we interviewed.

The challenge, according to Halamka, is that until the system pays for quality instead of quantity, there will be little incentive for providers to collect the sort of information that is essential to managing patient health rather than just that used for billing for patient care. Referring to the International Statistical Classification of Diseases and Related Health Problems (ICD) codes that are used for medical billing, he observed that "there is no ICD code for 'cure.' There is no ICD code for 'maintained a healthy weight' or 'kept blood pressure down.' " Halamka and his colleagues are engaged in a project to change that: by 2011, there will be twenty-nine standard quality measures on which doctors must report electronically in order to qualify for the highest Medicare reimbursement rates.

This sentiment was echoed by Kimberly Costa. A nurse who works both in the emergency room and on the maternity ward, she commented to us that the feedback she heard relative to technology was much more about reimbursement, than about quality. "We hear, 'great job, reimbursements are up,' not 'great job, infection rates are down.' "

Eddie Erlandson, a former vascular surgeon and chief of staff at St. Joseph Mercy Hospital in Ann Arbor, Michigan, sees a deeper problem in that the current system is largely a "left-brained machine: transactional and delivery-focused." He notes that no one gets paid for helping a patient avoid a hip replacement, for example, whereas many people get paid for replacing a hip. The system is proficient at designing advanced replacement hips and innovating ways to improve the replacement procedure and move the patient to home-based recovery more quickly. "But," he says, "it falls down completely on avoidance—the right steps to take before replacement is required." Another example is that the rehabilitation regimen prescribed for a patient suffering a broken leg would most likely be framed as "number of visits" to a physical therapist rather than "percentage of mobility restored." "That's where the real opportunity for improvement resides," he told us. "Technology can help but only if there is a fundamental shift in the mind-set of caregivers, payers, and patients to focus on quality of health and not just quantity of health care provided."

Introducing technology or purchasing new machines alone does not solve the enterprise-wide problem. Technology innovation, paradoxically, is much more a problem of people than of machines. Fears are likely to overcome benefits. Benefits, unless they speak to the motivating self-interests of those expected to embrace the change, will not move the masses. For enterprise-wide technology to be accepted and adopted, the enterprise itself must change. That can be a slow and tedious process. If it is to succeed, there must be deliberate, intentional, and persistent leadership to guide the change through the necessary steps over time.

What Iris Inkwater appreciates most about the Tuesday morning kitchen cabinet she has assembled is that it is hers: it is not a standing committee with an agenda, an elected body representing constituencies, or a group with a tradition. She has all that in other bodies, and what she needs in her cabinet is a flexible sounding board, her very own focus group. Although she means it to be an informal, unofficial body, she knows that the first meeting has already caused some chatter throughout the medical center: the implications of who is in the group and who is not, speculation about what they have talked about, and tea-leaf reading regarding her larger intentions for the place. Inkwater doesn't mind the talk. What might bother other people she views as a sign of life. People still care deeply about this place. She's taken steps to counter unproductive rumors about Oppidania Medical Center's future but thinks it is important that what's said in the kitchen, stays in the kitchen.

She decides to devote the second meeting of her kitchen cabinet to technology. It was not long ago that she found herself resistant to the wave of new gizmos, software programs, and digitally enabled capabilities that have been hitting health care and OMC like a tsunami. She had tuned out most of the sales pitches, because it seemed that the vendors were unrelenting with their promises of reduced costs, improved efficiencies, and market dominance, and eager to guarantee whatever it was they thought you wanted to hear. She knew they were too good to be true, but she now regrets not spending more time to get through the hype and understand which changes would really matter. "Maybe it's an age thing," she thinks, "or just a penchant for keeping health care about the people."

However, something changed for her after she got her most recent smartphone. She was genuinely impressed with its ease of use and its capacity to keep her remarkably organized and in touch. She became an overnight tech convert. Today, she believes that many of the most vexing problems in health care have technology as part of the solution. She's ready to climb the learning curve and wants the kitchen cabinet to join her for the ascent.

This second meeting of her Tuesday group starts with a much more upbeat and friendly tone. The coffee and her homemade zucchini bread help.

"Welcome to the second kitchen cabinet meeting," Inkwater begins. "I again really appreciate your taking the time for these informal discussions. I took the liberty of inviting our chief information officer, George Grant, to join us today. He and I have been doing a lot of talking lately—more so than ever before—about our technology investments. If I were to summarize our conversations in one phrase, it would be about getting the most technology bang for our buck. What has impressed me is that there is a lot of bang to be had out there, not all of which is worth our time and attention. There is a lot though that could be very helpful to our mission here, and I have asked George to help us sift through this. The point is not to decide on one program or another right now. Rather, I think we need to have a strategy for technology that matches and uplifts our strategy for moving the *new OMC* forward in a very different health care marketplace."

George Grant has been with OMC for more than five years, rising to the CIO position two years ago. He is a geek but a pragmatic one, with a sense of humor and a deep commitment to health care. His boyhood interest in computers overtook his interest in medicine, which he reluctantly did not pursue, and he finds that his work at OMC satisfies his enthusiasm for both fields. When excited by a new tech challenge, Grant lights up.

"Iris told me you are talking about a new OMC and asked if I would share some ideas about what this could mean through my lens. Now, this is a bit revolutionary but let me lay it out for you." He pauses for dramatic effect. "I would blow the walls off of this place. Literally—boom!" His eyes are wide as he illustrates an explosion with his hands. "And then what is inside and what is outside would meld, one and the same. Imagine what we could do for patients if we were as connected to them virtually as we are physically. Rather than just being with us on our campus, they could be with us—so to speak—all the time. Together with them we would be able to do incredible things to monitor and improve their health and their ability to live independently and, let's get to the bottom line, to better link them to us and our business model."

He takes his smartphone from his pocket and slides it to the center of the conference table. "That device—you and your patients all have one or will in the not-so-distant future—is about the size of a slice of Iris's zucchini bread. It has more computing power and connectivity than the clunky computer you had at your desk two years ago. This is the wave of the future. We can monitor, diagnose, and take action—all through electronic linkages between the patient at home or work and our information infrastructure here at the hospital. Rather than knowing what is happening with your patient during the narrow window of a ten-minute visit, you can know what is happening 24/7. This is the transformation going on in health care, and we are in a position to be a leader here in our community. If you think of its implications, it will change just about everything we do in one way or another. Connect outside capabilities to our electronic medical record and to the linkages with our medical practices and then OMC is the only place you would want to be. People would feel protected and cared for even when they are not here. For at-risk patients we could detect the first signs of a cardiac arrest automatically—even before the patient experiences discomfort—and trigger appropriate care. On the whole we can certainly save lives, reduce costs, and create a lot of very loyal customers. We can leverage technology into a productive business model with just a bit of imagination and some smart negotiation."

Grant has grabbed their attention, in part with his animated presentation style and in part because what he described so diverts from the group's experience with health care that it is as if he were talking about some strange make-believe world.

Larry Lumberg plunges in first: "So, George, you're talking about home monitoring, Web linkages, and remote diagnostic technology, right?"

"That and a bit more, Larry: I am talking about an overarching strategy that redefines care of our patients as well as our business model. Think of the continuum of care. You probably think of it as beginning when the patient arrives here at the hospital and ending following discharge. Yes, we do discharge planning, though that usually means sending the patient to additional providers in the community. But what if the patient was connected here even before arriving at our doors? We can get the capability to do that now, though we would have to design, internally sell, and then externally market a very different kind of health care platform."

"I dread it every time my phone or computer gets upgraded," Fred Fisher laments. "It just seems to get more confusing and harder to use."

"I always thought the same thing, Fred," says Inkwater. "But I think the software people have turned a corner. My new device really is easy and intuitive. I can't believe all the things that it can do—and that I can figure out how to make it do them."

"There's a rumor going around that you and that phone are an item," Lumberg chuckles. "You never seem to be without it."

Arlan Abbington is enthusiastic about what he is hearing. "What George is talking about for OMC we did in banking. How many people here use online banking?" Everyone but Fisher raises a hand.

"Never ask a doctor to balance a checkbook," says Fisher, explaining his abstention. "My wife does our banking."

"You're lucky, Fred. But for us ordinary folk," Abbington continues, "we can do a lot through our computers that used to require a stop at a bank. Though there are significant up-front costs in setting up online banking, the per transaction basis is much, much lower, it runs 24/7 with minimal employee time, and most important, it pulls customers the bank's way. It is what people are expecting from the service industry, and let's admit it, in its own way, health care is a service industry. And look at the demographics: people are growing older, health expenses are getting bigger, and everyone's looking to save money, remain independent, and live a longer, healthier life. Let's ask ourselves, 'What is successful aging?' and we could be a central part of the answer in this town. Technology is not the answer to every problem, though it is going to help shape the future, and Iris, if you want to be thinking *new*, this would be an exciting direction in which to take OMC."

"Arlan, I know that banking has done a lot with computers," Janice Johnson, retorts, "but let me tell you, as a nurse, when there is a searing pain in your back, you need the comfort of a caring hand. No fingers on a computer are going to help you feel better. 'ON-line' is not 'hands-ON.' I watch young people with their instant messaging, glued to some screen. Is this making people more connected? I don't think so. It is making people more alone and isolated. I think we should be very careful before we turn over patient care to some computer programmer. Let's think long and hard about what this would really mean for our patients, or even more, for people in general."

Perry Pudolski has been examining Grant's smartphone. He spins it back across the table to Grant as he enters the conversation. "You know, I don't think this falls into the category of really new. The introduction of successive generations of technology is part of an evolutionary process. One machine, one capability leads to the next, one step at a time. We could jump two steps ahead instead of one, though I don't see that this is the revolutionary thing you are suggesting, George. Quite frankly, we just have to do this to keep up with other places, including independent specialty facilities that are going to focus on the most lucrative procedures and treatments and leave us holding the rest. It's happened to us before with day surgery and office-based procedures. OK, so let's expand our thinking with some new programs and capabilities. Most everything else, though, will remain the same."

"Perry, I could not disagree with you more," Lumberg says, with an indignant wave of his hand. "What George is talking about really is new, both for the experience of the patient and for the work of the health practitioner. It is actually downright revolutionary. Mind you, I don't think we should talk about it in terms of tearing down the hospital walls. We still need to be here. There are accident victims and hysterical parents and stroke patients that we can't treat via computer. That said, there are also a lot of worried well people, folks who end up in the emergency room but who could be calmed and checked through a home-based remote monitoring system. What is most compelling to me is that being able to keep these people cared for and at home would be financially advantageous in a capitated system. We could be ahead of the trends, marrying new technology with reimbursement incentives on top of a strong base of clinical services here in the hospital: that combination sings and if put together properly could reflect something genuinely new here."

Fred Fisher is laughing as he starts speaking. "Well, I am going to be a bit out of character here this morning. I know I can barely use a cell phone, but I have seen how these new developments can transform care. My sister back east takes care of our mother, and she has set up some pretty marvelous capability and care. Mom is monitored around the clock. The equipment is simple, and they taught my mother how to do everything herself. She has a call button, and she is very motivated to make this work so she can stay in her own home. I don't think we have a choice here. We're either on the high-tech train or under it, because this is the way that every industry is going. If we don't start paying attention, there will be a lot of other entities taking our patients."

"I've also had some personal experience with this in my family," agrees Rajeev Rao. "There is tremendous potential, though we are going to have to be very entrepreneurial, seeking partnerships and alliances. I don't think we have to go out and buy or invent a lot of this on our own. We can, though, link up with companies who could view us as a powerful strategic partner. An alliance with OMC might be a big marketing plus for them. We would have to find or recruit people internally who would be part of what would be a new line of business. And Iris and everybody: I think this is a great thing, even a must. It's not, though, an instant remedy to all our woes. The major danger in this is that other places take a leap forward and we are left behind. Then we look out of date, and given all that is changing, that could be a death sentence."

Grant is feeling somewhat defensive as he responds to all these comments. "The knocking down the walls thing was a metaphor, but I think it an apt one. If we really do this, it will be a shift in our business model and in our clinical model. It's not just adding a machine or a program: it's making technology integral to our overall strategy and a much bigger part of our operations. That's huge and it's not easy. I do think, though, that it can be done, and it can be done for all the right reasons. In the end, Fred's experience and Rajeev's experience are part of a much larger and growing trend. And we could be a leader in moving it forward."

Iris Inkwater is getting a lot of information from just listening to this discussion. It is like going through a mini Walk in the Woods. There is a logical next question, and Inkwater puts it to the group: "OK, now I know where you are coming from and what you disagree on. What is it that you all agree on?"

Fisher is enjoying his status as a voice for the cutting edge and so is eager to answer this question. He turns first to Grant: "I think, George, you were being a bit provocative, though you make an important point. People are going to expect something different from health care, from hospitals, and from our whole array of services. And you know what, at the same time, they are also going to expect the things they like to be the same. That's just the way it is. And I think someplace in the middle there is that sweet spot, where we get the balance just right. And if we can find a way to be really smart about that, we'll do very well because we already have a solid track record. We have to maintain our same high standards of care for the people who do come here for care and cure, and we have to extend those standards to the people whom we can serve in alternative at-home arrangements.

Does that make sense to everyone here?'' Fisher makes a gesture with his hands asking for agreement.

Johnson responds: ''That's nice, Fred, but you can't be everything to everybody. We're already talking about a pared-down system, and what happens when things are readjusted? I'm afraid that all the new sexy stuff with the fancy bells and whistles will get the attention and those left behind to clean out the bedpans will have more pressure and fewer resources for coping with it. I'm just saying that we have to be careful, that's all. Yes, of course, let's do it. Just be careful, because the dirty work is necessary. It isn't going away.''

''I have another idea,'' said Grant. ''Janice, I fully understand what you are saying. It's important. Iris, if it is OK with you let's do a quick map of the patient experience on the whiteboard. What are all the touch points? Where can a human deliver a superior experience, and where can a machine do a better job? Where do you need both?''

''Well, it starts when the patient walks, or is brought, into the hospital and ends when he or she leaves,'' offers Pudolski.

''I disagree,'' counters Abbington. ''It begins at the first moment a potential patient realizes she needs a hospital's services and it ends with her last follow up.''

''It ends when the patient pays the final bill,'' adds Rao, with a smile.

''You're thinking bigger, Arlan, but not big enough,'' says Lumberg. ''I think that the relationship begins at birth and continues for as long as that person is in our service area—until death.''

''See, this isn't as easy as you think,'' says Grant. ''For now, let's use Arlan's starting point and Rajeev's end point, because the whiteboard is only so big. Larry, we can expand the scope later, OK?'' Lumberg nods his assent, and for the next twenty minutes Grant stands at the board adding comments and suggestions from the group. What emerges is a complex map of a multitude of touch points that shows the connections and interdependencies between the various parts of the hospital, other agencies and organizations, and the larger community necessary to successfully treat a single patient. With a glance at the clock, Grant brings the mapping to a close. He snaps a photo of the whiteboard with the camera in his phone. ''I'll re-create this in a virtual work space online and give you access so that you can add to it and comment. This is a great start.''

Inkwater has continued to glean a great deal from the discussion. She realizes that one big part of creating a strategic direction for OMC will be to understand where the push-back is going to be and to work to mitigate it early, before it becomes an overwhelming obstacle. She also understands that new technology is not simply about the machines and the dollars they cost. The changes embedded in their introduction also evoke strong emotions, that's the human side of change. If she does not pay attention to those real feelings and that resistance, these new systems and their opportunities will be at best delayed and at worst lost. And after all, at the end of the day, it's still about the people.

System-Based Technology: Conflict and Negotiation

Negotiating the adoption of new technology and resolving conflict on the systems level within a large organization is different from what happens on the enterprise level because it provides the opportunity to meet and plan with the people who are directly affected. You can organize meetings and forums, conduct instructional sessions and evaluation surveys, develop strategies, and formulate a deliberate timeline. Each of these activities allows you to directly negotiate fears and concerns while identifying the motives and incentives that will encourage or discourage technology adoption. Most important, you can reap the buy-in that is necessary to move large groups of people in the same direction.

Within your system you can organize multiple Walks in the Woods. The goal is not to force the issue but to engage the range of stakeholders so that you can learn about and work with the resistance. From this, you evolve a plan for implementation that takes the range of legitimate interests into account. Through this process you not only win allies for the short term but also build a mind-set about technological change and innovation that can define the culture of your organization in the long term.

What is the starting point for introducing and negotiating technological innovation within a large health system? Experience with other large-scale change initiatives suggests that approximately 20 percent of the people affected will be on board right away—they are the early adopters. Another 20 percent will be against the proposed changes, either actively or passively—they are the resisters. The remaining 60 percent will take a wait-and-see attitude and may ultimately wind up for or against the change. You want to build an active negotiation strategy with each of these groups, cognizant of the distinct ways in which they approach questions of change. As you hear and respond to their different concerns, provide them with information and training, and engage their involvement, you build momentum and support for the innovations you seek to bring into the system. It must be a two-way process—you too will learn and may very well modify what you hope to incorporate into the system and your process for introducing it. Exercising intentional meta-leadership, you grow the momentum that yields the cross-system support for integrating new thinking and methods into your organization. This is the essence of leading at the edge of technological innovation in health care.

While focused on the macro negotiation involved with incorporating new technology into your system, recognize also the micro negotiations and conflicts that are taking place. People's responses to technological innovation often reveal a generation gap. Some of those strongest in their resistance to change may hold senior positions and command an established power base within the system. They of course were schooled on the existing technologies, are comfortable using them, and enjoy the status of being the experts about their operation. These senior leaders may have the wherewithal to build compelling alliances that counter efforts to exercise change. The younger and more junior staff may then find themselves in an awkward position, embracing the innovations and being eager to work with them yet having to avoid openly undermining their bosses' position.

What are the sources of such vehement resistance to introducing new technologies in a health organization? In the case of the electronic medical record or other information systems that require universal system adoption, senior clinical leaders may cringe at the notion of replacing what is for them an already satisfactory arrangement. They may regard the proposed change as fostering a new set of problems rather than resolving old ones. And it is true that technology alone is almost never the solution to a problem. Technology is a tool that can be deployed to increase speed, reduce variation, and open up vast repositories of knowledge and expertise. However, if not deployed wisely and strategically, technology can increase inefficiencies, spawn a multitude of work-arounds that increase variation and conflict in various parts of the system, and erect walls between users and nonusers. Its effectiveness is dependent upon the design of the overall system of which it is a part and the acceptance of the very people whose work will make it a success. This is why forcing adoption is not the objective. Recruiting input into design after negotiating participation is the ultimate negotiation objective. As Andy Wiesenthal, associate executive director for Clinical Information Support for the Permanente Federation, explained to us, "automating a non-system doesn't make it a system."

Even integrated systems such as Kaiser Permanente (KP) have challenges when implementing organization-wide technology applications. Wiesenthal observes that it took the vertically integrated KP some five years to deploy the EMR across the system, simply because of the sheer size of the organization. It had to be a staged rollout and KP learned throughout the process. Deploying the system was one challenge; getting everyone to use common content within the system was another. "Specialties that already had documentation standards, like pediatricians, were easiest," he recalls. Nurses also came together systemwide rather easily according to Wiesenthal: "Their 'true north' was quality, safe care, and they were open to change so long as it brought them closer to that goal." Doctors were more resistant. "Doctors had more issues with control. They were more attached to the way they were used to doing things." With them, Kaiser leveraged peer-to-peer interactions: "The people from the different regions would meet each other at conferences and share best practices. The success stories spread doctor to doctor, which was more effective than a directive from the central office."

Peer-to-peer persuasion is one way to encourage adoption of new technology. Tangible reward is another. "Medicine responds to cash flow very quickly," says Kaiser Permanente CEO George Halvorson. Scott Ransom agrees: "Doctors will do what pays." For that same reason, rivalries can also be motivating. "Information-enabled health care will soon be the standard of care," says Cindy Ehnes, director of California's Department of Managed Health Care. "Organizations like Kaiser Permanente have changed the game. They have used information to create competitive advantage."

The two largest health providers in the United States, the public Veterans Health Administration health care networks and the private and nonprofit Kaiser Permanente Health Care System, were the first major systems to employ electronic medical records across their vast national organizations. Other regional and local medical and health systems are now following. The conflicts and negotiations surrounding the use of an EMR or other systemwide technology do not end when the computers are plugged in and the systems deployed. Technology evolves and with each evolution, there must be further negotiation to ensure that what is on the screen and in the memory fits with the work to be done and the people who are doing it.

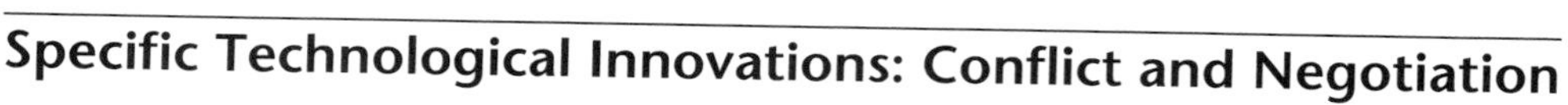

Specific Technological Innovations: Conflict and Negotiation

Our discussion of enterprise-wide and systemwide technological innovation addressed changes that will affect everyone in this country or everyone working in a large health care system. Most technological innovation is not that wide in scope and scale. The decision to upgrade diagnostic and treatment capacity through the purchase of specific new equipment is the direct or indirect subject of a large portion of the day-to-day negotiations and conflicts in all health care settings. Debates over whether to buy a new piece of equipment or software revolve around who pays, who benefits, who loses, and most important, the implications for each stakeholder of acquiring or not acquiring the latest technology.

Given the fast pace of technological innovation, negotiations and decisions on technological issues are a regular part of discussions. Perhaps the most difficult elements of these negotiations are the trade-offs implicit with each decision. Decision making is not simply a matter of choosing to invest in one innovation over another. It also requires calculating the revenues that any investment will reap and the amount of operating time it will take to pay off that initial expense. The question of whether the next generation of technological advance will occur before there can be a reasonable return on today's investment is always looming.

Frequently in these circumstances, on one side of the negotiating table are the clinicians who are advocating technological innovation: the latest diagnostic machine, surgical robot, or advance in information software. Of course every medical department and clinician wants the most up-to-date technology and will bargain with hospital or clinic administrators to purchase it on their behalf. The case will be made for the market growth possibilities as referring physicians and patients are attracted by the lure of the newest bells and whistles. The cost of any new piece of equipment will be confidently placed in light of the increased volume and the financial benefits expected to accrue with its purchase. And having the latest equipment quenches, for a time, the desires of clinicians to be working in a state-of-the-art atmosphere. These technological champions will expect the money, space, and personnel required to acquire and then operate cutting-edge technological advances.

On the other side of the table are the hospital or clinic managers. They must balance the decision about any particular purchase with other purchase decisions necessitated by the overall institutional budget, for which they are responsible. Market position, costs, and return on investment weigh in on any choice. These managers contemplate a much broader scope of practice than do the advocates of any particular piece of equipment. Whereas the department chief on the other side of the table has only to worry about his or her department, the hospital manager must worry about the well-being of every department and the institution as a whole. He or she must consider the many different ways to spend the limited dollars that are available. Many factors will push and pull on the parties at the negotiation table. The relative power and influence of the different department heads will weigh in. Who brings in the most money? Who is a favorite of the board of trustees? How does any one purchase fit into the overall inventory of technology in the hospital? And what are the downsides of not making a deal? These are complex questions, and the stakes can be very high.

There are many ways to frame the negotiations regarding technological innovation at the institutional and group-to-group level. Financial incentives and market pressures can be compelling drivers of influence and change. Christopher Crow was passionate about electronic medical records even before founding Legacy Medical Village in Plano, Texas. His primary care practice adopted a policy of referring patients only to specialists that used an EMR compatible with the one in Crow's practice. The lure of more referrals spurred specialists to go electronic, and now all the practices at Legacy Medical Village use interoperable EMR systems.

Technological innovation will also reshape the contours of medical practice, opening up heretofore unimaginable opportunities for practitioners. New and innovative uses of technology at the practice level could even uncover creative ways to increase the human touch that is so valued in the clinician-patient relationship. When physician Gordon Moore decided to leave his salaried position to start his own practice, simplicity was one thing he was looking for, and achieving it included removing barriers to communication with patients. "I decided to strip away all of the junk," he says. "I decided to launch a practice by myself: no administrator, no receptionist, no assistant. Just me. By keeping it simple I found that I was able to see my patients when they needed to see me and that my communication with them was more meaningful. I could have a smaller patient base and still be profitable. I had a Norman Rockwell practice in the twenty-first century."

Moore is not the only physician we found following this model. Pamela Wible in Eugene, Oregon, set up a one-person practice after burning out as an employee of a larger practice. We also met Richard Donahue, in the Boston area, who is now trying to replicate in an urban area the primary care setting he described as "perfect" when he was the sole year-round doctor on the island of Vinalhaven, Maine. Both echoed much of what Moore told us, and we will explore their practice models in greater detail in Chapter Fourteen.

"I found that giving my patients direct access to me—they have my cell phone number for use after hours—boosted their confidence in our relationship," Moore told us. "They were much more respectful of my time regarding after-hours calls than what I was used to when I had been on call covering a number of physicians' patients in my previous role." Moore's example demonstrates that removing barriers to access caused his patients to self-filter the information they communicated to him. In addition he was available for same-day appointments, so his patients felt less need to call him in the middle of the night unless they had a true emergency; they knew they would be able to get in to see him the next day, when it would be more convenient for them and for him.

Technology was central to Moore's approach. He knew that he would have to simplify the administrative back-end of his practice, and he chose what he calls "elegant" tools for doing so: applications and interfaces that were easy and pleasant to use and that involved no more complexity than was absolutely necessary. His practice grew to about four hundred patients and was financially viable (he did eventually bring a registered nurse into the practice).

As of the time of this writing, Moore was president of Hello Health University, which is part of Hello Health, one of the companies helping primary care practices use technology to improve patient relationships. Moore says that "studies have shown that great primary care is a key differentiator that creates a high-performance health system, and there are four critical features of great primary care: access, relationship over time, care coordination, and comprehensiveness of services. Technology has a role in each of these."

Hello Health facilitates patient-doctor interaction through instant messaging and Web-based video chats in addition to calling or scheduling an office visit. The company's Web site (www.hellohealth.com) states that one of the primary benefits offered by this multichannel approach is time saved by both the patient and the doctor. These elegant interfaces try to match the channel with the need to make the communication as efficient as possible. Insurance reimbursement policies, however, will often not yet pay for video or Web-based consultations, and this has been a significant barrier to adoption of these communication technologies. This lag by payers will often cause new technology to be passed over initially yet become adopted when payment practices and schedules catch up.

Hello Health is not the only company in search of an elegant solution to managing information. For example, Alta Point's mobile application gives access to medical records, patient notes, scheduling, and even images and X-rays on a provider's smartphone. Clinically Relevant Technologies offers an iPhone app that delivers "musculoskeletal diagnosis in your pocket" and is just one of a number of similarly specialized applications. There are tools for prioritizing and grouping e-mail messages and for automatically aggregating information on topics of interest. Forthcoming are programs designed to determine how "interruptible" a clinician is, based on keyboard and mouse patterns, and that then hold or deliver e-mail accordingly. Thousands of these innovative applications will be released in the years ahead. Of course, they are like a microcosm of the health care system itself in that most will address just a small part of the problem and many of them will add more information to the mix. And whether they are more help or burden will be a question for each new program and application.

Technology innovation is and will ever be a topic of negotiation and conflict resolution in your practice and work in health care. This fact speaks to the advantages of building routine mechanisms and methods for reconciling the inevitable tensions between bursting enthusiasm and overbearing resistance that accompany each new technological gadget and capability. Beyond responding to the strong emotional reactions that new technologies can evoke, leaders must also answer pragmatic questions of expenditures, revenues, and markets, judiciously incorporating all this information into the decision-making mix. Technological

Heather Harriford parks her car in the off-site parking lot and takes the shuttle to the hospital, as most nurses do on the evening shift. She is sitting way back on the left side of the van, staring vacantly out the window as it slowly makes its way about the lot, picking up employees. From the corner of her eye, she notices Gail Gonzalez making her way up the stairs. She pays no attention, content to be alone. She activates her tablet computer and stares intently at the nursing news feed to which she subscribes. She notes a new study on remote monitoring of outpatient EKGs for later reading.

Without looking up, Heather senses someone taking the place beside her. She turns to see Gonzalez, who is looking timidly in her direction. They haven't spoken since Heather left the intensive care unit.

"Checking your Facebook page?" Gonzalez asks meekly. She is obviously holding something she needs to get off her chest.

Heather rolls her eyes. "No, I've been staying away from the gossip mills. Just catching up on my professional reading."

Gonzalez nods knowingly. "Heather, I just want you to know how much I admire what you did with Cummings," she says. "There are a lot of nurses who think your making a stink was a bad idea. It took a lot of guts. Most people would have just put up with it. You need to know that I really respect you for what you did."

Gonzalez finishes her speech and sinks back in the seat. The sentiment has weighed heavily upon her, and now that it is out, she relaxes. She has felt guilty in the past about not protesting when the same thing had happened to her. She feels a comforting sense of atonement in lending encouragement to someone who did.

Harriford, sensing Gonzalez's confusion, is unsure how to respond. She retreats to what feels safe. "Thanks a lot." It is a lifeless statement.

Gonzalez feels Harriford's discomfort. She wants to explain. "I know that you and I haven't always seen eye to eye in the past. Sometimes it felt like we came from different planets, you know, very different approaches to what we do and how we go about doing it. I guess I just wrote you off—even worse, became annoyed with you, really. I just thought many times you had too much of, what do they call it?—*chutzpah*, saying what was on your mind and going against the grain."

"And then when this whole affair with Dr. Cummings happened—I mean this whole issue—well, it was that same boldness that let you stand up to him and his kind. Maybe you needed that self-confidence in order to handle it the way you did. I don't know how many times I have been in your shoes, with the same thing happening to me. You know, you put up with things. Or you play games to get what you need to get. And then afterwards, even if nothing really terrible happened, you still feel cheapened, like you were used. So to see someone stand up and say, 'Hell, no,' why that gets a lot of admiration in my book.'' Gonzalez is smiling: it takes guts for her to make even that admission. And she has said it. She feels good about herself.

Harriford smiles back. ''I really appreciate your saying this. I can't tell you how much self-doubt I've been feeling about this whole thing. I mean, on the one hand you're right, I did the right thing and I'm glad I did it. Some of the nurses have been great, supporting me and everything. Then on the other hand there have been a lot of people who have come out against me. The debate popped up on a couple of nursing blogs, and even though people were discreet enough to omit my name I feel like this is happening in a fish bowl. I guess it's just human nature that you hear those voices the loudest, because they speak to your own sense of uncertainty. It's scary bucking the system, going against one of those gospels of good nursing behavior.'' She pauses. She hadn't expressed all these feelings to anyone else. And now to open up to, of all people, Gail Gonzalez. Maybe it is fitting, because she had assumed Gonzalez was one of those gabbing the loudest against her behind her back but saying nothing to her face.

Harriford continues. ''I guess a lot of things flash through your mind when something like this happens. You get really practical. I have rent and my student loans to pay. What if I lose my job? How might this affect my getting into school again? And what would my family think? Once something is on the Internet, it is there forever. Privacy has become a quaint notion. Courage is a great thing as long as everything works out OK in the end. It just gets rough when there is no guarantee of a happy ending.''

''So, Gail, I guess that I really appreciate your saying this.'' She can feel her self-respect and self-confidence building. ''You're right, it took a lot of guts. Even as I was going through it, it felt like I was watching a movie about somebody else. And I think in the long run that it was even a good thing for Cummings. He wasn't mortally damaged, and actually, he would have gotten hit by this behavior eventually. He's just lucky that it hit him here and now. I realized that. He's a good doctor and he really cares about his patients. He learned his lesson and he'll go on. There was no need to cut off his . . . I mean, you know what I mean.'' Gonzalez nods, smiling. ''Anyway, I guess it all worked out in the end. You have guts too, now that I know how you feel. I know that I'm not always the easiest person to approach. The world sends you such mixed signals. It's nice to be reassured sometimes.''

Gonzalez realizes that her support for Harriford is far more important than she has ever imagined. She wants to make the point very clear. ''Heather, you taught me an important lesson about speaking out. If you don't have the backbone to state your mind, then the world does in fact become lopsided.'' She mimics the movement of a balance, lifting her hands up and down. ''That piece of what you have to offer simply is not on the scale if you don't express it. So part of our obligation is speaking out. The question should not be *whether* you do it. The question is *how* you do it, and when and to whom. Somehow, Heather, you got it right. I admire you for that."

The van stops in front of the hospital, its squeaking brakes punctuating Gail's last comment. The two nurses quietly make their way down the narrow aisle and into the hospital lobby. Before going their separate ways, they hug each other. Gonzalez whispers to Harriford, "You should feel very good about yourself. And if anything erupts on Twitter, you can count no me to leap to your defense."

Harriford whispers back, "Thanks a lot. I needed that. And let's just hope this whole thing doesn't go any more viral than it already has."

innovation is an evolving process that naturally transpires through successive steps of change and ultimate acceptance or rejection. The smoother that evolution, the fewer the distractions along the way and the better your focus on what your organization can do and do better. It is working through these people processes that will allow you to help the new machines to do their jobs.

Negotiating Trade-Offs in Technological Innovation

Nothing is perfect. The good old days weren't. The future won't be. And certainly there is no such thing as technological innovation without trade-offs. That may be hard for some to accept.

Although new technology will provide you with greater access to information, it will also demand greater standardization in how you enter information into a program and what you get out of the program on the other side. Information technology will make it much easier to access data and run analyses to inform your decisions, whether they are about which drug to administer or how many people to schedule for a Saturday afternoon shift. Evidence-based counsel will be more available as you make decisions, reducing your need to rely on rule of thumb or anecdotal acumen.

Standardization may irk some people. Specific questions will need to be asked in a precise order. Form may not always fit function. Discretion and flexibility may be sacrificed for the good of the whole. Standardizing questions and data is not as easy as it may appear. John Halamka told us that one of the first bits of data that the Health IT Standards Committee he serves on tackled was gender identification. "We thought that should be relatively easy," he said with a smile. However, the group found twenty-seven variations in how different systems collected even that basic information: "We got people to agree to use four: male, female, other, and unknown."

Halamka also noted that technology can smooth out some disparities in data gathered by different systems. Filters between the individual systems and the aggregator of the data can act almost like language translators: so long as the aggregator knows and understands the "language" each system is speaking, it can compile all the input in a consistent form in a master database.

Entering data can be time consuming. Martha Crowninshield O'Brien, a hospital-based nurse with twenty-five years of experience commented to us, "All of this technology is great but it can be cumbersome. It can take time away from patient care—and what is more important than that?" This was a sentiment echoed by Winchester Hospital's chief medical officer, Richard Iseke: "Increasingly, doctors and other caregivers will have to balance the time they spend with the patient and the time they spend entering information into the system—and that is a dilemma that must be solved."

Mary Bylone, assistant vice president of patient care at William W. Backus Hospital in Connecticut, brought forward another concern: technology-induced tunnel vision. She explained that in the "old days" a nurse would scan a patient's chart not only to see what tasks she needed to perform but also to double-check what had or had not been done by the doctor and other caregivers. She was able to spot anomalies, omissions, or mistakes. In the new tech-centered care environment, Bylone sees her nurses much more closely focused on just what the system identifies as the tasks for the nurse. "Tasks 'to do' are pink and turn to black when completed," she said. "The nurses are fanatical about turning the pink to black, but they tend not to worry about the tasks color coded for someone else. If it's not pink, they don't notice it."

Andy Wiesenthal counseled, "Get people to use the system first and worry about standardization later. People are wedded to how they do things, so you have to accept that certain aspects of adoption are going to occur through incremental change." He recommended negotiating and building the system on a consistent underlying platform and allowing each specialty to decide on best practices within the parameters of the platform. This gives power and a sense of control back to the caregivers and allows the "ideal" system to evolve over time and with input from stakeholders.

One common mistake made in the design and implementation of an enterprise-wide system is the *blue sky paradox* (McNulty, 2003). In order to get buy-in for the significant investment of time and resources necessary for such a system, advocates may ask people to "blue sky it": dream big and imagine their absolute ideal system. This discovery process is useful for uncovering what stakeholders really want, where their pain points are, and what objections they will raise. Expectations, however, must be managed carefully between discovery and delivery, because a host of factors—budgets, timelines, security requirements, legacy system integration issues, vendor design limitations, and more—shape the final system as much as the initial brainstorming. The delivered systems will not match anyone's ideal, and people will be disappointed, and in some cases hostile unless the process has been transparent and each stakeholder understands why and how the design decisions were made. Using the Walk in the Woods to frame such a conversation, a group can move constructively from their creative enlightened interests to their more pragmatic aligned interests, working in a manner that explicates complex trade-offs.

Care options will become more standardized as technologies are introduced, though there may be controversy over how those options are selected. A compelling argument can be made for ensuring that quality measures are paramount. Others may argue that other criteria should be in the mix, such as cost and convenience for the patient. You will have to negotiate the subtle choices, especially when the advantages of one option over another are ambiguous. Overall institutional utilization patterns may enter into decisions regarding a particular patient's access to or use of advanced technology. Some decisions will be afforded room to be negotiated whereas others will simply be put through standardized decision protocols. According to Paul Levy, former CEO of the Beth Israel Deaconess Medical Center in Boston, "Ninety-five percent of what patients need can be standardized. Doctors remained well intentioned but we face a battle of individual medical mythology—the doctor as artist—versus evidence-based medicine."

Although the adoption of the EMR in this country has been slow, its evolution will likely follow that of information technologies in other fields. In its early days, the EMR was an electronic replacement for the paper that came before it: its function was to document past actions and to be a reference and reporting resource. In time the EMR will become an increasingly robust, real-time decision support tool that will even be able to systematically predict future outcomes. Corporations call the combined capability of data collection, reporting, and analysis *business intelligence*. The predictive capability is called *analytics*.

More than ever, people in health care will practice their professions in glass houses. Each of the players in the health care system is likely to draw on various analyses to achieve his or her objectives: administrators will be able to monitor costs more closely and correlate expenditures to revenue, outcomes, and patient satisfaction; doctors and nurses will not only be able to make better clinical decisions but may be able to negotiate their compensation and perhaps even their access to facilities based on their performance; insurance companies may be able to exert more influence on care choices by setting reimbursement rates based on evidence of the efficacy of various options; and patients may be able to mimic their caregivers by becoming knowledgeable about their own conditions and treatment options (we will say more about that in Chapter Thirteen).

"You had better know the basic tools of negotiation because every conversation is a negotiation," advised Paul Levy. "What is your desired outcome? How do you get better at achieving it?" As we have discussed in previous chapters, not only will specific decisions proceed through a negotiation process but even the question of who participates in making the decision will be a matter of negotiation.

In the "good old days," diagnosis and care decisions rested with the doctor. He or she was master and commander, the sole keeper of the information. Patients deferred to the knowledgeable authority figure. Insurers too would generally bow to the doctor, so long as the course of treatment proposed fell within the parameters of clinically proven options. Administrators would also tolerate extra expenses because it was assumed that the doctor, operating under the Hippocratic oath, was always acting in the patient's best interest. And nurses labored in a hierarchical setting that put the doctor on top.

Now it is different. "It's all about influence," Eddie Erlandson, told us. "Physicians don't tend to see themselves as influencers but rather as repositories of knowledge and skill to turn knowledge into direct action. However, it is through influencers that they can have the greatest positive impact on patient outcomes by helping shape patient behaviors and the broader range of activities from prevention to rehabilitation. Influence creates a ripple effect of impact beyond the physician's direct actions."

The best news, according to Erlandson, is that influence is a learned skill. "The activities that lead to influence tend to be prefrontal activities," he said. "We know that we can grow brain cells throughout our lives so, in essence, influence all comes back to neuroscience and neuroplasticity. However, the trick is to use those cells or lose them."

Increasingly, health care is becoming a team sport, with the information technology portal holding a powerful seat at the table. In today's flattening hierarchies, more stakeholders expect to have input on decisions throughout the process. "The missing link to better health care isn't economic," said Kaiser Permanente's George Halvorson. "It is functional care delivery. 'Team' is the missing ingredient." In his book, *Health Care Will Not Reform Itself*, Halvorson (2009) argues that the vast majority of costs in the U.S. health care system come from chronic conditions and that the key to managing chronic conditions is coordinated care. Technology makes it possible to form care teams (which may be virtual) and share information, and it also provides the tools for oversight of those teams. If you are a primary care physician, you will be able to learn about the care received by your patients from the specialists to which you referred them. You will be able to compare the aggregate of your patients to those of the partners in your practice and across your region. But you will not be the only one who knows what percentage of your diabetic patients had their annual eye and foot exams; that information will be shared with your peers, your supervisors, your patients, and the general public.

The upside of these emerging technologies is they will exponentially unleash the potential for truly personalized medicine. If Moore's Law (Moore, 1965) holds true, computing power will continue to double approximately every two years, and it is predicted that we are rapidly approaching a time when mapping an individual genome will become affordable for the average person. Rather than acting based just on the evidence from a particular class of patients, doctors will be crafting a truly individualized treatment plan based on an in-depth analysis of each specific patient. Technology will be essential to this advance. It simply would not be possible for a caregiver who lacks information technology to master each patient's vast data set and to then optimize in a timely manner the many treatment variables available. As this evolution continues, even in your lifetime possibilities will become available that today can barely be imagined.

Living and Negotiating in an Evolving Health Care World

As technology grows so too will the mountain of information and communication available to you. As Mary Bylone reminded us, "Technology never stops." Reports and analyses like those outlined in this chapter will generate an almost endless stream of data. The struggle will be to give each participant in the system the information he or she needs, when and where she needs it. You may or may not have been born a "digital native" (Prensky, 2001). Nevertheless, you are likely only too familiar with the continual flow of information in most areas of your life, delivered via phone calls, text messages, e-mails, social networking site updates, tweets, RSS feeds, and many, many other media. You may even revel in it. As your professional life evolves, you will see this multiply by an order of magnitude. Your ability to make life-or-death decisions correctly will rest in part on your ability to master this torrent of data. In its 2008 annual report, Kaiser Permanente lists not only its key financial and clinical data but the number of patients using its online health management tool (2.7 million), of lab results viewed online (16.7 million), of secure e-mails sent to physicians and clinicians (6 million), and of online requests for appointments (1.4 million).

Information overload is a term coined by futurist Alvin Toffler to describe a flow of information so voluminous that it is difficult to differentiate what is important from what is not and therefore difficult to absorb and act on that which is important. Your professional challenge in this world of continuous and consistent technological innovation is to cast a net wide enough to capture all the vital information—news, developments in your field and with your patients, and even office gossip—and at same time to manage the total flow of information so you are not overwhelmed by the extraneous. The implications of succumbing to information overload are many: increased cardiovascular stress, confusion, impaired judgment, overconfidence, and decreased benevolence toward others (Shenk, 1997, pp. 37–38) along with adverse effects on decision making, innovation, and productivity. One study of knowledge workers distracted by phone calls and e-mails evidenced an average 10 point drop from normal in their IQ scores (Hemp, 2009).

In his classic study on urban stress published in 1970, Stanley Milgram laid out a number of responses and adaptations people make to deal with overload: they (1) allocate less time to each input; (2) disregard low-priority inputs; (3) redraw boundaries to shift burden to other parties; (4) block reception (using such tactics as unlisted phone numbers and unfriendly facial expressions); (5) employ filters to diminish the intensity of inputs; and (6) create specialized institutions to absorb inputs that would otherwise overwhelm the individual (Shenk, 1997, p. 39). Each of these adaptations is valid when applied intentionally, skillfully, and in the right context.

One can also learn to live with and manage technology so that it becomes less of a burden and more of a manageable tool. Learn to negotiate with yourself about the push and pulls that infringe on your time and attention. For example, you can set specific times of day to answer nonurgent e-mails or schedule a *devices-off* afternoon each week so that you have time for concentrated work and thinking. You can require yourself to put a quarter in a jar for each e-mail or text message you send so that you have a visible, if only relative, measure of the cost of the time spent. Find what works for you, always remembering that it is possible to preserve your very human control of technology.

Conclusion

When historians analyze the impact of the current wave of technological innovation on the evolution of the health enterprise, they likely will note that technology served to demystify and decentralize what before had been the province of the few and the privileged. Doctors were the fountains of knowledge and skill, and others were kept out. The World Wide Web opened the doors to that knowledge. Machines became more steady and reliable than the hands they replaced.

Medical records leapt from the confines of their file cabinets to the fingertips of their subjects, who could match their medical histories with emerging innovations in diagnosis and treatment.

Is it possible with all this change to imagine that the people who work in the system will be replaced? Some will, though all won't. Will the work, roles and responsibilities, and relative status shift? For all who remain, the answer is most certainly yes.

One example of this is what many physicians used to call the "tyranny of the image." Not too long ago, physicians were beholden to radiologists' and their reports about diagnostic images because radiologists owned the films. Now, those same images are captured digitally and can be transmitted and viewed on a computer screen anywhere. They can even be accessed by the patient remotely, one of a myriad of examples of just what decentralization and demystification can mean.

So what then will be the role of the humans in this quickly changing world of health care technological evolution? There will always be tasks and techniques that the machines cannot perform. Those jobs will be left to humans. There is the humanitarian quality of health care, which can never be assumed by a machine. And there is the day-to-day negotiation and conflict resolution that will drive the decisions regarding the course of this technological innovation. Unless the science fiction notion of the machines one day taking over comes to pass, it will be left to human leaders to chart the course of this history. There will be negotiation and conflict resolution aplenty. And should you take it: that is your seat at the table.

CHAPTER 13

THE NEGOTIATING PATIENT

At one time, health care operated in a neat "command-and-control" environment. There was a respected pyramid of roles, and everyone seemed to know the rules and how to play. Doctors were on top and had the power of the *doctor's orders*. Nurses and other professionals in the clinical chain of command put those orders into operation. Health care administrators kept the organization humming. And at the bottom of the pyramid—the object of all this clinical work and business—was the patient. Patients were expected to accept a subservient role, no matter their social or economic status outside the hospital gown that adorned them. To the same degree that those on top of the pyramid felt *in charge*, patients felt *powerless*.

A more knowledgeable patient is now emerging and changing that equation. Although the increasingly popular moniker of *empowered patient* would seem to indicate that all has changed, in fact it hasn't. Vestiges of the old order persist alongside a new and expanding set of expectations. As expectations change, conflicts emerge and negotiations occur between those who *get* services, information, and guidance from the health system and those who are on the *giving* side of the equation. Patients now expect to get something very different from before, as demonstrated by their interest in participating in decision making, sharing information, and having their unique personal needs and intentions accommodated. If all these patients formed a monolith, it would be relatively easy to devise and implement a strategy for negotiating with this universal template that we could call *today's patient*. Unfortunately, not only are these patients different from who they were before but the variations in what they

---

Unless otherwise noted, quotations and summaries of comments from James Conway, Kimberly Costa, Martha Crowninshield O'Brien, Cindy Ehnes, George Halvorson, Richard Iseke, and Paul Levy are taken from interviews conducted by the authors in 2009 and 2010.

expect are also spread across a much wider continuum: different patients are counting on different relationships with their caregivers. And for every force, there is a countervailing force.

In Chapter Twelve, we noted that one of the benefits and constraints of technology is that it pushes its users to standardize protocols, information, and communication. Common standards make it easier to make evidence-based decisions and to move and process data, procedures, and people in ways that reduce variability, mistakes, and the expenses of customizing work to fit unique circumstances. Improving efficiencies and reducing the variations that can prompt mistakes are compelling purposes and pressures. The question is whether the new technologies and their powers of standardization will reinvigorate the old pyramid of command and control or open it up. Will the mechanics of a system that relies on all-purpose protocols serve to dehumanize patients and the caregiving process?

These two seemingly contradictory forces—the emerging expectations of patients and the standardizing demands of technology—could very well fuse to foster a healthier set of expectations and relationships that enriches both caregivers and those cared for. Wise clinicians and hospitals could make this emerging set of expectations and relationships part of their marketing appeal. Patients do not want only to be cured. They want to be treated as distinct and assured individuals traversing a difficult period in their lives. Protection and personalization offer an exceptional and compelling allure when you are sick and in need of support, whether momentary or long term.

Changing Roles and Relationships

We can locate a number of sentinel turning points that mark changes in patient identity. At the beginning of this century, the Institute of Medicine (2001) produced a hallmark report, *Crossing the Quality Chasm: A New Health System for the 21st Century*, that clearly embraced the empowered patient. The principles of the proposed system call for an approach that will (1) respect patients' values, preferences, and expressed needs; (2) coordinate and integrate care across boundaries of the system; (3) provide the information, communication, and education that people need and want; and (4) guarantee physical comfort, emotional support, and the involvement of family and friends (pp. 52–53). It is intriguing that this document so moved the health system with a set of principles and recommendations that one might have assumed were already firmly in place. In fact they were not.

It is hard to imagine a health care professional who would not see patient care as the ultimate mission. However, beyond that core principle, there is significant variation in opinions about how patients should be treated and involved in their care. At one extreme are the traditionalists who believe that patients should simply do as they are told and leave the decision making and work to the professionals. At the other extreme are the champions of patient-centered care who picture the patient deeply involved and perhaps even acting as captain of the health care team. This distinction is not simply a matter of different camps that coalesce in different corners and around distinct strategies and mechanisms for treating patients. This battle can play out daily during hospital rounds, patient care conferences, discharge planning discussions, and in the direct interactions with patients and their families. And this is not a profession-specific set of battle lines. Doctors are arranged across a spectrum of opinions, as are nurses, physical therapists, social workers, and others who directly engage patients in their care. The different templates that are brought to the table then translate into the distinct frames used to understand and then either direct or negotiate patient care.

The starting point for engaging differently with patients is engaging differently with colleagues. What set of questions at a patient care conference or team meeting might help you to engage a brief Walk in the Woods as you and your colleagues traverse patient care considerations or recommendations? Once everyone on your floor or you and your colleagues make it a given that different patients and families want to be treated differently, you all can check in together and develop a strategy for most effectively constructing roles and relationships. Are you and your colleagues working with a patient and family who want to be actively involved in decision making? Do they have the wherewithal to assume a highly independent level of responsibility? Are you all working with a patient and family who are more passive, preferring a more directed approach and anxious when given too much information or too significant a role in decision making? As caregivers around the table briefly exchange their experiences with a patient and his or her family, as well as their opinions about which course will be most effective, they are presented with the opportunity to develop a strategy and plan that best suits the unique circumstances of each clinical encounter. With time, a rhythm and culture develops that informs both general principles regarding engaging patients and the efficient accomplishment of specific strategies.

Do these questions and this negotiation require a bit of extra work in the short run? Yes, they do. Will they save time and effort in the long run? Yes, they will. Negotiating care and activity is not only an interface with the patient. It begins with an appreciation for patients' overall experience with the people and providers they will encounter in the course of their care experience. Whether the patient is facing an acute episode or a longer-term, chronic care situation, charting the best course of patient involvement should be as much a part of the care plan as the medications and treatments prescribed. This requires looking at the individual not simply as a patient but as a complete human being for whom the encounter with the health system is one side of a much larger life. It is the person and the life that health care providers should consider, not simply the period that categorizes this human as a patient. In the long run, if the caregiving decisions chart well and appropriately leverage the active involvement of patient and family, what is done more accurately and thereby more efficiently matches the wishes and capacities of the patient, allowing the system to complement rather than unnecessarily supplant or miss what the patient can do on his or her own.

The Evolving Patient

The evolution of today's *negotiating patient* dates from developments that occurred during the last two decades of the twentieth century. This evolution arose in part from shifts in the availability of information and knowledge and from a growing suspicion of institutions and professions. The more people came to know and understand, the less trusting they became of the systems and caregivers directing their care, and the more in charge they have wanted to be. In health care as in other fields of endeavor, information technology opened new horizons and expectations. The economics and politics of health care and its reform leapt from the background and into the headlines, prompting new questions from consumers about what they were buying and getting in the way of services and guarantees. All this occurred alongside the country's changing demographics, and as the aging and activist-minded baby boomers turned with increasing need to the health system, they were disappointed in what they found. A less passive and more activist patient presented at the health care doors, carrying new frustrations and the conflicts that abide them.

Over this time frame, seven significant sets of change have continued to unfold: (1) the increasing availability and democratization of information resulting from the growth of Internet accessibility and content; (2) the growth of direct-to-consumer advertising by pharmaceutical companies; (3) a general shift of responsibility across society from institutions to individuals; (4) the negative reaction to the cost-containment practices of health maintenance organizations (HMOs); (5) the wider acceptance by the general public of nontraditional treatments as alternatives to conventional medicine; (6) the rise in the understanding of health literacy and its impact on population health; and (7) the growing acceptance of the impact of behavior, social determinants, and the environment, including foods, on individual health and well-being and, with that, acceptance of individual responsibility for one's health. Each of these areas of change will be individually discussed.

A.

The Internet and Information

August 25, 1995, may not be a date noted in many health care textbooks, though it should be. On that otherwise unremarkable day a sixteen-month-old Silicon Valley start-up called Netscape went public. Netscape was the first commercially available version of the Mosaic graphical user interface for the Internet. This innovation set in motion the Internet revolution that followed. It enabled any company or any individual to post and retrieve information on the World Wide Web. The volume of information available to anyone with a computer exploded when that computer became connected to the Internet.

Another noteworthy date is May 20, 1999. This is the day on which two companies, Healtheon Corporation and WebMD, Inc., merged. They established an enterprise that provided Web-based health information to both physicians and the general public. There are now a multitude of medical information providers online. At the time though, this merger was newsworthy because both medical professionals and the lay population were being served on the same information platform. Portending the future, the merged companies attracted investment from heavyweights like Microsoft and Intel.

We now take for granted the Internet as an information resource and communication tool. Searches for medical information are among the most frequent, with studies reporting that from 40 to 80 percent of U.S. adults have searched for health information on the Web (Sillence, Briggs, Harris, & Fishwick, 2007). The majority of patients who conduct searches do so before a clinical visit—to determine if one is necessary—and after a clinical visit—either for reassurance regarding the information that the clinician's provided or because the patient is not satisfied with that information (McMullan, 2006). And yet, in many ways, we are just beginning to tap into the Internet's potential to transform the relationships between patients and their caregivers. Doctors and nurses are learning to embrace e-mail and online video linkages as ways to communicate and interact with patients, encouraged by the fact that insurers are beginning to compensate for these virtual interactions. Patients at Kaiser Permanente and their doctors now receive clinical test results at the same time. That availability and transparency is likely to spread as patients, caregivers, and insurers become more Internet savvy.

In the previous chapter, the potential impact of emerging technology was explored. Extending that question to the changing expectations of patients and negotiations with those patients, how might these new technologies affect relationships and the patient experience? Consider, for example, how a method used in a different sector could migrate into the health system, if for no other reason than that it has attracted market demand and, with it, business interest.

LendingTree.com is a popular Web site that allows consumers to post their loan needs and lenders to bid for their business. It reverses the traditional arrangement of the borrower performing the research and coming as a supplicant hoping to be granted an audience by a bank loan officer. Instead, LendingTree allows the consumer to review up to four competitive loan offers. It assumes that the consumer, not the bank, is the scarce resource. It thereby *empowers* consumers, allowing them more choices, more leverage, and thereby a more competitive marketplace in which to select a lender. The company provided the platform and consumers created the demand. LendingTree recast the negotiation process.

Now imagine a similar site where a consumer could upload her electronic medical record and the pathology report from a biopsy and then receive competitive offers from physicians to treat her. Instead of comparing interest rates, the consumer could compare outcome measures, cost, and patient satisfaction scores. This puts the comparative bid and the information transparently in the hands of the patient. Who knew before what procedures cost, what the track record of the doctor was, and how well other patients rated their care experience? It would likewise recast the negotiation process in keeping with genuinely patient-directed health care.

Though health care institutions have been slower to realize its full potential than many other fields of endeavor, the Internet is a game changer. And it will continue to be so as long as there is progress in the data it can process and information it can provide. In time, virtually everything that the health care giver can access will be available to the patient: medical journals, lab reports, and medical records.

The problem of course is that data in the hands of the unschooled may prompt as much confusion and misdirection as it does illumination. For example, researchers from Microsoft have studied *cyberchondria*: the escalation of medical concerns as a result of information found on the Web (White & Horvitz, 2009). This is all the more problematic when such information is put in the hands of someone who is facing a health crisis and emotionally in the basement. Data and outcomes at the margin can climb to front and center in the mind of a person unused to discerning subtleties in medical information and fearful of what the data might mean. The fact is that for some people, ignorance truly is bliss. That is why they go to any expert for any piece of advice. Despite that, the Internet may have an allure they or their lay advisers cannot resist. Knowing more does not always make someone a wiser or more discerning decision maker. Even though the genie is now out of the bottle—we can never go back to that naive and compliant patient of yesteryear—negotiating with patients about what they have learned or concluded from what they have found on the Internet is simply a factor with which medical professionals must work.

Medical knowledge has evolved through a rigorous process of ferreting out fact from fiction. Publication in a medical journal is a validation of the research processes and reliability of the findings. No such filter exists for what patients find on the Internet. Fact, folly, and fantasy seamlessly coexist, and it can be difficult if not impossible to convince a suspicious and frightened patient that the side effects of a life-giving medication are not as reported on the Internet. Negotiating with patients about scientifically valid and rigorously researched matters is one thing. Negotiating about opinions based on hearsay and unsubstantiated claims is another. The latter phenomenon tests a caregiver's patience.

It is not simply the information explosion with which caregivers must contend. There is also the device explosion. Smartphones and other tools enable a patient or that patient's family member to gain access to information via the Internet from virtually anywhere in real time: from an office or exam room, an emergency room, or a hospital room. The patient is able to research caregivers' recommendations almost as fast as they make them.

Health care providers will also encounter a converse problem: some of the patients they treat, particularly the elderly, may have little understanding of or comfort with online information resources and tools. These patients are used to looking a doctor straight in the eye, with no computer in between. One patient complaint often heard is that "it is so hard to talk to a person anymore." Patients not caught up in the technology revolution may experience significant frustration and alienation and this may compromise the caregiving process. The lesson is to not assume the technological proficiency of your patients. As technology rapidly evolves, each generation will display a very different expectation about and proficiency and comfort with incorporating information technology into their health care experience. This necessarily is another point of negotiation.

Direct-to-Consumer Advertising by Pharmaceutical Companies

In 1997, the U.S. Food and Drug Administration changed its regulations to allow pharmaceutical companies to market prescription drugs directly to consumers. At this writing, only the United States and New Zealand allow this practice. According to a study published in the *New England Journal of Medicine*, from 1996 to 2005, spending on consumer-directed advertising for pharmaceuticals grew by 330 percent (Donahue, Cevasco, & Rosenthal, 2007). Remarkably, some researchers have estimated that in the year they studied, 2004, the pharmaceutical industry spent almost twice as much on promotion—including advertising and

Artie Ashwood's discharge conversation with Oscar Ortiz covers more than just the usual instructions for his posthospital care. Not only does Ortiz give him the sort of personal attention that he appreciates as a patient—and he is immeasurably grateful for that—this unusual nurse goes above and beyond the call of duty, helping him to resolve the conflict between his mother and girl friend about where he will recuperate. That is huge and as far as Ashwood is concerned: he'd like to nominate Ortiz for the Nobel peace prize.

Now that Ashwood has been home for five days and is feeling much better, his old college roommate, Sal Schwartz, stops by for a visit. "So, all your buddies are hoping this is going to be a wake-up call for you, Artie. You're too young to be acting like some old-timer. You've got to get in shape."

Ashwood's response is a mix of shame and hope. "I know. Some of this I did to myself," he says sheepishly. "I am promising everyone that I will be losing weight. I am shooting for forty pounds."

Schwartz looks at him with skepticism.

"No, really," Ashwood replies. "I talked with the nutrition specialist at the hospital. She helped me put together a plan I can live with. From now on, celery and low-carb dip when we get together to watch a game. No pizza and no beer for me—at least until I get to my target weight. Then, I go on maintenance. Maybe I'll inspire some other people to cut down with me," he says, gesturing with a laugh to the few extra pounds Schwartz has put on since their undergraduate days.

"Celery, huh? OK, I can do celery. I'll match you, two to one. I need to take off twenty myself. You know, if the two of us start a trend together, we could tackle the whole obesity problem in this country. We'll start some sort of thinness infection."

"It would be great having some company, Sal. If my lousy experience helps someone else, then it will have been worth it." Ashwood appreciates the support—something the nutritionist told him was important to diet success.

"What else did you pick up in the hospital, other than a big bill?" Schwartz asks.

"A couple of things. Besides feeling more compelled than ever to get healthy and stay out of there, I became impressed with how little I know about my body and what I can do for myself to keep it healthy. I never really paid attention. But I spent the time in the hospital surfing the Web and found some really good sites. It takes some of the mystery out of diagnosis and treatment." Ashwood flips open his laptop and logs into a site to show Schwartz. "Most important, the more I learned, the better the questions I was able to ask."

"How did the docs and nurses feel about that?" Schwartz asks.

"I got a mix of reactions from the people who were caring for me. Some respected that I had done my homework. I really appreciated that because they took the time to answer my questions and make me feel comfortable. There were others though who acted like I was about to take their jobs away, like I was invading their turf by trying to understand what was going on with my own body. It was incredibly frustrating because they wouldn't answer my questions. One guy outright told me to act like a 'good patient' and let him ask the questions. Can you believe that?"

"Dude, that's rude. Of course there's a lot of information out there—you can't believe everything you read though. There's a lot of rubbish out there too. I'm not sure I could tell the difference."

"That's why you read more than one site, check who's behind each, and read the comments to figure out which are the most reliable. Just like getting the details on a new phone before you buy. After awhile it gets easier to pick out the quacks and loonies."

"So do you have to get back to the hospital?" Schwartz asks, hoping that his friend will declare his freedom from a return trip.

"Don't know yet. Depends on how I am doing. They gave me this little setup to keep track of my vitals. There is an online site where I send the numbers. Some computer and a nurse at the hospital monitor what I send, and if anything is out of line, they are in touch to check on what's happening."

"That's nice but a lot of extra tinkering. One of my work buddies out west, a bit older than you, had a similar tour of the hospital himself. He came out with an incredible setup. They put an app on his cell phone that is linked wirelessly to a monitor on his wrist. It automatically keeps track of his vitals and sends the info back to the hospital and his doc. If there is anything out of the ordinary, they get in touch with him to alert him to come back to the hospital. And if he doesn't respond, the GPS in his phone alerts emergency personnel to his location, and they can go get him. And he doesn't have to input anything to make it work. It all just happens. I mean the guy is protected 24/7. They're making it harder and harder to die these days."

"That's incredible," Ashwood responds, "They must have tagged him or his insurance company for some extra cash to cover that upgrade."

"No, it's just part of how they do things at his hospital. Let's face it, Artie, once you've set up one of those systems, the marginal cost of adding one more patient is pretty small—especially if you can avoid the cost of someone coming back to the hospital. The programming—that's where guys like me come in—that's where the bucks are. Look at it though: put all that technology together and you can do good things for people. We're living in a new world now, my friend."

Ashwood opens a box of whole wheat crackers and a bag of organic carrot sticks for a snack. They moved on to more mundane topics, girlfriends, sports, and their jobs. Both are impressed though with both the primitive and the high-tech sides of their health picture: taking responsibility for keeping themselves healthy while using technology to protect against the downturns.

other activities—as on research and development ("Big Pharma Spends More on Advertising Than Research and Development," 2008).

There is great debate about whether this advertising is beneficial or detrimental. Those in favor view electronic and print marketing as an educational tool that foments important patient advocacy. For example, it informs patients of treatments for conditions that they may have not realized were curable and encourages their pursuit of a remedy. Those against believe the volume of advertising encourages unnecessary demand and overuse. Consumers are lured by promises without understanding other options and side effects, despite the warnings and admonitions, delivered in fast talk or small print, with every ad.

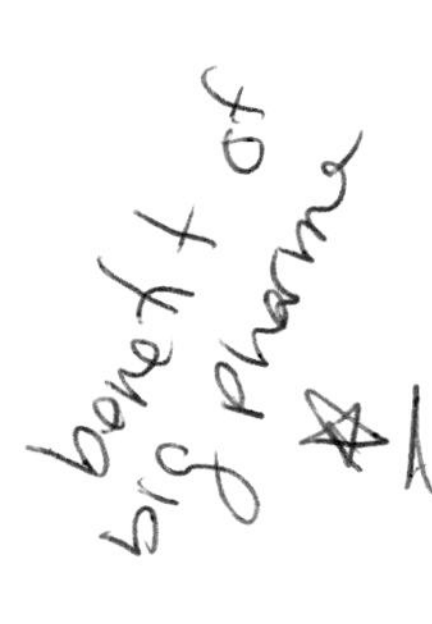

Whatever your take on this debate, the profuse presence of pharmaceutical marketing campaigns has, to be sure, changed the flavor and content of patient-physician discussion. According to Julie Donahue of the University of Pittsburg Graduate School of Public Health, early pharmaceutical advertising campaigns "pursued a marketing strategy that depended on consumers taking a more active role in prescribing decisions" (Donahue, 2006). In very real terms, the advertising changes the negotiations about clinical care, in part because the patient, rather than coming to the doctor with a problem, is more likely to come with a solution. Not only are patients eager to self-diagnose and self-prescribe, they likely will resent the medical opinion that a particular drug is not suited to their particular condition. That will lead to conflict, especially as patients cite anecdotal evidence from satisfied friends or enthusiastic Internet sites. Medical know-how often takes a backseat to the beautiful and happy people depicted in well-crafted and seductive advertising.

Donahue et al. (2007) note that "advertising increases classwide sales" and that "direct-to-consumer advertising has a significant effect on demand for prescription drugs." Advertisements for pharmaceuticals religiously include the admonition to "ask your doctor." In essence then, physicians are not really negotiating with the patient. They are implicitly negotiating with an envoy, single-mindedly dispatched on a mission to them by the drug company, with a message: "Give me this [brand name] drug. They told me to tell you and then to ask you." Two studies have shown "a significantly increased trend in the prescribing volume of drugs that had been the subject of DTCA [direct-to-consumer advertising] campaigns" and another has shown that patient requests for specific prescription drugs increased with DCTA and that physicians were more likely to prescribe the drug even if they were ambivalent about it (Gilbody, Wilson, & Watt, 2005). Physicians are more likely to prescribe a medication when they believe that the patient has an expectation of receiving that medication (Gellad & Lyles, 2007).

Of course, simply concurring is one conflict resolution strategy. If a physician agrees with the patient on symptoms, diagnosis, and the appropriateness of the advertised drug, there will be no conflict. After all, time with patients is precious: face-to-face time in the average outpatient visit is about ten minutes and involves engaging on care options for three to four problems (Stange, 2007). The patient leaves satisfied. The physician may have other considerations though. This may not be the best treatment for the patient's condition. The drug may not be on the formulary of the institution, meaning that this prescription may attract unwanted attention from others at the physician's workplace. If the patient is part of a capitated care plan and the drug is not appropriate, the cost comes, so to speak, out of the physician's hide. If the physician disagrees with the patient, the two of them enter a negotiation.

As of this writing, some of the most advertised drugs fall in the categories of treatments for heartburn, insomnia, high cholesterol, asthma and allergies, nail fungus, blood clots, and erectile dysfunction. A physician may recommend that a patient's heartburn is better addressed through dietary changes. She may be reluctant to prescribe an allergy medication just so another patient can keep her cat. She may have concerns that the heavy advertising soon after FDA approval may not have allowed time for a convincing safety record to accumulate. She may also worry that her patient will seek out a more compliant physician if she denies his request for a particular drug.

Each of these concerns requires caregivers to assess what they hope to achieve in negotiating with a patient. They will do best going into the conversation with an open mind. Their bias on the debate about the wisdom of drug advertising—whether for or against—should not weigh into their calculations about a particular pharmaceutical or particular patient. This process is not an ideological conflict: it should be an honest assessment of the patient's condition and the best treatment for it. First, caregivers must listen to the patient. They will get clues on the reason for the request, how best to frame the discussion, and what they can hope to achieve. They may learn something they otherwise would not know, certainly about this particular human and perhaps about other matters as well. As they consider the best course of action, they will be noting that for any drug there are both benefits and risks. These can be discussed with attention to the specific health profile and needs of the patient. There must be patience with the arguments brought by the patient: some may derive from sources with far less credible authority than the physician has, and some may center on concerns not readily solved by any drug. For example, ads promising to resolve erectile dysfunction may have changed the patient's concept of what it is to "be a man." In the end, if the patient better understands what the physician has said and he better understands the patient, he will have improved the likelihood that a balanced decision will arise from the conversation. He may then have to deal with the patient's disappointment, though that outcome will be easier for the patient to accept if he or she believes that the doctor listened. The bottom line is that pharmaceutical ads are now a part of the negotiation equation. And with the right template for engaging in the discussion and the proper understanding for framing it, clinicians can turn annoyance into an opportunity for better patient understanding.

The Responsibility Shift from Institutions to Individuals

Technology has allowed us to become a self-serve society. We pump our own gas, make our own airline reservations, buy and sell our own stocks, manage our pensions, and check out our own groceries. At one time all these activities required someone else to do them for us. Yes, there were initial concerns: Left to our own devices, we could blow up the gas station, book the wrong flight, lose our life's savings, or cheat our grocer. And yet the benefits and the savings have overcome the risks. Consumers have become more independent, and they like the convenience, flexibility, and control that self-service affords them. Could the same phenomenon arise in health care?

As pressures to contain costs grow, technologies advance, and consumers seek a more independent role in their own care, home health monitoring and telemedicine for postdischarge care will assume a growing presence. Additional factors that will make self-serve health care a must are the expanding aging patient population and the shrinking workforce. There will simply be too many patients and too few workers. Far-flung, smaller, and busier nuclear families will not be able to fill the gap in care needed by grandparents and other kin.

Technologies are moving beyond phones, faxes, and Internet communications to allow more robust links between patient and clinic. New technologies allow patients to be watched and cared for remotely so that a face-to-face encounter is not routinely required. Smaller and faster processors and sensors offer home and mobile health monitoring, imaging, and video conferencing. These products and services are attracting companies that see market opportunities in the quest to achieve successful aging despite both acute episodes and chronic illnesses. Treatment that used to require hospitalization and clinical attention can and will be accommodated by the emerging self-serve culture.

What are the trade-offs and how will this phenomenon affect negotiations and spur conflicts? On one hand the independence of individuals in the self-service culture reshapes their expectations. People who are used to being on their own increasingly insist on an active role for themselves. Martha Crowninshield O'Brien, a hospital-based nurse with twenty-five years of experience, explains that "patients no longer think of themselves just as patients; they are 'clients' and don't expect to simply do as they are told. They expect to have a voice and be listened to." James Conway, senior vice president at the Institute for Healthcare Improvement, notes that "consumers are declaring that the current state is unacceptable." They expect a voice in shaping their future. Conway observes that when wisely framed, this more activist and involved patient provides a quality of care advantage because "a satisfied consumer is more engaged and gets better outcomes"—an argument for more intentionally reframing roles and relationships.

Is there, however, a downside in reducing the human touch that has been so much at the heart of what health care has been about? Much can be learned and communicated in a simple gesture. Eyes cannot really meet through a computer monitor, and the subtle manipulations, clues, and insights of face-to-face contact are lost in the distant whir of monitors and telecommunications. One day when we are ill, we may wake up and miss the real people. Our negotiations will have become less robust and our conflicts less sharply targeted. Patients will become subjects in a data pool and their contact with a provider will be an automatic beep on a monitor. Finding a proper balance and maintaining humane values amid the allure of all these bells and whistles will require the human qualities to remain, reassuringly, at the table.

The HMO Backlash

The health maintenance organization (HMO) moniker rose in popularity on a health promise and descended precipitously when the business imperative changed the game. In a typical HMO, care is provided through a network of doctors, other caregivers, and hospitals that the HMO employs or owns and through a series of contractual arrangements. HMOs have their roots in the early twentieth century and expanded significantly following passage of the Health Maintenance Organization Act of 1973. That law required employers with more than twenty-five workers to include an HMO plan as one of their health insurance options.

The promise of these integrated networks was stated in the name: a commitment to provide linked and connected decision making and services on the premise of keeping people healthy. The business opportunity derived from the notion that keeping people healthy would hold down system costs. The concept of a package of high-quality, cost-efficient care for subscribers—care that did not exceed premium revenues—attracted both consumers and the employers who paid the bill. Over time, however, the compulsion to control cost increases overcame the commitment to open-access care, and HMOs became associated more with restricting care than providing it. As cost management overrode care management, the allure of the HMO and anything that resembled it was tainted in the public's mind (Coombs, 2005).

HMOs have made important contributions to the overall health care system: they set new standards and models for reining in wasteful spending and elevated the importance of evidence-based treatment protocols. However, in the words of Bradford H. Gray (2006), "HMOs were the object of the most bitter criticisms of American health care at the end of the 20th century." And in October 1999, a special issue of the *Journal of Health Politics, Policy, and Law* was dedicated to what its editor called the "managed care backlash."

How did this come to pass? According to Jan Gregoire Coombs (2005), the HMO movement introduced intense economic competition into U.S health care and that led to the rise of administrators and managers more focused on financial returns than patient outcomes. They found that the most efficient way to achieve their organizations' financial objectives was by reducing services to subscribers and refusing to enroll individuals with significant health problems. According to Cindy Ehnes, director of California's Department of Managed Health Care, "The HMO concept was never well articulated to the consumer, and the industry did some things that were not smart, like mandate what became known as 'drive-through maternity care,' that gave the impression that profits came first, not patients."

What are the lingering effects of this backlash? Many consumers have come to believe that they must approach the health care system armed for battle. Getting care requires a fight. They recognize doctors and nurses less as their advocates and more as agents of a system trying to save money on the back of their insurance premium and their health. As clinicians explain the rigors of getting approval to order a test or make a referral, the reduced clinical autonomy and system authority of caregivers has come into full light. This can turn a clinical encounter into an emotional and escalated conflict. Demanding patients can yell and scream until the system relents and they get what they want. The bottom line from the patient's perspective is that if you are not willing to self-advocate, negotiate, and if need be fight, you may very well not get the care you need.

Martha Crowninshield O'Brien echoes this, saying: "Patients need an advocate to get the best from the system. Historically, nurses have in part played that role but they cannot always do so. The patient—or someone from the patient's family—needs to know how and when to push." As the system becomes more complex, the patient is best served by having an advocate to accompany him or her on the arduous journey through a landscape often difficult to comprehend. If you work in the system, then you are on the other side of that negotiation, frustrated by the fact that those advocating are often unfamiliar with what reasonably can or cannot be provided, given the constraints of the system.

As we have seen in earlier chapters through the examples of Kaiser Permanente and other managed care systems, the managed care model has much to offer, especially as technologies emerge with the potential to make getting services a less personal and more fragmented experience. You will note, however, that none of these systems has adopted the HMO moniker: the bad association and reputation lingers.

E.

The Growing Acceptance of Alternative Treatments

"How does acupuncture fit into my treatment plan?" This is a question and a negotiation for which caregivers should be prepared. Acupuncture is just one of a number of complementary and alternative medicine (CAM) therapies. David Eisenberg, of the Harvard Medical School defines a CAM therapy as "any form of therapy not widely taught in medical schools or generally available in hospitals." Included in the list of CAM therapies are acupuncture, yoga, chiropractics, massage therapy, herbal supplements, and more. Marking the rise in CAM's popularity among patients and also clinicians, Eisenberg and his colleagues published an overview of trends in alternative medicine in *JAMA* in 1998 and observed that increasing numbers of patients were seeking alternative treatments. Indeed in 1997, Americans visited alternative medicine practitioners 628 million times, 243 million more visits than were made to all primary care physicians ("Alternative Medicine Goes Mainstream," n.d.; Eisenberg et al., 1998). A follow-up article looking at trends through 2002 showed that about one-third of adult Americans had used CAM in the previous year, which was consistent with the 1997 findings (Barnes, Powell-Griner, McFann, & Nahin, 2004).

David Edelberg, founder and former chair of the integrated medicine clinic WholeHealth, has found that most of these users were not looking for a substitute for conventional health care. Rather, as he explained to *Discovery Health*, they wanted "physician-supervised alternative medicine . . . . They wanted a center that had two toolboxes" ("Alternative Medicine Goes Mainstream," n.d.). Given that, woe to the orthopedic surgeon who is willing to prescribe physical therapy and yet denies his patient chiropractic care.

For those working in conventional care systems, this means that they will field questions and negotiate decisions about these alternative and complementary therapies. These therapies will enter into care recommendations and caregivers will have to balance how they will interact with the conventional care they are prescribing. There are many sources of information to help in making informed decisions and recommendations, including the National Center for Complementary and Alternative Medicine at the National Institutes of Health. Some of these sources will meet the standards of peer-reviewed journals to which medical professionals have become accustomed and many may not. The alternative care field emerged as a movement that was counter to traditional

Iris Inkwater is concerned about noise: there are so many distractions from outside the hospital that she's afraid her people will lose their focus on what is needed inside. She is afraid she may unintentionally be escalating that diversion because at every one of her standing meetings—of department chiefs, the board's executive committee, administrative staff, medical staff—everyone is asking and talking about the latest news in the Community Health Plan and Arena Health Insurance struggles and the impact on the Oppidania and Urbania Medical Centers. She needs to get refocused herself, and so she decides to use her Tuesday morning meeting to shift the conversation. She has invited Dr. Rusty Rice, who is chief of the hospitalist program, to participate in the conversation.

"I asked Rusty to join us today because I think one part of our assessing what this *New Oppidania Medical Center* will be," she says to open the meeting, gesturing to those words that still adorn her office whiteboard, "is figuring out how we will better manage the patient care experience in the future. When we started the hospitalist program here, it was considered cutting edge. There were a lot of people against it, and I have to admit, I couldn't fully understand the level of resistance we met. I know that we were treading on some long-standing and lucrative turf, though I underestimated just how fierce the push-back would be. Despite that, the program has shown itself to be a plus for patient outcomes, patient satisfaction, and cost containment. That's impressive. And given the volume of capitated care we are seeing, those numbers are extremely helpful to our financial health. We all know," she says with a wry smile, "that we have to be attentive to that these days."

"So," she continues, "I asked Rusty to sit in with us today. Imagine that this is the enlightened interests step of a much larger Walk in the Woods and we are here to do some creative and imaginative brainstorming. What might we do with the hospitalist program, what sort of resistance would we get, and how can we marry the opportunities and genuine and legitimate concerns that are embedded in that push-back in order to come up with a plan that will work? If we have something good going for us, I want us to be able to leverage and nurture it. Rusty, anything you want to say to start us off?"

"Thanks, Iris," Rusty says. "We appreciate your interest. As you know, it has been an uphill battle getting this effort off the ground and despite that, I think we have made significant progress and the numbers—which I follow closely—bear that out. The hospitalists, because their whole focus is getting the best care for the patient within the hospital and doing it as efficiently as possible, have been able to bring down costs and have achieved notable improvements in our patient satisfaction tracking. We are, however, not nearly as big as we could be. We're still a small group, and I think the question for the hospital is whether leaders and staff want to grow what we are doing, and if so, figuring out how we are going to do that."

Inkwater turns to the group and asks, "Well, what do people think?"

Dr. Fred Fisher had been among those with the greatest reservations about the hospitalist program when it was first proposed and launched. Everyone waits for his response now, as it will certainly color the remainder of the conversation. "Iris, you know I have been a reticent fan of the hospitalist program. My reticence comes from focusing on what patients and their primary care docs want when they come here. Those community doctors are our customers, and even more important, they are a critically important factor in our business. We depend on their referrals to keep our volume up—they are our life blood. If they all were of one mind about how they wanted to manage the care of their patients within the hospital, this would be an easy discussion. They are not. There are some medical practices that want to continue to manage their patients throughout their time here. From their perspective the time in the hospital is a brief stint in the overall experience of their patient. It makes no sense for them to be on top of everything on an outpatient basis and then to walk away when their patient is hospitalized. That is just when you as a patient want your personal doctor by your side. These doctors, and I might say they tend to be more the old-school docs, feel that turning care over to a hospitalist is tantamount to abandoning their patients at their time of greatest medical need. The idea is foreign to them. There is of course another school of thought—especially among physicians who find that coming to the hospital to do rounds and figuring out who's who here and how to get things done—is all too much bother for a large and active practice. These doctors are tickled pink to have someone else assume hospital duties for them, as long as they know what is going on with their patients so that the posthospital care coordinates with what happened while the patients were under our care. And I know that hospitalists are doing a great job of improving care and lowering costs. That's why I am reticent and that's why I am a fan. I don't know. So what do we do with that? Or, how do we get creative about that, as you would say, Iris."

"Fred, I have some thoughts," Rice adds. "But first I want to first hear what others have to say."

Janice Johnson raises her hand, "I for one am a huge fan of the hospitalist program. It has been a real boon for getting things done and has made the lives of our nurses much, much easier. Patients get better care. Coordination with other departments and services is so much more seamless. And we spend a lot less time running after, waiting for, and holding the hands of outside doctors who don't know our processes. The hospitalists know the place. They know us and we know them. We've developed a rhythm. My suggestion is that we get, as Larry said a few weeks ago, more intentional about coordinating the work of the hospitalists with that of others here."

"What do you mean by that?" Inkwater asks. "Say more."

"Well, we could assume more of a team approach to patient care, so that what the hospitalists are doing is part of a team effort with nursing, occupational health, social work, physical therapy, and whoever else is on board for a particular patient. If a patient could be guided through her care here by a team from the beginning, getting things done and done well would be significantly easier. And that has to be what we are about. Is that what you are looking for, Iris?''

Larry Lumberg adds, ''And the primary doc could be part of the extended team, so that the patient doesn't feel like she's been handed off to strangers.''

''Interesting,'' Inkwater replies with an encouraging nod.

Rajeev Rao has a question. ''Fred, I don't quite get the reservations of the community doctors, I mean from a pure business perspective. They don't get that much money for doing rounds here and it takes them away from revenue-generating time in their offices. They're paying for the people and overhead back at their offices while they are traipsing through here. Why wouldn't they want to let us do it for them?''

''Rajeev, it's not just about the business,'' Fisher answers. ''They believe they have an ongoing commitment to their patients. It's not uncommon for a physician to have a thirty-year-long relationship with a patient they are seeing here during their rounds. They feel, as do their patients, that the relationship is even more important when serious illness takes over. If you want to see this in business terms, think of it as an ongoing customer loyalty program.''

Arlan Abbington breaks into the conversation. ''So I am going to admit that when I was in here for my little episode, Fred and everyone else treated me like a king, which was much appreciated, though I know that a board chairman sometimes gets a little extra attention,'' he says with a smile. ''That said, I think we can inspire creative thinking if we explore what it is about that relationship that is important, what we should preserve, and what we change. That's what we do at the bank—and for anyone here who pays attention, the banking industry has gone through tremendous changes in how we handle our customers in the past few years. Let me be a focus group of one: I wanted my doctor to see me face to face. He knows me, my history, and my family. I wanted him to know what was going on with me and my care. And I wanted him to keep an eye on how that care was progressing. I assumed he knew how, in general, this place worked. I didn't need him to personally order every test or interpret every result—I trust the specialists here who do this every day—but I wanted my doctor in the loop. Looked at from that perspective, you can maintain the patient-physician relationship, the guidance, and the knowledge while readjusting the expectations. If you preserve what's important and then transfer what's not in a way that is convenient, cheaper, and better, people will drift in that direction. And looking back on it, a call from my doctor some days would have been just as good as a visit. And if he has good-quality access to information online or through periodic consults with someone on the phone, that could satisfy everyone's concerns while buying you the efficiencies you are looking for.''

Lumberg leans forward in his chair and points dramatically at Abbington, "That is exactly what I am talking about, Arlan, when I say we have to be intentional. I like the idea of people 'drifting,' as you say, in the direction we would like them to go. If we make sure both the doctors and the patients are getting what they need and it is easier, then people will migrate naturally to what makes sense to them."

Perry Pudolski is encouraged by Lumberg's line of thinking, "That's simple economics theory. Give people what they are looking for and they will come. I think there has been a haughty attitude in health care that says what we do is so mysterious that we don't have to treat people as if we really want their business. They'll just come to us because we have anointed ourselves into a special role. I think we need to map out what everyone wants and figure out a way to deliver it to them."

Fisher rubs his chin. He is getting annoyed, "Perry, if every patient was the same, that formula could work. This is not some fast-food joint with a limited menu that assumes the masses all want to eat the same cheap french fries. We are a hospital. Patients are all different. Their conditions are different. The system is going through a lot of change and not everyone is on the same wave length. It's a lot more complicated than that. Jumping at simple solutions will simply create a whole new set of problems." There is an uncomfortable silence in the room as Fisher finishes speaking and takes a long drink of his coffee.

Iris Inkwater waits a moment before she speaks. "The solution here is not a simple formula, and at the same time, we can't be all things to all people. Fred, how do we find that sweet spot that you once described, and Perry, how do we build systems that account for variations in what different people—patients, physicians, and other caregivers—need while they are here?" Abbington is impressed with how Inkwater is handling the conversation: engaging, acknowledging, and then challenging both Fisher and Pudolski without humiliating either. The tense mood continues though no hostility erupts.

Pudolski takes up the challenge, speaking with an air of authentic respect. "Fred, I am not suggesting that we treat people who turn to us with anything less than genuine and individual care and concern. However, the more variation we build into our system, the more costly it will be, the higher the likelihood that we will get something wrong, and therefore the more difficult it will be for us to be competitive. My point is that I think we can find a balance because we have some really smart people here." Pudolski knows that he had gone a bit too far before and that alienating Fred Fisher is not a good idea. He wants to get his point across but doesn't want to win the battle only to lose the war.

Fisher too wants to be perceived as conciliatory. Being combative is not the spirit that Iris is hoping to achieve, he knows that. OMC is at a critical point, and he understands that he has to be a team player. "Perry, I hear what you are saying and appreciate it. I think we have to be careful if we try to run faster than we and others are prepared to adjust. We can make a lot of mistakes that way, and they will be the most costly of mistakes."

Rice sees his opening: "I think what everyone is saying here is important and has to be in the mix. That doesn't mean being all things to all people. And just so you know, this is what we hospitalists talk about at our national society meetings all the time. Actually, a group of my colleagues had a conversation about this very topic around the pool at our last meeting. Though OMC's hospitalists will need buy-in from those of you around this table and more, I am confident that they will be happy to step up to the plate. They can play an even greater role in leading efforts to improve coordination between community physicians and the work going on here in the hospital. Several things can help. One, if we build patient care coordinating teams in the hospital, then there will be better and smoother linkages of information and decision making that we can provide to a patient's referring physician. The physicians will like seeing the whole picture and providing that purview to their patients. Second, a lot of this can be managed through our electronic medical record system by more aggressively engaging the outside docs, especially the relatively older generation, to use these online tools. Third, and I know this won't be popular, we need more hospitalists. You get a lot of value for this investment, as I have shown in my reports."

"We're not in a position to be adding personnel, Rusty," Rao says sharply. "We're looking to cut costs, not add to them."

Rice had seen this coming. He takes a file and slides it across to the CFO. "We have been tracking costs, satisfaction, and outcomes on a comparative basis, and each hospitalist produces excellent value. This is especially true in the pay-for-performance, accountability valued, and capitated environment in which we find ourselves. Take a look for yourself."

By the end of the meeting the group members have discovered some new ideas, developed a new set of understandings, and most important, come together. Once again, the Tuesday morning dialogue has been a good investment of time and effort.

belief and so there remains in that community a firm suspicion of conventional sources and methods for validating the impact of these treatments.

According to Kimberly Costa, a community hospital nurse, caregivers must be open to what works as long as there are no obvious serious risks. "If I see a patient with chronic back pain who is helped by acupuncture," she said, "I think that's great. We have to stop reflexively fighting against alternative treatments just because they are 'alternative.' "

As the field opens, know too that requests from patients may even fall outside of what now has become recognized as legitimate CAM therapy. Such requests might include making healing statements before closing a surgical incision. This will require a compassionate negotiation on the surgeon's part. He will have to balance the importance of these requests for his patient—and for some patients they will have extraordinary significance—with his confidence in their efficacy, their potential consequences, his own belief systems, and his time pressures. He will have to decide what he will embrace, to what he will acquiesce, what he will refuse. He may risk losing the patient to another caregiver or facility. As delicate and consequential as each of these decisions is, the way in which he negotiates and communicates a decision may be as important to his patient and colleagues as the decision itself.

The Role of Health Literacy

In its *Healthy People 2010* report, the U.S. Department of Health and Human Services (2000) defined *health literacy* as "the degree to which individuals have the capacity to obtain, process and understand basic health information and services needed to make appropriate health decisions." Rima Rudd of the Harvard School of Public Health has reported that more than eight hundred peer-reviewed articles have shown that most health materials are written at reading levels above the reading ability of the average high school graduate (Rudd, 2010). This means that a vast number of people in this country simply cannot understand the health care instructions and information they are provided. It is not that they are noncompliant. They simply lack full access to what they need to know. Given that those working in the health field tend to be well educated, that the field is crammed with technical terms and jargon, and that many materials have to pass legal as well as medical scrutiny, the existence of this language and comprehension problem is not a surprise. But understanding the reason for the problem does not make it less serious. Gaps in patient understanding can result in missed appointments, noncompliant use of medications, incorrect information entered on forms, and less than fully informed consent for procedures, to name just a few examples with potentially serious consequences. *Health Literacy in Canada*, a 2007 report from the Canadian Council on Learning, cites nearly one hundred studies that establish "a clear relationship between the literacy skills of patients and a variety of health outcomes" (Murray, Rudd, Kirsch, Yamamoto, & Grenier, 2007).

Extensive efforts have been underway to close this gap at the Institute of Medicine and other organizations. The objective is for patients to understand more, ask more informed questions, and demand more complete answers. It boils down to giving people information in ways they will fully understand. Navigating our complex, multiparty health care system often requires substantive literacy skills. The mismatch between the information provided and the ability to understand it and the link between literacy and health outcomes are well established (Rudd & Keller, 2009).

In the absence of easily understood information from the traditional authoritative health care sources, the public turns for advice to friends and family as well as to the popular media, Web sites, and consumer-friendly books. In turn, people will come to medical professionals with questions and opinions derived from that exploration, bearing misconceptions and inaccuracies collected along the way as well as legitimate concerns and questions. As a voice for the health care system, caregivers must break down communication barriers so they can meet their patients' *want to know* as well as *need to know* requirements. They may find themselves debunking myths or embracing new options that may require them to expand their own knowledge base about nontraditional sources of information.

Health professionals may also find that their patients are reading peer-reviewed journals, now much more widely available, for substantive information about proposed treatment regimens and alternatives. In the words of Paul Levy, then CEO of Boston's Beth Israel Deaconess Medical Center, "If you can't believe that the lay public can interpret clinical results, you'll never embrace this new transparency." Part of the caregiving job then is being that responsible interpreter—or making sure that someone in the organization is filling that role.

Health and Behavior, Social Determinants, and the Environment

When it comes to personal choices such as smoking or environmental contaminants, no set of diseases raises more concern than do the many forms of cancer. And no other set of diseases has been the focus of such intense research and advocacy. In May 2010, the President's Cancer Panel released its 2008–2009 report. This body reports on the progress in the fight against cancer and recommends priorities for future policy and funding by the U.S. government. In its latest report, the panel recommended a paradigm shift, moving from "current reactionary approaches to environmental contaminants in which human harm must be proven before action is taken to reduce or eliminate exposure" to a more "precautionary, prevention-oriented approach" (Leffall & Kripke, 2010). The report both raised the legitimacy of the claims about the risks of exposure to new chemicals and environmental substances and recommended a more proactive strategy of protection and prevention. The panel considered a broad set of contaminants, including those from industrial, agricultural, medical, and natural sources as well as from "modern lifestyles" sources, such as dry cleaning and air travel.

The report reflects the growing recognition of the impact of environmental as well as behavioral factors, including diet, on individual health and well-being. Parallel to that recognition is the mounting expectation that individuals, by virtue of their life choices, bear some responsibility for their own health. Some of this sentiment is driven by the high cost of preventable diseases that result, at least in some cases, from personal choices, including chronic conditions such as obesity, type 2 diabetes, asthma, and high blood pressure. DeVol and Bedroussian (2007) have calculated the annual cost to the U.S. economy of preventable diseases at $1.3 trillion, with the bulk of that cost in lost productivity. This expectation is also driven by considerations of fairness: should those who do not smoke, who stay in shape, and who choose to eat a healthy diet in effect subsidize the health care costs of those with less healthy habits?

The concept of personal responsibility for health has evolved and will continue to do so as policymakers and health care purchasers seek more effective strategies to limit the rise in health spending. When the notion of personal responsibility first surfaced in the 1970s, it was viewed as a responsibility to oneself: your health could be sustained through adoption of healthy habits, and this was a better alternative for you than getting sick with the hope that the health system would correct your infractions (Winkler, 2002). Over time, having healthy habits has assumed more of an aura of social obligation. If appropriate information and assistance is available, do you not have the responsibility—to your employer who is subsidizing your insurance and to other members of your risk pool—to stay healthy? Or is this all a matter of free will: are people not entitled to make choices about what they eat, whether they drink alcohol, whether they smoke, and how they care for their own body?

At the interface of free will, the efforts to reduce health costs, and the initiatives to improve well-being are health professionals. Whether they are dealing with individual patients or populations, the effort to educate and encourage healthy choices demands a complex set of negotiations. Caregivers can quickly find themselves in an ethical thicket. If they provide care through a capitated system, their patients' poor health choices are literally dollars out of their own pockets. It is costing the caregivers far more to provide these patients with care than it would cost to keep them healthy. What can one do though: accompany them to the fast-food joint and encourage the salad over the burger? What if patients refuse preventive treatment, such as those at risk for heart disease who are recommended to take a low-dose aspirin daily? A more dramatic, well-documented debate asks whether alcoholics should be eligible for liver transplants (Winkler, 2002). Although certain incentives and penalties are legal in the United States,

The hostilities between the major insurers and the two major hospitals in Oppidania have reached a deafening roar. Every health-related story in the local media seems to reference the struggle. It also provides a convenient local angle on the health policies being debated in the state capital and in Washington. They previously always had a productive relationship, but the current antipathy between the Oppidania Medical Center (OMC) and the Community Health Plan (CHP), aggravated by CHP's "take it or leave it" offer to give OMC the same rates that CHP negotiated with the Urbania Medical Center (UMC), has obviated any substantive discussions between them. Likewise, the people at UMC are riled at CHP for dropping a humiliating and unwarranted public relations nightmare on their doorstep. The timeworn rivalry between OMC and UMC, generally kept within cordial limits, has been ignited by the uproar. Urbania is resentful of Oppidania's status and recognition, and now disdains its foe even more; OMC's stance of superiority is only bolstered by the negative press its competitor has attracted. Many resent Arena Health Insurance's opportunism as that company exploits the disarray and anxiety of the situation to promote its own status and to grab market share.

And the public, including patients who frequent one or both of these hospitals, watch the fray like children witnessing the hostilities of quarreling parents. These are institutions that claim to care for the community, and this war is unbecoming to the respect they had both enjoyed. Patients were left wondering who to trust and whether the sparring would affect the quality of care they would receive.

The real predicament with this disarray, of course, is that no one is really in charge of health care. The federal, state, and municipal agencies that follow the skirmishes have quietly conceded that the standoff presents a political catch-22. In the public's eye, any agency that gets involved will assume responsibility for the issues, though it won't necessarily have the authority to remedy them. The bureaucrats also presume that the private sector hospital and insurance leaders, with their lavish salaries and perks, have always considered themselves superior to the heads of public agencies and therefore will be reticent to accept government input on the matter. There is also fear on all sides that government interference could create pressures for some sort of regulatory or legal action, which everyone, including the bureaucrats and politicians, knows is undesirable. As long as nothing illegal or overtly damaging occurs as a result of the standoff, there is really little for government to do.

Mayor Walt Wynn is aware of the political pitfalls that this standoff could create for him. He summons his public health commissioner, Manuel Mendez, to brief him on the situation. Would it be possible to arrange a private meeting to explore some sort of resolution? If it works, only then would the city take the credit. If it failed, the secrecy of the meeting would guarantee that no one would ever know Wynn had taken the risk. Mendez commends Wynn for his willingness to make an attempt, noting that in the long run, complete inaction on this issue could be a point of political liability in the next election. Standing idly by while a major health care crisis unfolds in town could rile the electorate, especially the large elderly population for whom health care is an important issue.

In spite of the potential pitfalls, Mendez is eager to get involved. He personally calls and invites Iris Inkwater, the CEO of Oppidania, and Pete Patterson, the CEO of Urbania, to a private meeting, just the three of them. He explains Mayor Wynn's hope of seeing these issues resolved. Mendez describes the session as exploratory, and he asks that the meeting be kept strictly confidential. To his relief, both Patterson and Inkwater agree to attend.

Though they belong to the same professional associations, Inkwater has never considered Patterson a peer. He represents the old mold of hospital administrator: he grew into his job without the training or background now expected of the leader at a first-rate institution. Inkwater fears he's not open to change. While Inkwater is still aggressively on the rise, Patterson peaked years earlier and is close to retirement. She thinks he is probably more concerned about his golf game than about going through the turmoil of running a troubled institution. Similarly, Patterson does not much care for Inkwater. In his mind she is a brash executive, somewhat cold and calculating in her moves, and not to be trusted. He feels she has "big elbows" and is not afraid to use them to get her way. He has always felt one-upped by Inkwater and Oppidania and he resents that Urbania is considered a lesser institution. He'll come, but he decides to play his hand slowly.

As the meeting between Mendez, Inkwater, and Patterson opens, the mood is polite and reserved. Patterson is in a charcoal pinstripe suit with a navy tie. His thick silver hair is carefully combed. Inkwater thinks that if you looked in the dictionary for the definition of a late-twentieth-century hospital CEO, you wouldn't be surprised to see Patterson's picture. This is, however, she mentally notes, the twenty-first century. She too is in a tailored suit but has been careful not to look too formal. She wants to project calm authority and the message that she sees this as a working meeting, not a ceremonial event.

Careful not to imply blame, Mendez carefully begins the proceedings. He fairly assesses the problem as belonging to more than just the institutions involved. To the extent that patients, jobs, and business relationships are affected by the standoff, the city has an interest in encouraging the parties to reach some sort of resolution. He emphasizes that it is not up to the city to solve the problem, though the city is prepared to do whatever it can reasonably do to help the two hospitals resolve the issues. Inkwater thanks Mendez, as does Patterson.

Mendez asks each of them to describe the situation from his or her own perspective. Surprisingly, neither sees the problem as being with the other. Each feels jostled into this predicament more on account of the machinations of the insurers than because of any interchanges between themselves. That revelation turns out to be significant. From that perspective, they each have shared problems and shared interests. They laugh themselves into commenting on the more bizarre aspects of the recent round of negotiations, and they note how they have been played off each other.

With the mood of the meeting turning, Mendez decides to pose a delicate question: have the two ever considered some sort of an alliance? The question is met with dubious silence. Inkwater finally says that the possibility has not been given any serious consideration at Oppidania. Patterson says the same is true at Urbania. Mendez pursues the question: has either of them specifically *rejected* such an alliance? They agree that they have not. Mendez then becomes bolder in his questioning: might it be in the realm of the conceivable? After some discussion, they each agree that it very well might, depending upon how one defines *alliance*.

The mood of the meeting once again swerves. Having concurred with something that only a moment before had been unthinkable, they retreat from their positions. An animated discussion ensues, during which each explains to Mendez the deeply ingrained and different histories, cultures, statuses, business practices, and positions of the two organizations. Though neither openly states his or her reservations, Mendez understands Inkwater to say that she does not want to affiliate with an "inferior" institution. He discerns Patterson as saying that he does not want to get gobbled up by a behemoth.

"So you each have legitimate organizational concerns," Mendez says. "Yet, as I have watched your organizations over the years, I see more in common than I see differences. You are both by-products of this city, and you are both very committed to our citizens. Because of your competitive edge, you each have invested and continue to invest in expensive equipment in order to remain competitive. You have two of too many machines, when one could do for this town. Essentially, the competition has become expensive for both of you. Might there be an option?"

Inkwater feels stunned. There is something so obvious about what Mendez is saying that she is baffled why she has not thought of it herself. Pete feels differently. He isn't sure where Mendez is going with this line of questioning.

Inkwater turns to Patterson. "You know, Pete, the two of us have acted more like competing high school football rivals than two major health care organizations. I think Manuel has raised an important question. The fact is, we are both overbedded and overequipped. We are each trying to be a full-service institution, and that is, as we know, a very expensive proposition. There have been consolidations in other cities between the most unlikely of bedfellows." Inkwater turns to Mendez. "You know, Manuel, we have been so caught up in preserving our competition that we—well, I'll speak for myself, I—never even considered this possibility."

Patterson appreciates Inkwater's candor. He smiles as if he has just gotten the punch line of a joke he had heard some time before. "Actually, Iris, there has been talk about discussing some sort of a relationship with Oppidania. It was rejected outright on the assumption that you people wouldn't hear of it. Quite frankly, we didn't want to become your stepchild. Instead, we decided to put all our marbles in with CHP. We thought we could become that economy airline that would attract such large volume that it would redefine the market. Wow, did that ever blow up in our faces," he says with a shrug.

Inkwater feels her shoulders relaxing. Patterson's openness and his sense of humor are welcome. "Look, Pete, through the grapevine, you know enough about what's going on in my shop and I know enough about what's going on in yours to figure out that we are both being squeezed hard. On one side it's the insurers and on the other side it's the staff. If by working together we can share some expenses and defer some costs, then it's worth at least exploring the possibility."

Patterson is a bit surprised by her enthusiasm. Is she thinking alliance, he wonders, or takeover? Whichever it is, Urbania is no longer in a position to enjoy the luxury of full independence as a full-service facility. "Iris, I agree with you. It is at least worth exploring the possibility."

Mendez feels a sense of cautious optimism. He suggests that they each give the idea forty-eight hours of considered thought. He recommends that these discussions remain confidential: if word leaks prematurely, it could derail any potential progress. He further offers that if there is continued interest, he will remain available to help move the process along. He also has to consider the implications of what he has launched: what will happen if a merger results and Oppidania becomes a city with just one health care organization?

they have met resistance from those who claim that they impinge on individual rights and discriminate against the unhealthy (Crossley, 2005). Health care providers may find encouragement from employers. According to a 2010 study (Hewitt Associates, 2010), under pressure to control health costs employers are showing an increasing appetite for using penalties. An increasing number of self-insured employers are leveraging financial rewards or penalties (for physicians and individuals), wellness and education programs, and other methods to tangibly promote healthy behavior and limit the costs of health treatment (Pearson & Lieber, 2009).

This is in essence a multiparty, enterprise-wide, negotiation in which the desired outcome—healthy people—is subject to a complex array of conflicting forces. It is in part a matter of individual behavior, and a volume of research and experience catalogues just how hard it is to change behavior and encourage healthy habits. It is in part a corporate marketing matter, as fast-food chains and other businesses offer food and encourage behaviors that are not health friendly—though that is changing. In addition, while the health care system espouses health, insurers compensate and reward healing the sick, not keeping people well. For individuals wending their way through life, this mix of contradictions primes lifestyles that detract from population health, no matter what miracles the health system conjures up to fix the mess.

Some health providers are better at encouraging healthy behaviors in their patients than are others. Such encouragement involves negotiation that calls for the application of dimension 5 of meta-leadership: building and using influence with people over whom you have little or no direct authority. It is a subtle, delicate, and very personal process. As a care provider, you have few explicit sticks or carrots. You must skillfully encourage patients to embrace personal responsibility. To help you, there is information, the feel-good result of that lost weight, the improved body image, and the exciting opportunities that a healthy lifestyle can offer. Doing a mini Walk in the Woods with a patient does take time: to listen to his reservations, to engage what he sees as better living, to generate new and exciting ideas that motivate change, and then to agree to a plan and its monitoring. And if you can make it work, it is time well spent.

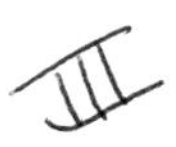

When Things Go Wrong

Inspired in large measure by Lucian Leape and other health care pioneers, the quality and patient safety movement that took hold in the late 1990s and launched into the new millennium with the publication of *To Err Is Human: Building a Safer Health System* (Kohn, Corrigan, & Donaldson, 2000), and *Crossing the Quality Chasm: A New Health System for the 21st Century* (Institute of Medicine, 2001), strives for error-free delivery of health care services. Through the leadership of Donald Berwick, his colleagues, and the network that has been established by the Institute for Healthcare Improvement, the 100,000 Lives Campaign has sought to challenge hospitals to eliminate that number of patient deaths in U.S. hospitals each year, and the 5 Million Lives Campaign seeks to protect that many patients from medical harm. These campaigns seek commitment to eliminating conditions that can lead to errors, to learning from errors so they will not be repeated, and to implementing systems that reduce the likelihood of making a mistake or make it impossible to make a mistake.

Despite that, the work of health care, public health, and population health institutions and professionals is rife with possibilities for disappointment, unexpected consequences, and miscommunications. When things go wrong, what is said, how it is accepted, and what the result is determine whether a difficult situation will escalate further or begin the process toward a reasonable resolution. The choice is yours. What will you do?

The time to start working on a strategy for when things go wrong is not the day of the calamity. What happens that day will depend on the relationship building, communications, reputation, and negotiations that preceded it. If a caregiver has built a mutually respectful and trusting bond with a patient beforehand, the consequences of the problem will evolve from that starting point. If the patient resents the caregiver, does not feel respected, and has become suspicious, whatever unfortunate incident has occurred will just confirm preconceived notions. The standoff will become a battle and every misstep another piece of evidence. At that point, reconstructing the relationship is near impossible. The caregiver is stuck in the mud and it did not have to be that way. Many brilliant careers have been toppled by the arrogant notion that preparing for the possibility of things going wrong is unnecessary.

Many states have adopted laws that protect apologies and explanations given following an unexpected outcome. These laws hope to debunk the notion that medical professionals make themselves vulnerable by admitting that something went wrong. What is the rationale for communicating? In many cases patients or family members are aware that there is a problem. Yet just when they are most impatient about knowing what is going on, everyone about them turns silent for fear of a malpractice suit. Although information and an apology may not be able to correct what has happened, when well done, they can calm people's initial emotions and help them in understanding what, if anything, comes next. Because different states have different specifications for defining the statements are or are not protected, check with state law to guide what caregivers can say and what they should avoid saying. Remember, in the moments after an unintended outcome, the caregiver and the people with whom she is talking are all in the basement. Getting up and out of the basement, speaking calmly and clearly, and listening, even though it may be difficult, are that caregiver's best tools for getting through what will be among the most difficult and consequential conversations of her career.

In Chapter Nine we described a situation in which the daughter of a patient who had died and that patient's physician met with a mediator on the recommendation of a state board of medical registration. That example is based on our own experience in the 1990s in developing and then executing a voluntary mediation program with the Massachusetts Board of Registration in Medicine. The program provided a mediation option for patients, or patients' families, and doctors in situations where a physician had not engaged in egregious substandard care or inappropriate behavior and yet where there was the potential for corrective actions that would improve the physician's quality of care going forward. Approximately 90 percent of the cases over a three-year period were settled with a mutually agreed upon resolution between patient and physician. Those involved in the settlements included a urologist who agreed to taking a refresher course on oncology after a failure-to-diagnose incident; an allergist who agreed to change office procedures after a child was pricked by a carelessly disposed of syringe; and two physicians who agreed to change informed consent procedures at their hospital after a patient was endangered by a potentially fatal drug interaction during a clinical trial. What we learned through these mediations is that after a problem in the course of care, patients or family members want primarily three things: (1) they want to know what happened in detail and in a way they can understand, (2) they want an apology or acknowledgment regarding what went wrong, and (3) they want to know that it will never happen again. We found the third item to be poignantly meaningful, especially when what had happened could not be reversed. People longed for a sense of meaning or purpose from a terrible experience that for them could never go away. The belief that others would not suffer the same tribulations gave them peace and comfort after what occurred. When money came up as an issue, it was only to compensate for direct expenses that derived from the experience. One woman wanted her money back so she could have a different plastic surgeon fix her misshapen nose. Another wanted the physician to make a charitable contribution, as also illustrated in the case detailed in Chapter Nine.

If none of what we have discussed so far succeeds, a caregiver may find himself on the painful side of a malpractice suit. At that point the provider is in someone else's game. The civil justice system is not about corrective actions and apologies. It is about money. Unless the action can be diverted from the courts to an alternative dispute process such as arbitration or mediation, compensation is the end point that is being negotiated and judged. And as evidence is brought to bear on the case, much will focus on technical matters of substandard care and negligence. Some may focus on communications as well, and any clear negotiations and information sharing that the provider long ago incorporated into his professional operating system may assume an important point in his defense.

Conclusion

Although some in health care will consider negotiating patients to be a nuisance or a distraction, their involvement is essential according to Kaiser Permanente CEO George Halvorson, who told us: "Change will come [to the health care system] when consumers refuse to accept suboptimal outcomes." In regard to the work of doctors, Richard Iseke, chief medical officer at Winchester Hospital, near Boston, observes that "patients question more and that's good. But in many cases that may take more time. We need to be innovative in how we provide information to patients so that time with the physician can be focused on matters that can be best addressed by a physician. Traditional relationships between patients and physicians are, and will continue to be, recast."

There are many sides to this recasting of roles and responsibilities. New arrangements also require that patients be open to innovation and embrace new methods for making the system work for them. There is a learning curve on this adaptive way of being. The challenge for those in health care is how, with a deft understanding of conflict resolution and negotiation, they become a positive force in the transformation.

We humans a long time ago crafted different languages and communication forms that vary greatly from group to group. Working between groups, translators became a powerful source for fostering understanding and productive interactions. Although patients today are certainly more knowledgeable than in the past, there is still much they do not understand and cannot decide on their own. Without appropriate training and expertise, it is impossible for them to translate what can be found on the Web and Internet into their unique life circumstances. Health care decisions are emotionally powerful, and at times it is not information alone that is needed to translate facts and research into life-changing decisions. That interpreting function increasingly is and will be a significant role that clinicians will play.

You may wonder why the term *negotiation* is used here to frame the clinician–patient link and not simply *communication* or *relationship building*. The reason is that caregivers are with their patients not simply as a friend or information provider. This is a working connection in which an objective must be achieved: discussions and actions that promote the patient's healing. Both parties have something to contribute to the cause. And if they are not working together toward a mutually understood and accepted set of objectives, the chances of getting there are greatly compromised. There are *gives* and *gets* for the chain of caregivers, payers, patients, managers, and others who are part of the equation. Those ideally are dynamically exchanged so that patient and provider are truly working together.

With this as caregivers' clinical template, their tone and tenor are reframed in a way that engages both patients and others in their circle. On the table is their clinical knowledge and vast experience in understanding treatment options, the risks along with the benefits. Doctor's orders are not part of the equation. Patient compliance is recast because it is not a matter of the patient complying or not with your orders. Patients understand and adopt the plan forward because they have been part of its development. Caregivers have then reaped the buy-in that is the intent of the Walk in the Woods. With this buy-in on board, their chances of getting it right with their patients are greatly enhanced. And at those rare times when things go wrong, they will be in a much better place to handle the difficult situation.

So who is this *negotiating patient*? In the good old days, it was the doctors and the system that defined the patient. In the future, it will be more and more the patients who define the contours of the health enterprise and how they want to be treated. Each of your patients is different and each will want different ingredients as part of his or her care package. Your ability to treat patients as different people, to be the translator as they traverse an increasingly automatic and self-serve system, is the essence of what they need and what you will do. Even though machines may be smarter than you at times and robots may do some of your job more precisely, nothing can replace the human qualities you bring. As long as health care providers keep those human qualities on the table, they keep for themselves a place in their patients' lives.

And that bottom line is what negotiating patients want most: the knowledge and comfort that they are being treated as valued human beings by a system that can lose that quality in the pursuit of its many layered agenda.

CHAPTER 14

CHANGING WORK AND A CHANGING WORKFORCE

THERE ARE stark differences between what the health care enterprise did in the past and what it will do and how it will do it in the future. As noted in prior chapters, these changes result from innovative technologies, shifts in demographics and patient expectations, and also important, developments in the politics and economics of health. As a result, the work to be done and the people needed to accomplish it will navigate through a series of potentially awkward adjustments. The question is whether there are workers prepared and ready to fill the new requirements, and if not, what will be done? There are implications for you and your career just as there are consequences for your organization and how it operates. And the path is crowded with inevitable conflict and abundant negotiation.

There are many sides to the complex questions regarding the changing workforce because one problem or solution often affects or prompts another. If demand for services increases and the supply of workers ready to supply those services decreases, what will be the effect on the population's health and the cost of labor? What adjustments must or can be made to fill the likely gaps that will grow? If you are in the workforce, how will you evolve in your own career—so that you are less likely to become irrelevant or, even worse, unemployed or underpaid—in light of rapidly changing work requirements and resultant compensation? If you are an employer, what will you do to maintain a qualified, motivated, and sufficient workforce for your organization?

The answers to these questions will distinguish institutions that are able to employ and retain a top-notch collection of professionals and an ample supply

---

Unless otherwise noted, quotations and summaries of comments from Kimberly Costa, Richard Donahue, Patrick Jordan, Derik King, Gordon Moore, Scott Ransom, and Pamela Wible are taken from interviews conducted by the authors in 2009 and 2010.

of skilled labor from those that are not. They will distinguish those professionals who are able to adapt to changing opportunities—by keeping pace with the latest technologies and methods—from those who are not. And from a strategic perspective, they will determine whether a shrinking workforce will be able to serve a ballooning population of people in need of attention. In other words, these are the distinctions between success and failure for you, your organization, and on a much larger level, society as a whole. Will the least advantaged, the first to suffer in times of scarcity, be neglected amid the shortage of people to provide necessary health care? Will the middle class be forced to make compromises in the care that they have come to expect, and will that care cost them more?

In the "good old days," graduates of nursing, medical, health care management, and related schools of higher learning could look forward to a fairly predictable career trajectory. With time and experience, status, salary, and recognition would grow in step to provide increased autonomy, independence, and professional satisfaction. There were career ladders to climb and opportunities that would surely lie ahead. And if there were any doubt, you could follow in the steps of mentors ahead of you, gleaning from their experiences in the hope of replicating their successes.

Not so today. What you have learned as you accept your graduate degree could very well be passé by the time you step into your second job. In the 1970s, there were approximately 500 clinical trials annually. By the 1990s, that number had grown to 10,000 each year (Schrock & Cydulka, 2006). In 2011, ClinicalTrials.gov had information on more than 102,000 clinical trials in 174 countries (NIH, 2011). This is just one example of the exponential advances in knowledge. Keeping current with the innovations in medical and technical understanding is almost a full-time job of its own. Especially for people who go into the most specialized practice fields, the pace of change will render today's expertise rapidly outmoded. New capabilities, such as quick and inexpensive genetic testing, will create the demand for new skills and services. A thriving career trajectory in today's environment will demand significant flexibility, a heavy load of continuing education and training, and a willingness to continuously invest in your own professional evolution and relevance. You may find that negotiating your "learning package" is as important as negotiating your financial package when you explore an employment opportunity.

As the work has changed, so too have the expectations of those entering the health care workforce changed. Once, professional elders insisted that each new crop of inductees go through the same trials and apprenticeship learning processes as they did to earn their stripes. This included seemingly endless on-call hours to the less-than-stimulating clerical work necessary in the routine care of patients. It also meant intense competition between individuals for valued assignments. Each generation, however, introduces its own needs and desires. For example, research on the Millennial generation (those born between 1981 and 1999) has shown that in general they dislike working long hours and desire more family time. They shun conflict and prefer working in teams, a distinct outlook that will affect workplace interactions and negotiations as they move through their careers (Benko, 2007).

What are the trends in the health care workforce and what do they portend for your future and that of the health enterprise?

Evolution of Work and the Workforce

Health care is a growth industry. Even a slowdown in the economy that tempered the production and service sectors did not squeeze the size of the health workforce. During the recession of 2008 and 2009, deemed the worst downturn since the Great Depression of the 1930s, the United States added health care jobs, despite a national unemployment rate that reached more than 10 percent. Yes, specific organizations and departments trimmed their payrolls and dismissed staff. Overall, however, a reliable stream of cash from government and private insurers and a steady supply of patients kept the engines running and revving.

In the midst of this growth are well-documented shortages of clinicians that are projected to swell continuously for years to come. One study projects a shortage of 260,000 nurses by the year 2025 (Buerhaus, Auerbach, & Staiger, 2009). The ensuing pressures are not simply on nurse managers trying to fill shifts. There are also tangible implications for patient care. According to estimates from one study, 6,700 patient deaths and 4 million days of hospital care could be averted annually by increasing the number of nurses (Needleman, Buerhaus, Stewart, Zelevinsky, & Mattke, 2006).

The situation is not much better on the physician front. One estimate warns of a deficit of approximately 200,000 physicians in the United States by 2020 (Cooper, 2004). In addition, with higher-paying specialty careers luring doctors away from primary care, the overall percentage of physicians ready to meet growing demand is decreasing: 2009 marked the twelfth consecutive year that the number of U.S. medical school graduates who chose primary care residencies was "dismally low" (Bodenheimer, Grumbach, & Berenson, 2009). The explanations include higher debt loads from medical education weighed against primary care's lower compensation and higher workloads leading to work-life imbalance (Reuben, 2007; Bodenheimer et al., 2009).

Responses to this development may generate battlegrounds of conflict within the profession. In 2009, the Medicare Payment Advisory Commission, an independent federal panel, recommended that payments to primary care physicians be raised by 10 percent (Pear, 2009). However, because the panel also recommended that the increase be funded by reducing payments for other covered services, specialists lobbied against this change. "We don't have enough doctors in primary care or in any specialty," U.S. Representative Shelley Berkley explained to the *New York Times*. Ultimately, the subsequent legislation addressing Medicare payments included a 10 percent increase for some primary care services and for select general surgeons for a five-year period beginning in 2011 (Robert Wood Johnson Foundation, 2010). Efforts to adjust incentives and compensation to redirect practice patterns will continue to prompt conflict as veterans rally to hold their ground.

The United States has long relied on immigrants to populate a portion of the health care workforce, particularly in primary care (Hing & Lin, cited in Steinbrook, 2009). Lured by the chance for greater earnings, security, and in some cases political freedom, these individuals became valuable contributors as doctors, nurses, technicians, and administrators. However, a *reverse brain drain* is emerging as immigrants who are students and professionals in a variety of fields decide to seek opportunities in their native countries rather than in the United States (Webber, 2004; Wadhwa, 2007, 2009). The 2009 HSBC Bank International Expat Explorer Survey found that 23 percent of other countries' expatriates working in all fields and living in the United States are considering returning home versus 15 percent of U.S. expatriates based elsewhere. The most commonly cited reason is diminished career prospects in the United States. There are now more attractive opportunities in China, India, and Eastern Europe than there were a generation ago (*Expat Explorer Survey*, 2009).

Worker shortages in the health care enterprise are part of larger shifts in the overall U.S. workforce. In their book *Workforce Crisis*, Ken Dychtwald, Tamara Erickson, and Robert Morison (2006) state that the growth rate of the overall U.S. workforce will slow from 12 percent in 2010 to just 4 percent in 2020. The exact effect on health care is not well known; however, in general, approximately 80 percent of the native-born workforce growth between now and 2020 will come from workers aged fifty and older (Dychtwald et al., 2006, p. 8). Dychtwald et al. present nine "trends to count on." The workforce (1) will get older, (2) will have more women, (3) will have more ethnic diversity, and (4) will display increased lifestyle and life-stage variety. In addition, (5) labor markets will tighten and (6) shortages of educated candidates will arise. This will lead to (7) pressures on training and development systems as organizations try to bring undereducated candidates up to standard and keep their existing workforce fully abreast of new knowledge, skills, and technologies; (8) tensions over the human resource (HR) policies and practices applied to adapt to these changes; and (9) strains on organizational coherence owing to the adoption of flextime and telecommuting and greater use of contract and contingency workers. Each of these factors is discussed in the following sections.

The Aging Workforce

The graying workforce has been cited as a primary factor in the projected nursing shortage: in a *Nursing Management* survey, 55 percent of surveyed nurses said they intended to retire between 2011 and 2020 and, after 2020, more than 25 percent plan to retire (Hader, Saver, & Steltzer, 2006). There is likely to be a similar trend among the ranks of physicians, as they are subject to many of the same demographic forces (Salsberg & Grover, 2006). Ironically, those same population trends will increase demand for health care as aging baby boomers, the seventy-eight million people who were born between 1946 and 1964, reach their most health care intensive years. These are also the years when much of their care will be paid for by Medicare, traditionally the lowest dollar payer in the market. This all combines into more patients, fewer caregivers, and diminishing reimbursement: a perfect storm for conflict and discontent. The one saving grace in this picture could be a trend away from routine retirement at the age of sixty-five. As people live longer and expect to be healthy and productive for a longer period, many may opt to keep working, encouraged by the satisfactions of a job and career. As sixty becomes the new forty and centenarians become more commonplace, clinicians may opt for longer careers, though what they do may shift as they become less nimble and perhaps less current with emerging knowledge and methods.

More Women in the Workforce

The neat divide of most of the twentieth century when most doctors were men and most nurses were women continues to blur. This is leading to significant changes in the tone and tenor of health services, as female doctors have been shown to be more likely to actively engage patients in their own care, to be more team-oriented as leaders, and to have a more sympathetic view of the need for a work-life balance (Levinson & Lurie, 2004). These changes could well change the flavor of long-standing conflicts, especially those between nurses and physicians regarding patient care decisions and authority. This is not to imply that these conflicts will disappear. Rather it is to suggest that conflicts among men and women—especially when men are in the dominant position—are different from conflicts among women. In addition, women have traditionally gravitated toward primary care roles, which offer lower compensation than specialty care.

Nick Norton, Oppidania Medical Center's chief of orthopedics, and Rusty Rice, head of OMC's hospitalist program, took just three days to find the time to meet and review the numbers on the surgical checklists: it is a priority for both, though for different reasons. Rice is a champion for putting checklists in place. Norton is looking for the hole in Rice's argument. Norton is clever enough to know that you can't kill something unless you first understand it. Rice is discerning enough to know that Norton is a tough character and resistant to anything new and disruptive. Rice can't be confident that he has convinced Norton until he watches this surgeon make checklists part of his routine in the operating room (OR). These are tall orders for both.

Norton has distributed Rice's numbers to members of the surgical department's executive leadership committee in preparation for their next meeting. He expects that this very smart group of people will find some way to mount a decisive defense.

Dr. Frank Farwell, chief of the surgical department, opens the meeting and then graciously turns the floor over to Norton, thanking him for his efforts. Norton is ready. "As you all know, the patient safety committee, which has long been on our backs, has made surgical checklists their latest battle cry. Although I am all in favor of patient safety, I think we have to hold the line on this one. There are three very sound reasons. First, this is going to take time, and as we all know, time in our business is big money. It's not only money out of our pockets. It is going to cost the hospital, a matter that I think is in our favor because it will put the administration on our side. Given the current climate, they are ready to run after every dollar. Second, I think it will have a marginal benefit for patient safety, if that. We all have our personal techniques and ways to make sure we are concentrated and grounded in the OR. Bill, you have your music, Tom, you have routines, and I do my mindfulness stuff. Every individual has his or her own way of making sure we get things right. I think what this will do is get in the way of all that, make us less grounded in what works for us, and actually disrupt rather than aid our concentration. And finally, my next-door neighbor is a commercial pilot. He went into aviation around the same time I went into surgery. He says his job simply is no fun anymore. When he first entered the cockpit after coming out of the military, he used to actually fly the plane. Now with autopilot, the array of machines, and rules on top of rules, he is basically baby-sitting the computers up there. And he hates it. He warned me that they'll try to do the same thing to us. There is an art to surgery, and each person around this room has perfected it. That's why we made it onto this team, it's what gets us up in the morning, and it's what makes us good. I think this checklist business is a fad and a move in the wrong direction. I think we should resist it. The question for us to figure out today is how to put this whole thing to rest."

Farwell thanks Norton and then turns to the other surgeons around the table and asks, "Well, what do you all think?"

Dr. Bill Bentley speaks up first. "You're right, Nick. Without my music, I couldn't concentrate. Mozart has been my surgical companion for years now. But I don't think that the surgical checklists get in the way of that. I actually think this is a good idea. First, I think it will unite everyone in the operating room, which is a good thing. Second, it's a good modeling technique for our residents, who come in overwhelmed anyway. It will give them a map and get them ready to roll. And finally, over our careers, we all have acquired that short list of things we wish we had remembered to do and or not do in the OR, and we all probably would be willing to do anything to erase them. If a couple of minutes will make it less likely that I or someone else will mess up, I'm prepared to do it."

"Actually, I don't see this as such a big burden," said Dr. Tom Thrush, nodding in agreement with Bentley. "I don't even quite understand why it is seen as so revolutionary. It's just common sense to me. I've been doing checklists in my own way for years now. I do it verbally and from memory, though I don't find any problem in making it a bit more formal. I have checklists for everything in my life. I pack with a list, I go shopping with a list, and I do surgery with a list. What's the big deal?"

Frank Farwell takes up the beat from Thrush, "I think we also have to consider the legal environment. This checklist thing has really taken off. A lot of places are doing it, and they have shown improvements in outcomes. If we don't take it on and have an unexpected problem or outcome, some personal injury attack dog is going to come after us, saying that if we had checklists just like everyone else it wouldn't have happened. Then they'll get some clown on the stand testifying how checklists saved the world, and the jury will be scratching their heads about why we didn't require them here. I hate to say it, but that's the world we live in nowadays. And I dislike that world, Nick, more than I dislike the world of your pilot friend. On top of that, in the overall scheme of things, I don't think this will take that much extra time."

Norton feels downright deflated. He can't believe that his own people are turning against him. Bentley, the more interpersonally sensitive surgeon on the executive committee, senses Nick's discomfort. "Nick, we all appreciate your watching our backs on the patient safety committee. And I think you've given us the chance to consider this and a whole lot of other measures that have come our way." Bentley sees that Norton is hurting and wants to not only ease that but give him a way to save face. "However, I think you can use this as a clever negotiating chip. Let the safety committee know that we have reasonable reservations about the checklists and are considering all the arguments you've presented. I think we all heard them, and everything you mentioned was also on my mind. Then come across as a really nice and accommodating sort of guy. We can win brownie points for this, so that when they hit us next, you can put those good behavior points on the table. As far as the hospital and costs go, this whole thing cuts both ways. You are 100 percent right that this will have costs attached. Now though, with pay for performance and other mechanisms that are tying outcomes to reimbursement, the hospital can't afford a single foul-up. It costs too much in the long run. It also can't afford to get dinged by those Internet sites evaluating hospitals and outcomes—once something is on the Internet, it's there forever. So this is ultimately good for the hospital, it's good for the department, and as Frank points out, it leaves us a tad less legally vulnerable. Just one thing, Nick: when you tell the committee that we're willing to go along, make it a home run for us."

Norton feels a sense of relief, though he is not quite sure why. He thanks the committee members for their input and scribbles some notes to himself as the meeting moves on to its next item of business.

This factor could raise a gender inequity theme in the existing conflicts over compensation between primary care providers and specialists. And although they have made progress in reaching the highest echelons of health care management, women still achieve the role of chief executive officer at 63 percent of the rate for men (American College of Healthcare Executives, 2006), leading to resentment and friction.

The desire to attract and retain women in the workforce will lead to the renegotiation of traditional career paths, allowing, for example, more seamless incorporation of maternity leaves, without adverse impact on a woman's career. More men may also expect to follow nontraditional career paths, with women blazing the trails for them.

Sylvia Ann Hewlett and Carolyn Buck Luce (2005) introduced the concept of *off ramps* and *on ramps* in their seminal 2005 *Harvard Business Review* article examining the challenges that face professional women who confront career interruptions on account of care responsibilities for young children or elderly parents. They argue that organizations need to make it easier for workers to come in and out of the work world if they want to leverage the fullest range of contributions from valued individuals. Since then the concept of a nonlinear career path has grown and is now being seen as a viable career option for both women and men. No longer is study-work-retire-die the formula. Instead, people might choose to study-work-break-work-study-break-work-break-study or some other combination best suited to their skills, talents, family demands, and preferences.

More Ethnic Diversity in the Workforce

An ethnically diverse workforce is a valuable asset for providing culturally competent care to an equally diverse population. However, ethnic minorities have historically been underrepresented among health care workers (Cohen, Gabriel, & Terrell, 2002). The overall shortage of qualified workers along with the continued growth in well-paying health care jobs—fully half of the occupations projected to grow fastest over through 2018 are health care–related (U.S. Bureau of Labor Statistics, 2008)—is likely to both push and pull a broader population toward employment opportunities in this field.

A more diverse workforce also affects the delicate balance of culture and expectation among those operating in close quarters and with the day-to-day stresses that are typical of health care. On one hand it is a simple fact of life that different cultures handle hope, joy, disappointment, anger, and frustration in different ways, and those differences themselves can prompt their own frustrations and anger. A greater potential for misunderstanding, miscommunication, and at times even outright animus exists when ethnocentrism and differences in language, custom, values, and history are present (Mighty, 1991). On the other hand, when led and managed skillfully, a diverse team can bring broader and deeper perspectives that can enrich the work environment and the delivery of care, especially when the patient population mirrors the workforce.

Changing Lifestyle and Life-Stage Expectations in the Workforce

For prior generations, work was life's central activity. Long hours, steady and long-term employment with the same organization, and a predictable career ladder melded into one's personal identity. Those expectations have changed. Generational differences, the increasing presence of women in all roles in health care, and the need to remain current with professional knowledge are combining to breed demands for flexibility in roles, schedules, and responsibilities. Workers with young children or aging parents will want—and expect—consideration to be given to those demands in addition to traditional professional duties. Those pursuing advanced or continuing education will see their supplementary training to be as important to their performance and professional development as their on-the-job experience. These developments will put new stress on managers and colleagues and will generate conflicts of priorities and preferences as the work-life balance is negotiated. No longer will it be assumed that work comes first. Rather work will be part of an individualized blend of work, family, education, and leisure, as what Benko (2007) terms the *career lattice* replaces the career ladder.

Tightening Labor Markets

In its projections for the U.S. labor market through 2018, the U.S. Bureau of Labor Statistics (2008) shows health care and social assistance as adding the greatest gross number of jobs, more than four million. Younger segments of the workforce (aged sixteen to thirty-four) will either shrink or remain relatively flat as a percentage of the total workforce. The greatest growth, in percentage terms, will be among workers fifty-five and over. Thus the average age of the workforce is rising. Both the overall population and the workforce are projected to grow at a slower pace than they did from 1998 to 2008. The result will be an intense competition for workers of all ages—to attract new nurses, doctors, and technicians or to retain those already in the system—that will tip the negotiating table in favor of the labor force.

Shortages of Educated Candidates

According to the authors of *Workforce Crisis* (Dychtwald, Erickson, & Morison, 2006), there is a growing disparity between the skills needed by organizations and those possessed by workers. The demand for highly educated workers is increasing as the economy as a whole and medicine in particular become more knowledge based. Despite that demand, the pace at which highly trained workers enter the market has been slowing since the 1970s. In California, as just one example, it is projected that the demand for workers with at least a bachelor's degree will equal 41 percent of the workforce in 2025; just 34 percent of the workforce had a bachelor's degree in 2006, and growth in degrees granted was slowing (Reed, 2008). The education system is simply not producing enough college graduates to meet demand.

Many health care positions, of course, require advanced degrees. Even midlevel technical positions demand significant training as technology becomes central to more and more work. Therefore the shortage of college graduates has systemwide implications. This is another trend that will increase the competition for talent, not only between health care organizations but across all sectors that require technical and scientific expertise.

Pressures on Education and Training Systems

There is a basic pipeline issue underlying the shortage of both doctors and nurses. According to the American Association of Colleges of Nursing, almost 50,000 qualified candidates were turned away from nursing programs in 2008 for lack of capacity. Teaching nursing pays less than clinical practice, and this pay differential has been among the factors complicating recruitment of faculty to nursing colleges. The same is true for the training of physicians. Clinical practice compensates physicians far more generously than does teaching, despite the satisfactions derived from preparing the next generation of doctors. Proposals to expand class size in medical schools and residency training programs have been advocated to increase the supply of physicians (Cooper, 2007). As the demand for physicians grows, the entirety of medical education and training will need to be evaluated.

Medicine is also at a relative disadvantage in competing for top talent relative to other science- or technology-based sectors. Medical training requires both an extended time commitment and considerable cost. Thus young people may choose other challenging and rewarding careers that will be less demanding. There are plenty of opportunities, as Scott Ransom, president of the University of North Texas Medical Center at Fort Worth told us, and "insurance and pharma can be more attractive and lucrative than medicine."

H

Tensions over HR Policies and Strains on Organizational Coherence

As the work itself changes, so too do the organizations in which it occurs. An organization's human resource department is designed to provide a structure, a set of policies and regulations that apply to all organizational employees and that govern intervention when staff and employee problems arise. These policies and regulations must keep pace with the changes in the economic, political, and social forces that have an impact on the health care organization. Organizations will less and less be homogeneous entities operating within the neat boxes of an organizational chart that reflects long-term, full-time workers moving methodically up a predetermined career path. They will face strains, changes, and adjustments as they hire more part-time and contract workers; experience greater worker mobility, increasing turnover; and outsource specialized operations such as emergency or radiology departments. Physicians, nurses, technicians, and administrators will have increasing requirements for continuing education training, a budget item that is likely to grow as science and technology advance.

In a market of intense competition for the best talent, individuals will lobby for individual accommodations for flextime, time off, retirement packages, use of temporary workers, and other measures to balance work and lifestyle. There will be intense and ongoing negotiation to accommodate the needs of the organization and the people it serves and also meet the expressed desires of the workforce through which the organization fulfills its mission. Managers will be engaged in continuous recalibration to meet the needs of patients, the requirements of administrators and regulators, and the demands of workers who will have more bidders than ever for their employment. HR professionals will be more aggressively active in talent acquisition, retention, and advising rather than simply providing compliance-driven support. This adjustment will prompt its own conflict: a higher HR profile will be seen as useful by some and as meddling

Iris Inkwater knows this is going to be a trying meeting and she wants no uncertainty about its purpose and tenor. Rather than convening privately with Janice Johnson, the vice president of nursing, she asks Perry Pudolski, the COO, and Rajeev Rao, the CFO, to join the session in her office. As they take their seats around the table at the far end of Inkwater's office, heavy clouds threaten rain outside the window, eerily reflecting what each one of them understands will be a somber meeting.

Iris Inkwater believes in being direct. "Janice, I have some disappointing news. Rajeev has just put together a new report on the hospital's finances. Things now look worse than we anticipated, and they will probably get much worse before they get better. I know that you have been working on reengineering the patient care units and redefining roles for all the caregivers. That in turn has begun to reduce expenses. That effort is appreciated but the reductions are not enough. As we sign more capitated contracts with managed care organizations, we need to reduce staff further because our inpatient census continues to decline."

"What are we looking at now?" Johnson asks with trepidation. Inkwater turns toward Rao. That is planned. She wants Rao to deliver the really bad news, allowing her to play the role of option builder and not mere tyrant.

"Ten percent," he sighs with resignation.

"Ten percent?" Agitated, Johnson looks to Inkwater for confirmation. "Right away?" Inkwater nods. "That's too much change for the staff in too short a time," Johnson exclaims. "Just once I'd like to have one of those bean-counting insurance guys spend a shift with us cleaning bedpans and changing bandages. Comforting people in pain. They wouldn't last half a shift. How about one of you trying it?" She is red with rage. She looks with scorn at Pudolski and Rao.

"Janice, it isn't their fault. It's just the reality we face," Inkwater says. She is firm but careful to calibrate her tone so as not to further escalate her nursing chief's distress.

"The process we established will allow us to get there, but it will take time," Johnson pleads. Her shoulders sag as the news sinks in.

Johnson's descent to the basement is expected. Inkwater has seen everyone else who has been to this series of meetings go there in his or her own way. That's one reason why she wanted to position herself to be able to offer options: part of her job is to help her people climb out of the basement.

Rao carefully explains the figures. Inkwater watches Johnson as she stares at Rao while he reviews the overall reduction in the current and projected census, the overcapacity of the nursing staff, and the hospital's dire financial straits. He puts the situation in the context of the hospital's reengineering, case management, and quality improvement efforts. Inkwater knows Johnson is not interested in facts and figures at the moment: Johnson is thinking about "her" nurses.

Johnson is indeed pondering the painful human toll this will take on a dedicated and hard-working staff and the patients they serve. This is not how to reward people for years of round-the-clock devotion. How will she decide who goes? How will she tell them? When will it all have to begin? Rao has mustered as much energy as he can for his report. He too is thinking of the people, though he is also considering the jobs they will save if Oppidania survives these difficult times. Johnson is almost in tears. It is hard for anyone in the room to make eye contact with the others.

"Are other departments being asked to cut so severely?" Johnson speaks as if she were looking for some justice in the news. Inkwater explains that this has been a day of bad news for many of the department heads. Johnson asks if the 10 percent figure is negotiable. Perry Pudolski explains that it isn't. He adds, though, that how the cuts will be achieved and the criteria for deciding what to cut will be open to discussion. He assures her that he and the staff in the human resource department will be available to help implement the directive.

Johnson, with union rules on her mind, turns to Inkwater. "Iris, I have two concerns. I am concerned about the 10 percent who are leaving. Because of the union contract, these will be our youngest and most energetic nurses, and it will be a tragedy for them to start their nursing careers with this kind of a beginning. If they are flexible, though, they will probably be OK. There are numerous jobs opening up in home care, and these nurses are probably better able to fill these positions than their older counterparts. It is the 90 percent who remain that worry me most. When we close down the designated units, we will be dislodging people who have been working together in the same place for years. We will have to rotate shifts for a lot of people now accustomed to the routine of a day shift. And they will all have to work harder because there will be no slack in the staffing. What can we do for the 90 percent?"

Inkwater is impressed. All the other department heads had pleaded to keep the staff they were going to lose. Those meetings had turned into vain attempts to readjust Rao's figures, which simply left little room for adjustment. Though upset, Johnson has listened to Rao's numbers, and she recognizes that pleading would be a useless exercise. She has to be cognizant of carefully leading up to her boss, just as her boss has to be cognizant of carefully leading down to her.

"Janice, you raise a valid point, and I would like to work with you to address exactly that issue. We will do everything possible to accommodate those who remain and show our appreciation for their continued commitment." A few plausible ideas to do just that are exchanged, and it brightens the mood for a moment. The meeting concludes after forty-five minutes. As Johnson walks to her office, she is pale and shaken by the reality that she will be saying "farewell" to some valued colleagues and friends. Nevertheless she is buoyed somewhat by her confidence that she can work with Inkwater to find some reasonable solutions to the challenges that will remain.

by others. Though the love-hate relationship between HR and employees is not confined to health care (Hammonds, 2005), it will be a feature of the bidding and competition for health care talent.

If you are in a leadership position, all of this greatly increases the complexity of leading down to your organizational base. You must discern the motivations, desires, and capabilities of a mosaic of individuals and unite them behind a singular vision. You must craft a compelling organizational narrative in which each member of the workforce can see that they play an important part, understand their role, and become loyal, enthusiastic contributors. You must balance myriad demands without showing real or perceived favoritism or bias. This will require you to draw continuously on all your skills as a negotiator and meta-leader. It will be up to meta-leaders to stitch together what otherwise could become a motley collection of tasks, technologies, and skilled individuals. This is not simply a matter of effective management. Understanding and engaging the human dimensions of this evolution is becoming an extraordinary and critical leadership challenge.

Changes in Work Formats

Simply put, there will be more demand for certain types of work and less demand for others. New technologies and cost pressures will drive the shifts just as demands for improved and safer care will emerge from the marketplace. One example of such a recalibration has been in the field of noninvasive cardiology, which often provides better solutions to cardiovascular disease, is less risky for the patient, and is less expensive than open heart surgery, for which demand has declined. On other fronts there will be a greater need for translating and interpreting medical decisions and results, both for the more sophisticated patients and those lacking in health literacy. There will be less demand for memorization, note taking, and monitoring: computers will have more data and be able to analyze and cross reference it more quickly and more effectively than human clinicians. Patients will key in their own medical history or will carry it on a chip. Sophisticated sensors will be able to take readings from patients automatically and directly, allowing information to be transmitted from the patient in his home to the doctor in her office.

The decline of individuals' need for particular services and skills is not a painless process. People will have invested their educations and their careers in acquiring these skills and providing these services and in doing them well. To be replaced by a monitor, computer, or new technique is a frightening proposition.

The guarantee of lifelong employment and sustenance is no longer part of the promise of a health care education.

The rise in the demand for particular services is likewise not an easy process, though the discomfort is more an organizational phenomenon than a personal phenomenon. As a new procedure or method gains favor, there will be an aggressive struggle to find talent. Each practice, hospital, clinic, and laboratory will position itself as the preferred employer for its most desired candidates. Active employee referral and networking campaigns will be needed. Innovative practices will also be essential, and forward thinking leaders will have to understand that promises made in recruiting materials could backfire if the organization cannot live up to them. The following sections discuss a number of contingent strategies that may be deployed alone or in combination to find new reservoirs of talent or to reconfigure work to take best advantage of the talent at hand.

A

Outsourcing

One of the strategies to combat scarce labor is to outsource to another provider: for example, by having X-ray images read in India. Not only can these services offer cost-saving advantages, they also may provide twenty-four-hour service without overtime payments: the three shifts of your day could be spread across different global time zones. Digital records can be economically dispatched and returned from ready workers around the world.

Another strategy involves subcontracting the management of portions of an organization, such as a set of services or a hospital department. One such management company, Emergency Consultants, Inc. (ECI), has been staffing and managing emergency departments and hospitalist staffs at hospitals and urgent care clinics for more than thirty-five years. ECI does this through a limited liability partnership structure set up between ECI and the host facility. This can mean that doctors working directly for a hospital are collaborating on cases with physicians who are paid by another organization, such as ECI. Many of the ECI-contracted physicians will be people that the hospital once employed, because ECI retains as many of the existing staff in departments it takes over as is feasible. Although the legal agreement is designed to align interests and construct avenues for resolving conflict, this is complicated by workers with multiple allegiances related to money and control.

"We're often brought in as change agents," Derik King, the president of ECI, told us. For example, one hospital CEO we interviewed was enthusiastic about evidence-based protocols—he felt that almost everything needed by patients can be standardized—yet he had met resistance from the leaders of the medical staff, who resented the administrative staff interfering in their procedures. Physicians are used to independence. Thus the CEO could choose to turn to an outside resource to forcefully catalyze the desired change.

"A company like ECI can come in with better data capture and analysis than the in-house department because we can draw on an entire network of sites," said King. "We have a lot of experience implementing evidence-based protocols. We dedicate a lot of effort to bringing the medical staff on board but aren't afraid to make the changes necessary to deliver on the agreed-upon metrics. Ultimately, the best-run departments attract and retain the best staffs—and that's essential in a tight labor market."

Outsourcing may improve patient outcomes, decrease costs, relieve strain on other staff resources, or provide any number of other benefits. However, outsourcing to an offshore provider or in-house management company can breed resentment among an institution's staff. Those who remain or who are shifted from employee to subcontractor likely will resent the new arrangements. Respected experts may see in the move a swerve in their own status from that of valued professional to that of expendable laborer. The new arrangements, if not carefully negotiated with both contractor and staff, could generate paralyzing conflict, threatening the very advantages sought in the deal. When some health care providers are employed by an outsourced service but work in-house, there may be resentment and friction between them and staff who are directly employed. The outsourced workers may also have divided loyalties, feeling obligated both to the organization that pays their salary and the one to which they are providing services.

How can leaders best conduct outsourcing negotiations in order to reap the intended benefits while accounting for the very real concerns of existing staff members? As appropriate, genuine transparency will advantage all sides of the table. Conversely, if people are suspicious of ulterior motives and hidden agendas, they will overcompensate in their demands and expectations. To the extent that there are benefits to share or downsides to endure: ensure that they are fairly spread about the table. And although an arrangement may require some staff to leave the organization, know that how they are treated on their exit sends an important message to those left behind. An organization that demonstrates and acts upon its expressed values even when hard decisions must be made will have far more negotiation currency in the future than one that demonstrates little care for the people on whom it has depended and will continue to depend.

Insourcing

Another strategy for rearranging work and the workforce is to *insource* it to a group within your organization or network that has the capacity to get the job done though it has not traditionally performed the particular function. One current example of this strategy is having advanced practice nurses (APNs) perform specific activities customarily performed by physicians. There is logic to this arrangement when accomplished with the appropriate quality supervision; nevertheless, it could cause a cascade of further problems, exacerbating the shortage of nurses if the additional challenge, prestige, and pay draw people away from general nursing practice.

The use of insourcing could very well portend a trend of downshifting specific tasks to professions with less training yet equal skill to perform work at lower cost. Training itself could migrate to focusing more on functional preparation and less on acquisition of a broad knowledge base that applies to a broad range of tasks.

Insofar as individuals' status within a health care organization derives from what they do, their training to do it, what they don't do, and who reports to whom, the shifts in status that derive from this insourcing could spark difficult negotiations and bitter conflicts. The fights themselves could center on questions of risk—who bears it and who does not—and assumption of medical liability when something goes wrong. The legal equation could very well trump the efficiency line of reasoning, especially as the losers in the adjustment—specifically the doctors—demand legal immunity for oversight of services they have forgone.

Contingent Workers

The use of *contingent workers*—contractors, temporary employees, consultants, and the like—is another way that organizations can shift work from their employed staff. According to a brief from Manpower, Inc., a survey of 41,000 employers in thirty-five countries revealed that more than one-third of respondents said they view contingent labor as a key element of their workforce strategy (Rules of Engagement, 2009). Contingent workers have been traditionally used to cover a specific task or seasonal demand: for example, a hospital in a mountain town could expect a surge in patients during ski season and hire a locum tenans to supplement its medical staff. Temporary workers are also used to cover short-term absences. Now, however, organizations are also using contingent workers to fulfill core functions, to try out candidates before hiring them permanently, or to quickly find specialized skills.

Contingent workers are not a panacea. If they are not brought on board with the same care accorded regular employees, they may not assimilate well with the permanent staff, understand the larger context of their role, or fully embrace the mission of the organization. Long-term contingent workers may have the same needs and expectations for advancement, development, and recognition as regular employees.

News of the cuts spreads faster than a fire. No one in the hospital is spared from the anxiety. It is one thing to read about the massive shift the health care industry is undergoing and quite another to have it hit home. It is like an earthquake, with waves of impact rattling through Oppidania Medical Center. In their pursuit to cover and care for everyone, insurers and the government are desperate to cut costs by shifting care to the least expensive venues. Hospitals, the most costly point on the care continuum, are being further restricted by payers to providing only that narrow slice of services demanding their extensive—and expensive—facilities. This shrinking provides vendors in the health care market with new opportunities, including the promotion of technologies that can effectively keep people at home, engaged, healthy, and happy. If you work in a hospital though, the rattling tremblers don't feel good.

Heather Harriford stares listlessly at the cup of yogurt she's brought to work. She knows that she is right on the border line: she's been here a short enough time to be on the 10 percent cut list though long enough and productively enough to possibly be able to stay on board. She is nervous; after making the move to the general medical floor, she had splurged on a new car and those payments won't go away if she is laid off. She knows that there are many opportunities out there, including some that would actually advance her career. The problem is that she loves working in a hospital; it is her lifelong dream. Of course she can adapt, though she is finally feeling really good about working at OMC.

She decides that she needs more than just yogurt tonight and heads to the cafeteria. She is debating between a veggie burger and a salad when she hears a frightening voice from behind. Could it be Chuck Cummings? She feels a sudden chill. They haven't exchanged a word since the mediation session. She has been trying to avoid him and guessing that he has likely been trying to do the same. She realizes that she is shaking and grips her tray more tightly to steady herself. Maybe coming to the cafeteria wasn't such a good idea after all.

She reaches for the first thing she can—a prepacked tuna sandwich—and gets into line. She thinks that if she beats him to the cash register she can slip back up to Six West. She doesn't look back. She focuses on the cashier chatting with one of her coworkers and begins to tap her foot. Why can't they work faster? Can she just drop everything and escape? She hears the voice again. "Heather, how are you?"

She winces and then turns around to find Cummings standing directly behind her. "Oh, Chuck. Fine. How are you?"

"I'm doing OK. Crazy days around here, eh?"

"Yup," she gives him a tight smile, still hoping that the line will carry her away from him.

"Would you be willing to share a table? This, um, jerk of a doctor has something he wants to say to you."

No, actually, sitting with Chuck Cummings is the last thing she wants to do. But he is being polite and appears somewhat humbler than she's ever seen him. What's the worst that can happen? It's a sandwich in a public place. It will at least be a distraction from all of the gossip about layoffs. OK, she is feeling tough enough to take anything. Or at least she hopes she is.

Harriford agrees and they take a table by the windows at the far side of the cafeteria. They settle in uncomfortably, unwrapping their food.

"I didn't think I'd ever say this to you, Heather," Cummings begins. "I want to thank you. Now that I have had a bit of time to reflect and to get off the defensive, I have a different attitude about what happened. You were right on many, many counts, from the patient care side all the way to the how-to-treat-people side. And I was arrogant. It's something I guess I'd gotten quite good at and which I've learned is not necessarily a good thing."

Harriford laughs lightly. This self-deprecation isn't something she expected. Could Cummings really have changed? Or is he just playing with her?

Cummings moves his salad around on the plate. His voice cracks slightly as he continues: "All through med school it was about being macho. No emotions. Just tough it through any difficulties. It was all one big game for me and I'd been doing it so long that I couldn't even recognize it anymore. No one had the stuff to wake me up. No one. Except for you. It didn't feel good, that's for sure. I think, though, that if it felt good, it would not have been the wake-up call I needed. You are a good person, Heather, and I sincerely apologize for what I put you through. Anyway, I wanted to say that to you."

Harriford is shocked. She thought she was the one feeling uncomfortable. Here is this outgoing guy who looks like he walked out of central casting and he is the one feeling uncomfortable? Wow.

"Well, um, I am glad to know that it was helpful to you, Chuck." She thinks that sounds diplomatic. She really isn't sure of what to say although her defenses remain up. This may be an apology, but the conversation has so far been all about him. What is behind the compelling need to report his evolution? Will her approval somehow validate his emotional growth?

"You know, I took those classes at the Multicultural Institute," Cummings says. "They were OK, informative. What really hit me though were conversations I had with my dad afterward. Those classes got us talking about stuff we had never talked about before. You know he is a doc, at the tail end of his career now. I went into medicine because I wanted to be like him. And I wanted his approval. I got it, at least on the surface. He told me he had wanted to talk with me for many years, but he's not exactly the emotive type either. He saw that I was pretty well defended, and that meant I missed a lot of cues. He told me that if you are a good doctor and a good person, you simply don't miss those cues. He thought I'd learn eventually. You don't pay attention, and you get yourself in trouble. And he was right. He actually also appreciated your stepping up to the plate—you've really won his approval."

Harriford is moved by what Cummings has to say but is also still skeptical. This guy is a smooth talker, and this habit goes back long and far. This could just be another ruse, and she simply isn't going to fall for it.

Cummings continues, "You know, I have been able to flirt and engage with many, many people. It seemed to come naturally. I fed off it. And you know, if I ticked someone off, I didn't much care because there were still plenty of other people at my party. And if I needed to, I could easily go out and get more. I was pretty insensitive."

"My dad and I are very much alike in many ways. He is a really good people person. I thought I was being like him, but I've learned that people don't love him because he's chatty or a flirt. He's a giving person. He gives just because he loves giving, not as a means to get something. I had a great role model, and somehow I blew it."

"We never appreciate all that we can learn from our parents," Harriford says. "We pick up bits here and there, but sometimes it has to be a teachable moment if it's going to stick. My dad spent his last dozen years in a wheelchair. It never slowed him down and he never threw a pity party. Watching him taught me how to keep things in perspective."

"He sounds like an inspiration, Heather. My dad and I have been talking about the differences between his career trajectory and mine. When he was at my stage of life, doctors were smarter than the computers and their hands were more agile than the machines. You relied on your memory, everyone thought you were a deity, and you did the best you could. Good bedside manner was good for business. If you played it right, and he did, you could have a satisfying and lucrative career."

"It's a different world now for doctors, Heather. The computers may not yet be smarter but they are faster and they don't forget things. We can now do surgery with machines that we could never do with just our hands. So if you're going to make it as a doctor, you have to find your right place between the technology and the people who are your patients. My dad said that I have the smarts and the analytical skills to figure that out. But he reminded me that people skills are going to be more and more important and that not paying attention to other people's feelings is my Achilles' heel. He made me realize that if I didn't figure this out soon, I might jeopardize my career—and hurt some good people along the way." He looks into her eyes to gauge her reaction. Is he getting across what he intends? She looks sympathetic but also a bit confused.

"Chuck, your father sounds like a wise man," Harriford says. She appreciates his openness but remains firm. "I'm glad you've had a chance to connect with him. But I never set out to ruin your career. I simply stood up for my career, my patient, and for my dignity as a person."

"Exactly as you should have, Heather. I was wrong on many levels. And if I'm making inappropriate passes at an extremely appropriate nurse, if I'm not paying attention, and if I give a patient the wrong medication, then I screw up. And I screwed up. You called me on it like no one else has ever called me on it. You were brave—I know that not everyone thought what you did was smart or right—and in the end you were generous. I cannot tell you, Heather, just how much I appreciate both your tenacity and your kindness."

Harriford looks down at her plate to collect her thoughts. She fiddles with the wrapper from her sandwich. What does he want her to say? What does she really want to say?

Finally, she speaks. "Chuck, I don't know what to say. I'm really happy for you. It would be great if other doctors could figure this out. Maybe you can help spread the word, because I don't want another woman to have to go through what I did." She doesn't want him to ignore what she has had to endure so he can arrive at his awakening. She admires what he has said but she also doesn't fully trust it. Cummings still looks like a pretty boy—albeit a humbled pretty boy—and she never did like his type. She has to admit, though, that he does seem genuine. "I appreciate your sharing this with me. You didn't have to do it. And if you really mean it, Chuck, then this is important stuff. Your dad is right about the people side of things: who we are is as important as what we do. After all, we're *human beings* not *human doings*."

They sit together for another ten minutes and move beyond their confrontation to talk about the hospital and the many changes underway. Harriford is surprised by how comfortable the conversation has become. It feels as though somehow they have broken through a barrier. She is no longer afraid of seeing Cummings. As they part company, she realizes that it took someone who wasn't fawning all over him to put Cummings in his place. She feels better about herself for taking a stand and is gratified that Cummings seems to be making some significant changes. It is all intriguing, yes, very intriguing.

It is important to recognize that the perception of contingent workers is changing. Where once this talent pool was made up of people whose real motive was in seeking a permanent, full-time position, it is now a status of choice for an increasing number of workers. Some prefer seasonal flexibility. Others find it an advantageous alternative during child-rearing years or when other personal responsibilities are in the mix, such as when caring for aging parents. These contingent workers can be just as qualified and committed as permanent staff, especially when their host organization is intentional about how to best manage their unique status and circumstances.

Building and Shaping Talent Pools

At times the search for talent requires reframing the challenge from one of scarcity to one of abundance. Where can you find abundant talent, and how can you put that talent to work to meet your objectives? Some of the members of the large, exiting cohort of retiring nurses, for example, might welcome part-time adjunct faculty positions at nursing colleges. Most people are not only living longer but enjoying more physical and mental vitality during the period traditionally thought of as the golden years. These people are likely to seek new opportunities, especially if they face financial pressures that keep them in the workforce. Some of these people will want to stay in their roles beyond a traditional retirement age or move into jobs that are less demanding than their original full-time roles. Others will want to downshift into part-time or seasonal positions.

Of course many health care roles require specific skills and, in many cases, formal certification. Not every golden-ager will be ready to go back for this training. There are, however, numerous possibilities. An orthopedic surgeon could become a nonoperative orthopedist provided that he or she has support from a group that can handle operative cases. An intensive care unit nurse could assume a role in outpatient surgery with little or no training. A medical records clerk could be a useful addition to the information technology department following adoption of an electronic health record. These transformations require examining both what roles exist and what roles could be created through process redesign. When done well, these accommodations allow both the health care organization and the people working in it to take best advantage of the skills, talent, and opportunities that are available.

Kimberly Costa, a community hospital nurse who also teaches in the nursing program at a community college, says that about half of the students she sees now are older than traditional students and that many are career changers: "I've had people from business, education, and the hospitality industries in addition to emergency medical technicians and others who have some health care background."

Health care organizations may also have to create talent pools by training individuals who were previously underqualified. This demand could very well reinvigorate the training sector, as people and organizations migrate in search of skills and jobs in a highly volatile marketplace. There will be growing opportunities to build strategic alliances between talent pool builders such as educational institutions and talent consumers such as hospitals in order to shape workforce capability.

How then do you reshape and reorient the talent pool to create organizational success amid this workforce change?

One health care organization that has created competitive advantage through innovative workforce practices is Newton-Wellesley Hospital, a community teaching hospital with almost 300 beds (Facts and Figures, 2008), located just west of Boston. In 2008, Newton-Wellesley had more than 18,000 patient admissions and more than 500,000 outpatient visits. There were approximately 700 inpatient surgeries performed and about 56,000 visits to its emergency room (Newton-Wellesley Hospital details, 2010). The hospital operates in one of the most competitive markets in the nation: there are ten hospitals within ten miles, at least two of which consistently rank in the top ten nationally. Not long ago Newton-Wellesley was an organization on the edge: low name recognition, no distinctive identity, and a financial loss of $1 million a month.

We spoke with Patrick Jordan, the chief operating officer, brought in from Massachusetts General Hospital (MGH) to help lead a turnaround. (Newton-Wellesley is a member of Partners HealthCare, which also includes MGH and other operations.) "Our clinical operations were good, but we weren't differentiated in any way," Jordan told us. "There was no compelling reason to choose us over our competitors."

Jordan and his team felt that they had an opportunity if they focused on transforming the patient experience, and they developed an intentional program to create a service culture throughout the organization. They began the process by benchmarking with nearby organizations known for their customer service, including Marriott Hotels and, astonishingly, the Massachusetts Registry of Motor Vehicles, which had recently gone through a transformation similar to the one the hospital was seeking. They also looked farther geographically to other service-driven hospitals, such as Baptist Hospital of Pensacola, Florida, which proclaims, "You'll Love the Way Baptist Cares for You." They began by gathering relevant data. They also initiated a telephone follow-up twenty-four to forty-eight hours after each patient was discharged. The caller asked about the patient's condition, checked that the patient understood any postdischarge instructions, and inquired about the service the patient received while in the hospital.

Hospital leaders focused on how to communicate appropriately by identifying the most important messages at each step of the hospital experience. They instituted a program called Key Words, Key Times. This effort helped the workforce to understand, for example, when it is most critical to show "compassion and empathy" and when to be "friendly and helpful." Particular focus was placed on teaching staff how to say that they are sorry and how to become more adept at the interpersonal aspects of service recovery—the process

Janice Johnson lives for the annual meetings of the regional nurse executives association. Over the past ten years she has worked her way up the ranks of the organization and earned the place of a respected old-timer. She enjoys the camaraderie at the meeting and the chance to share war stories. She always feels she can comfortably let go here, far from her public leadership role at Oppidania.

Her favorite part of the meeting is connecting with longtime friends, especially Patty Pinkerton. Janice and Patty go back as far as nursing school and have stayed in close touch ever since. Patty directs a nursing department in a large urban hospital about five hundred miles from Oppidania. In size and complexity it resembles Janice's shop. Janice has a tremendous respect, and sometimes a touch of jealousy, for Patty's professionalism and her inspired thinking. Patty is able to take risks, to try new ideas and then make them work. Janice has never left a discussion with Patty without some new insight or approach that was both innovative and practical. That combination is Patty's genius.

They both are eager to talk and, after the opening plenary session reception, they rendezvous in a corner of the hotel lobby bar. They relax in two comfortable chairs, each with a glass of wine. A bowl of nuts sits invitingly perched on the small table between them. They chat about family, their kids, vacations, and the work Patty has been doing on her house.

Patty eventually changes the topic. "So, what's happening at Oppidania, Janice? I was reading about the fight between the insurance companies online. Seems like quite a dustup." They've shared work stories for so long that Patty feels she knows the people at Oppidania, even though she has met only a few of them.

"What a train wreck!" Janice says. "We were already struggling a bit financially—who isn't these days—and then our biggest insurance company walks. It sent everyone into a panic. Just before I came here I was told I have to cut the nursing staff by 10 percent. Ten percent!" Janice stares down at her wine glass and pauses before looking back up at Patty. "I had to think twice before coming here, so you know that the picture is pretty rotten back home. I was afraid to leave."

Patty gives her friend's arm a gentle squeeze. "So what are you going to do?"

"What can I do? Try not to drink too many of these, I suppose," Janice says, raising her wine glass. "I either go along or quit. I'll have to go through each section and tell the supervisors how many people they have to let go. We'll have to prepare the separation packages. There are legal considerations in delivering this kind of news. It's not going to be pretty."

"Are you going to be delivering any pink slips yourself?"

Janice gives Patty a look of incredulity. "No, I think it's better for the department heads and supervisors to do that. I don't think a nursing VP should be running around the floors with an ax."

"That's not what I meant." Patty says gently. "I mean, are you going to be eliminating any administrative or supervisory positions?"

"No, I have to keep my infrastructure in place. It's going to be hard enough to keep the ship afloat with fewer people around. I'll need those people."

"*You'll* need those people, Janice. The question is whether those people are really needed."

"What do you mean?" There is a touch of annoyance in Janice's voice.

"I think sometimes we get stuck on keeping our own nest feathered, that's all. You know, there is another way to do this."

"What's that?" Janice is feeling both defensive and intrigued.

"I got a similar message from my CEO. Our situation was a bit different, though. Rather than losing an insurance contract, we got one. The problem was that it became a do-or-die situation. There was some pretty heavy-handed bargaining going on, and to make a long story short, we ended up with a steady stream of patients and a meager stream of money. I mean, we're talking bare bones. Our CEO made a convincing argument that in the long run this was a better solution than losing the contract and starving. I mean, at least we're alive. I was told we had to 'readjust' to a 12 percent cut in nursing staff."

"More patients with fewer nurses. Show me the logic in that," Janice says defiantly. "So what did you do?"

"I cut my administrative staff and pretty much left everybody else in place," Patty replies. "The other thing I did is look for people who were ready to retire or willing to think about it. I needed my young people who had the energy and passion to get the work done. I convinced enough people to move on that I was able to keep my youngest and most dynamic nurses."

"So you flattened the organization?"

"Exactly. I flattened and I invigorated. I have to admit, it shocked a lot of people. But once they came around, it made a lot of sense. The hospital has a great nursing reputation in the community, which I did not want to compromise. I had two meetings with each shift, so I personally saw just about every nurse in the hospital. I told them that our commitment to patient care and quality nursing would not be jeopardized. I talked with them about professional autonomy, and trust, and their doing their jobs. And I said that in the bigger picture, this approach would be better for us all. I thought this was the way we had to go."

"So you're suggesting that I trim my administrative people over my staff nurses? Who is going to do the administrative work?" Johnson is already mulling the options in her head, reformulating processes, and calculating a different approach to her cuts.

"Janice, you know I never make stock recommendations, and I would never tell you what to do—it's just too risky for a good friendship if it doesn't work. What I am saying, though, is that there are some options other than cutting across the board and, in particular, cutting your fresh graduates. You'll find a way to get the administrative work done, but without enough frontline nurses you can't maintain the quality and vitality of your patient care. Without that, the game's over. It's not a perfect solution, but it is a viable option."

"I can imagine two groups that wouldn't like this kind of proposal," Janice muses. "Obviously, my managers would go into shock. I think, though, that even the staff nurses would hate it. They count on an ever-present supervisory infrastructure as well."

"Janice, there is a good deal of talk at these conferences about professionalizing nursing. Well, if that's ever going to happen, nurses are going to have to get used to working a bit more independently. Today's nursing school graduates are better trained and more professionally ready to go. I think there are a lot of people out there who not only can handle a bit more independence—they thrive on it. If you look at the bigger picture—and over the long run—a cadre of professionals who can drive teamwork with hospitalists and others will give you a stronger department and a stronger hospital. And mind you, I am not talking about no supervisory staff, I am just suggesting a leaner one."

"But, Patty, your situation is a bit different than mine. You have too many patients with too little money. I have too few patients on top of too little money."

"Janice, bottom line, what I am suggesting is not about patients and money. It is about your thinking and strategy and priorities. And it is about letting the people in the hospital see how you work. All that I am saying is that this is crunch time. The pressure is high. Be clear about the choices you are making. The usual answers get you the usual results. Just try rethinking those old assumptions, that's all."

They stay talking in the lounge too late for both of them, calling it quits only when they remember the 7:30 A.M. leadership breakfast the next morning. Janice returns to her room and dozes off, wondering what she will do with Patty's inventive ideas.

through which goodwill toward the institution is restored after a patient has had an unsatisfactory experience.

When a visitor arrives at the hospital's main information desk, a person is behind the desk ready to help. Greeters waiting in front of the desk are prepared to walk patients to their destination if it involves a number of twists and turns through the complex of buildings. If a technician has a hard time locating a vein when drawing blood, she may offer a parking voucher as an apology for the inconvenience and discomfort experienced. The hospital has empowered people to help patients and has given them tools with which to work.

According to Jordan, the most important element is that everyone on the staff shares the same values and a commitment to the goals of the institution.

"Selection and retention of the right people is paramount," Jordan told us. Newton-Wellesley has a goal of having no more than 8 percent voluntary turnover each year. The hospital conducts follow-up interviews with new hires at 45 and 90 days of employment. At 180 days each new hire attends a lunch with the president of the hospital. Each of these interactions centers around the question, "Are we helping you succeed?"

Recognition and reward begin with some decidedly low-tech efforts. Managers are encouraged to recognize outstanding acts of service with thank-you notes. In 2009, more than 3,000 handwritten notes were sent to employees at their home addresses. This is a hospital where being nice has been embedded in the institutional culture. That culture is, however, not only about coddling. Senior managers track low performers and move them methodically through a performance improvement plan. Staff members who cannot embrace the service culture and meet its standards are removed from the system. They are fired. "We were able to elevate ourselves from the bottom half of hospitals ranked for patient satisfaction nationally to the top quartile," Jordan said. "Now we have a more ambitious goal: to be in the top 5 percent nationally. We will only get there if everyone is pulling together."

Managers in all of the patient-facing areas are engaged in service recovery. Each is required to call patients who have reported a poor service experience and to take appropriate action to remedy the problem. Each of these calls is reported publicly at a weekly meeting of all the managers. "When you start talking to patients and have to share what they said and what you did about it with your peers, you come to understand our values pretty quickly," said Jordan. "Just having this group, the Service Operations Committee, meeting weekly sends a message." All of this activity rolls up into a *leader scorecard* report, which provides a detailed accounting of service performance throughout the organization. "We live by it," declared Jordan.

Will Newton-Wellesley Hospital make it to the top 5 percent nationally? We will be able to watch how it is being measured on publicly reported hospital rankings, such as those published by *U.S. News & World Report*.

Efforts to Personalize Care

As we have suggested earlier, amid current and forthcoming changes in the work to be done, changes in the workforce itself, and evolving ways to organize and manage the people doing the work, many people may be concerned that the personal side of health and health care will be lost in the fray. Likewise, they may fear that those practicing in the system will cede control of the hours they devote to work and of their very careers. There certainly will be significant change and many who have invested their professional lives into health care will be disappointed. Nevertheless, with every change there is also opportunity. We offer here several examples for how you might rethink what you are doing and how you go about doing it. Although these examples are about primary care medicine and the work of physicians, we offer them in order to encourage creative thinking well beyond these illustrations and across the continuum of health care.

Not all work and workforce change is happening and will happen in large organizations. The majority of medical care is provided by generalist, family, and general internal medicine physicians (Reuben, 2007). Therefore changes in that segment of the workforce have the potential to produce the greatest impact of all. Not only will these changes affect primary care. They will also cascade through other parts of the system, accompanied by fresh opportunities for collaboration and potential for conflict. After all, the primary care doctor and nurse are not the same today as they were fifty or one hundred years ago, and there is no reason to believe that stasis has been established now.

There are powerful financial and quality motives for shifting as much care as possible to primary care settings. For one thing, they can be more cost efficient than specialist practices or hospital settings. The transition cannot happen, however, without fundamental change to the current primary care practice. We have noted that there is a shortage of primary care doctors that shows no signs of abating. It is difficult to attract those entering the medical field to embark on a career in primary care medicine because the hours are longer, the pace is faster, and the compensation and prestige are generally less than that accorded to specialists.

It has been said that this field is on "death row" (Reuben, 2007). Yet it has also been noted that "the better the primary care, the greater the cost savings, the better the health outcomes, and the greater the reduction in health and health care disparities" (Epstein, 2001; Rosenthal, 2008). The conflicts over the future course of primary care are among the most vexing facing the system. Looked at strictly from a large-scale business perspective, one could argue that the future of primary care is in being the quarterback: coordinating care delivered largely by others. Three physicians we spoke with looked at that equation and dared to imagine something even more different. They refused to believe it is impossible be an "old-fashioned" doctor in the twenty-first century.

The practices of these three physicians have a number of common features: (1) each is relationship based rather than production based in that their patient groups are smaller than those in the average U.S. practice; (2) visits are longer than average, and the doctor provides a relatively broader range of services with little or no support staff; (3) each has a business plan that demonstrates how it can be financially sustainable; and (4) each uses its variation on the general model to offer greater satisfaction to patients as well as to the physician's own personal and professional lives.

Pamela Wible practices in Eugene, Oregon. She opened her solo practice after feeling burnt out as a physician employee of a larger practice. "I was ready to quit medicine and go back to waiting tables just so that I could be nice to people," she told us. Instead of changing careers, Wible convened a series of community meetings and asked her potential patients to help her design the ideal medical practice. They gave her almost one hundred pages of ideas, and she incorporated many of them into her "ideal clinic" (www.idealmedicalcare.org).

Community members told her that they felt rushed in a short visit and found the interactions with multiple people in a medical office disruptive. Wible decided that she could do everything herself—from blood pressure to billing—and does not employ a staff. She feels that this both lowers costs and enhances her availability for her patients. Rather than the typical fifteen-minute visit, she schedules visits ranging from thirty to sixty minutes—time that is uninterrupted as she and the patient are the only ones present. Her office resembles a living room more than a clinic. She refers to it as a "sacred space." "I don't know why it is perceived as radical to allow patients into the design process, but it is," she said. "We need to find ways to empower patients to tell us what they seek. When you do, your patients think you've been sent from Heaven."

Wible has chosen to work part time (although she is available to her patients 24/7 through her cellular and home telephones) and sees just over four hundred patients through her practice. She accepts insurance but notes that she treats patients across the income and insurance spectrum. She said that her income was comparable to that of a physician working in a more traditional practice, though financial rewards are not her primary motive.

Across the country, physician Richard Donahue, is embarking on a similar ambition. Donahue spent ten years as the only year-round physician on the remote island of Vinalhaven, Maine, before moving to Boston to pursue a master's degree in public health at the Harvard School of Public Health. He then practiced in one of the Boston area's university health systems. When we interviewed him, he was on the verge of launching a new practice, Personal Health MD (http://personalhealthmd.com).

On the island, "I had a large role in a small-town system," he explained. "I wore lots of hats: emergency care provider, end-of-life hospice caregiver, school doctor, and town health officer. I delivered a large slice of the health care pie for a decade to this population of about 1,200 people." Now working in an urban setting, he sees great differences in the patient culture. Primary care on an island is about providing comprehensive care. In the city it is quite different. It is more about providing referrals to specialists.

"My patients on Vinalhaven often said to me, 'Doc, you treat me or I'm going to live with it,' because getting to a specialist required a ferry ride and a drive on the mainland. It required a major commitment, and so my patients would much rather have me try to take care of whatever condition they presented rather than go to a specialist. High patient expectations honed my clinical skills, allowing me to meet a higher proportion of their health care needs. There was also a premium on having excellent clinical outcomes in this highly accountable small-town setting. On the other hand, the urban patient simply expects to be sent to a specialist and views the primary care doctor as a gatekeeper."

Donahue hopes to bring "island-style care" to the city in his new Personal Health MD practice. Even though fully admitting to being somewhat biased by what he recalls as the "perfect" primary care setting in Maine, he sees many benefits in transferring the model to other venues. "When you have enough time to negotiate a relationship and build a rapport with a patient, you get to know them better which can lead to earlier and more accurate diagnoses with fewer tests. The result is better patient care at a lower cost to the system. It's also easier to help a patient you know well stay well." This is a sentiment echoed by Pamela Wible, who also finds that she orders fewer tests and has less need to refer patients to specialists when she knows them well and has time to speak with them in depth. Donahue believes that a physician is more likely to use technology and tests when he or she thinks this is a one-time interaction with the patient, as is the case with many specialists. "I learned to perform careful physical exams because I had to," he said. "If I was wrong, everyone on the island would know it."

Donahue also sees important implications for his skills as a physician. When the primary care doctor is challenged to provide more care, he hones a greater range of skills and his job becomes more engaging. The specialists, in turn, are called upon to handle difficult cases and not the easy bread-and-butter procedures that are commonly referred to them in an urban system. The result is that all are more likely to be the best doctors they can be.

Donahue was still tinkering with the business model for his practice when we spoke with him. He wants to use a concierge model, where there is a membership fee to be part of the patient base plus a fee for service, but eschews the elitism that name implies. "I want to be able to serve an entire community," he said. "I want to be able to serve patients at all income levels."

The third doctor we spoke with is Gordon Moore, of Rochester, New York. (You can read more about his practice in Chapter Twelve.) Moore's work model was driven by cost factors: when he looked at what it would cost to set up a traditional private practice—with an office, waiting room, exam rooms, receptionist, billing clerks, nursing support, and the rest—he realized that he simply could never see himself having enough capital to make it work. He decided to investigate how much of that cost he could eliminate and still have a viable medical practice. He found that he could strip away quite a bit. He, like Pamela Wible, decided to practice on his own without a staff. He sublet an exam room in a larger practice that doubled as his office. He met his patients when they arrived and billed for his services when they left. Moore found that despite having these additional duties, he was able to spend more time with his patients and could practice the kind of medicine that was satisfying to him and his patients: focused, unrushed, and centered on making and keeping people well.

His practice grew to about four hundred patients. He added a nurse to the staff, as he was often teaching, along with more physical space (though at less than four hundred total square feet, the physical plant could hardly be considered excessively spacious). He reports that the practice was financially sustainable. He closed the office in 2008 to assume a new role helping other solo and small practices embrace technological tools that would cut costs and free up time. He felt that enabling others to discover what he had found was the most significant impact he could have on the quality of the health care experience for primary care physicians and their patients.

These three examples hardly constitute a tidal wave of change in the system. Nevertheless, they do illustrate what is possible when you think creatively about how to make your work more satisfying, for both you and your patients. And these cases also demonstrate what can happen when you refuse to believe that work must be accomplished in a way that many consider unsustainable for both the caregivers and those receiving care.

One could argue that these "renegades" of primary care are more aberration than model, given projections that there will be more patients and fewer doctors. Perhaps so, though we offer them here more as a model of innovation than as a panacea. If the problem were reframed less as a shortage of primary care doctors and more as question of how to attract physicians to primary care, such models and their variants could gain considerable currency. If such work were rewarding, satisfying, and a contribution to quality of care, the problem of shortages could be mitigated. The individuals profiled here demonstrate what bottom-up innovation and solution building might yield. They have renegotiated their roles in the health care system.

Conclusion

The conflicts over the changing workforce are being fought on predictable fields of battle. On one side are the clinical innovators, technological pioneers, entrepreneurs, and yes, opportunists who are responding to market, political, and technological forces that are changing health and health care in ways that were barely imaginable just a few years ago. On the other side are the traditionalists, clinical experts, professional leaders, and patients who want to hold onto the values, principles, and personal relationships that have been the foundation of the health system for years. It would be simplistic and unhelpful to merely see one set of characters as the "dark side" and the other as the "force for good." Some of the ongoing evolutionary changes are good, some are not, and many opportunities lie in between. And there you stand in the middle of this field, perhaps puzzled as you hope to maintain a steady career and professional trajectory when so much is changing and so much is uncertain. What will distinguish those who succeed in this arena from those who do not?

There are solutions to these workforce dilemmas. Those individuals and those organizations who assertively and confidently seek those solutions will find many opportunities for both success and satisfaction, though each will be measured in terms different from before. There are ways to discover professional fulfillment and financial reward as the health enterprise changes and builds to serve an expanding population with new tools and technologies to help.

There are also many problems in addressing these workforce dilemmas. Among the most difficult of the quandaries is discerning between what is valuable in past practices and should be kept and what must be discarded. Organizational and individual principles, quality of care, respect for patients, baseline financial imperatives, and standards of evidence-based practice will in varying ways persist as the health system evolves. Timeworn professional practices, hierarchical status, and organizational relationships will likely evaporate into the past. Their demise will be painful as adherents cling to tradition, become protective of their professional turf, and draw hard lines for holding their fort.

Progressive change in the makeup of the health care workforce will be replete with conflict and complex negotiation. There will be those with a satisfying health career and those left by the wayside. What will you strategically do to be on the better side of that dividing line?

First, be able to distinguish what is worthy and reasonable to hold onto from what is not. Protect values. Be cautious when it comes to clutching your turf. Significant differences can exist within each professional group, and those conflicts may be more intense than conflicts between professional groups. In defending the history, record, and accomplishments of the past, traditionalists may fail to distinguish what is truly valuable from what is less so, just as they may well confound the legitimate self-interests of a profession with selfish interests. Conversely innovators will promote the opportunities for getting ahead of the change curve and, in their zeal, may be too eager to abandon fundamental practices and ways of being that remain important.

Second, be open, honest, and transparent in your negotiations and expect the same from others. These conflicts will not manifest as didactic academic debates. They will be about people, jobs, salaries, and status—all topics that engender self-protective instincts and, with them, emotional basement behaviors. One side may want to cover or sweeten the bad news, and the other may want to exaggerate the consequences. Leaders and negotiators at all levels set precedent with every conversation. Integrity and confidence provide constructive currency for the difficult decisions and actions that are ahead, in both the short and the long run. Remember that evolution advances as a series of steps, and each move leads to the next.

Third, be flexible in what you do and how you go about doing it. Many signposts point to what lies ahead, and the more current you are with them, the less likely you are as an organization or an individual to head down the wrong path. If you make a mistake, find ways to recover and be resilient. There are investments that will lure you with their promise: some could reap value and others could prove to be costly mistakes. New technologies, training opportunities, strategic alliances, and organizational change represent just a few of these investment opportunities. Remember the old ice hockey adage: don't skate to where the puck is, aim for where it is going to be.

Fourth, anticipate the conflict along the way and be prepared to effectively negotiate. This conflict can be managed and resolved. If this is done so that you derive buy-in and greater support for what you hope to accomplish, that resolved conflict and the deals it reaps will become important assets as you advance yourself and your organization. Conflicts can also become significant distractions. They can drain out your energy and attention, seeming to be the problem when they are in fact only a manifestation of a larger and more significant phenomenon, one that will not be resolved no matter who wins the internal organizational or professional war. You will have many opportunities to rehearse and practice the Walk in the Woods.

Finally, there are many opportunities for meta-leadership in this fray. Seek them. You could find yourself leading and doing things you had never imagined. There will be a premium on leadership that shows the way, integrates a broad base of involvement, and thereby builds solutions others could not see. Therein may lie your most exciting opportunities.

PART
FIVE

SHAPING PURPOSE

CHAPTER 15

CRAFTING THE ESSENTIALS

HEALTH AND the health care system are in the midst of a massive reinvention. What you do and how you go about doing it are being redefined by political reform, economics, business imperatives, technology, know-how, demographics, history, the future, and the very people who are now part of the system: yes, an extraordinarily complex mix of factors. These are moments of great possibility and significant challenge—a time begging for meta-leadership. If history is the best instructor for the future, we can reflect on notable past changes, celebrating the important advances and lamenting the shortcomings represented by particular actions that shaped the evolution of the health enterprise. Each step in that evolution was marked by both conflict and robust negotiation. The same is true for what lies ahead.

As noted in the discussion of the Walk in the Woods (Chapter Seven), your most essential tool in any negotiation is a compelling set of questions. What are you trying to accomplish? What are the trends in the field that will affect your work? Are your efforts and investments compatible with those trends? What might you do to influence those factors? Do your actions and decisions enhance your objectives? Do the answers to these questions fit one another? Do your results and outcomes resonate with what it is you are trying to accomplish? If not, why not?

Generating compatibility among the extensive cast of characters affected by these forces of change is a vital and compelling undertaking. The presence or absence of compatibility is reflected by the intersecting pieces of the puzzle that constitute our health system. The better-tuned the fit, the more closely aligned will be our shared objectives and our capacity to achieve them. When purpose and action mesh, we optimize our aggregate capacity. That is what effective collaboration is all about (see Susskind & Cruikshank, 1987; Carpenter & Kennedy, 1988; Gray, 1989).

Wanting to keep the Tuesday morning kitchen cabinet meetings truly ad hoc, Iris Inkwater realized that the group would have to be suspended before it became deeply rooted in the participants' calendars. As the fifth meeting concluded, she had thanked each participant and handed out small gifts in appreciation of their time and thinking.

However, she didn't want to let go of this "think time," so she reserved this, the next Tuesday morning time slot, for another private session for herself. She perches alone on the couch in her office, with her green book, pen, and trusty mug of coffee.

What is the essence of what she needs right now? She is looking for just the right word to jot on the top of her page. "*Smarts*?" she thinks. "Too obvious and doesn't say enough. *Money*? Wouldn't that be nice? That would only bandage and not solve the problems. *Focus*? Maybe, though there's plenty of that to go around these days. It fosters the bunker mentality and wouldn't really add value. What could it be?" She continues thinking.

"*Curiosity*! Yes, curiosity. Questions. Wondering. Asking. Probing. Exploring. Experimenting. Yes, that fits. You can lead with curiosity. Challenge. Inquire. Inspire. Imagine. It works."

"OK, that was the easy part. How best to do *curious*? There are so many unknowns. The political process is such an unsatisfying method for changing and improving the health system. What emerges out of the push and pull is more a map of which lobbying group has the most money and influence than it is a guide to how to foster a healthier population. The market too produces odd outcomes, again, more a reflection of what money and opportunity motivate than the most efficient way to take care of people. Put the lobbyists together with the opportunists and, wow, can we waste a lot of money in this country. And my job is to run a hospital under these conditions? What am I, nuts?"

"Is it really possible to make a go of it? The obvious answer is yes, as in, I am in this to keep my job, aren't I? And I do want this institution to play a positive role in this community. Maybe it's not possible to make a go of it in our current form. Maybe we need to let the mission drive the structure. So what form do we take? What does health care look like if we are really curious about what it could become? What if we started all over? What would we be?"

"What will be different? Computers and machines are getting smarter, faster, and cheaper. It's won't be long before they become better than us humans. Aren't they already in so many ways? What does that mean? How do we humans let go of what can be surrendered? How do we figure out what can't—and then how do we hold onto it?"

"And patients. We will find cures for the diseases that now kill people before they reach a ripe old age. Will there be new diseases and ailments that wouldn't have emerged had people died younger? How will we care for and treat an aging population? Maybe we need to rethink the way we build and organize health services. Are there completely new ways of doing this that we haven't discovered because we want to sustain our old models? People will want to age successfully through the different stages of their lives? How do we help them do it?"

"What if I lead with questions? I could encourage and motivate people to really use their imaginations. Wouldn't that be fun? I would cultivate new and bold thinking. We could uncover problems and explore solutions that we would never otherwise find. We could be a leader as an institution and a groundbreaker as a community. That would make this job endlessly exciting, encouraging people to wonder and, most important, helping them to discover."

"So how do I catalyze curiosity into the people around here? What does it mean to encourage curiosity? The Tuesday group, what about them? Fred: OK, he's old school yet he's got rock solid values and principles. And he is more open to new ideas than he would ever admit. How do I keep him current and hold onto those values and principles that we have to preserve? Janice: nursing can be so much more. Can I prod her to think widely and encourage her to persuade her nurses to be more and do more, and even do it differently? Larry: that fellow's got leadership promise. How do I help him grow? He has great potential to help lead this place toward imaginative understandings and possibilities. Perry: he could use a hearty dose of curiosity. He jumps to conclusions too quickly. Hard to be curious when you are so attached to the basement. He is smart though. Combine his smarts with a greater openness and willingness to question, learn, and discover new opportunities? Yes, that's possible. Rajeev: that guy gets what's going on, though only in the most tangible ways possible. His common sense attached to a thirst for wonder and exploration? He could help us find pragmatic solutions linked to new opportunities. We could make things work that others couldn't even imagine. Arlan: that guy really cares about this place. Heart of gold. He is very good for our curiosity. Given that health care seems to be behind every other industry in changing, incorporating technology, and being more customer oriented, it's lucky that Arlan is a fount of knowledge about the mistakes and successes of other sectors. He has been a great spark for curiosity around here. Not always focused in the right direction, though curiosity doesn't have to be. Sometimes a bit of wandering for the brain is a good thing. Having him around is good for us."

The time has flown. Several pages of the green book are filled with notes. The coffee cup is long empty. Iris feels energized. "OK, *curiosity*. It's got legs. I'll buy that. More important, I can sell that."

The challenge facing us in these moments of reinvention is that for a long time, our health system has been out of balance. What we have been doing—our purpose—has not been clear. How we have gone about doing it—the process—has not been working as well as it could. And people in general have had only mixed satisfaction with the outcomes we achieve. On the whole, society is clear that it is unhappy with what the health system costs. The priorities have not been right. And even though we are able to dazzle with new technologies and capabilities, the population's overall health status and statistics do not reflect well upon what the U.S. health system has been able to accomplish.

The problem is that the very people responsible for fixing the balance are the same people who will benefit or lose by the necessary adjustments. That is why the imbalance has for so long been both tolerated and unyielding. Things, however, are changing. Why? In part, it is because efforts to provide universal access to insurance present new imperatives and opportunities. It has become generally accepted that those who create and offer a well-aligned response to these changes are most likely to advance in the emerging health care environment. The people who pay for, receive, monitor, and regulate health care—the *market*—are demanding changes. There are tangible choices and clear consequences.

Amid this emerging new balance, the negotiation and conflict resolution method presented here offers you a vital toolbox: a reservoir of skills, techniques, and behaviors. Meta-leadership practice offers you and others an inspiring perspective on what you can leverage, link, and achieve. Your task is to contribute to this process of defining and refining the balance. In so doing, you foster fundamental understanding, cultivate pragmatic concurrence, and generate the necessary collaboration to make the system work. You understand others better. You are able to help them better understand you. And you are able to engage your colleagues and others in a manner that is mutually constructive and beneficial.

Meta-leadership, negotiation, and conflict resolution are, however, only methods if practiced without purpose. Like the adept aircraft pilot, you may be able to fly the plane; however, if you don't know where you are going, chances are you are not going to get there. Or even worse, you might take the passengers to a destination where they don't want to be. The human and financial stakes are too high in health care to tolerate mindless wandering.

Some might presume that this process of grappling with purpose is merely the domain of legislative policymakers, corporate leaders, and major purchasers of health services. This is not so in health care. Because of the close interpersonal nature of health care work, this theme is implicitly manifest in every interaction between coworkers, patients, providers, and the many organizations and departments whose work must be orchestrated. Defining purpose is an interactive process that spans all levels, from you as an individual to the web of countless individuals who constitute the system. It must be done—in keeping with the organizational dimensions of meta-leadership practice—up, down, and across the enterprise.

How do you understand and align all the varied perspectives, types of expertise, and values? How do you synthesize motives, incentives, and actions? How do you promote better health and better health care?

What You Do

The work of health care, and therefore negotiation about it, embodies circumstances, choices, decisions and actions, and consequences.

Circumstances blend the needs of patients and populations, the considerations of professionals and policymakers, and the possibilities and the side-effects of science and technology—along with the ambiguous mystery of just what wellness and illness are. It is this changing context in which you and your organization practice: the macrocosm never remains the same. Emerging discoveries, new diseases, innovative treatments, changing political winds, and redefined business calculations shape the shifting domains of your work.

Though health care rests on the work of science, its everyday endeavors dwell in the realm of the human. It is from this intersection that your range of *choices* emanates. Those choices derive not only from what is factual. Perception, preference, and philosophy, too, infuse what is acceptable to one person and what is reprehensible to another: a surgical or nonsurgical treatment; the purchase of equipment or the provision of vaccines; the appropriateness of a physician or the substitution of a physician's assistant? As long as you respect that right to exercise choice, a range of expectations will always be with you. That range of choices must be assessed, weighed, balanced, and counterbalanced until the parties are ready to decide. It is a field rife with conflict and searching for compelling negotiation.

Decisions and *actions* are the substance of what health care does and does not do. They are the programs you implement, the people you hire, the treatments you administer, the administrative moves you make, and the human attentiveness you render. It is that to which you commit and for which you are responsible and accountable. What you do is a measure of your compassion, tenacity, values, and vision.

Consequences are what you produce. Because you work in the most vital and intimate of human endeavors, that achievement is measured both for each individual patient and for society as a whole. Your challenge is to correctly balance the needs of each individual, whether patient or staff member, with the needs of the whole, whether professional group, organization, or populace. If you have successfully treated the few at the expense of the many, have you accomplished your purpose? And yet if you abandon the few in favor of the

In addition to functioning as Oppidania Medical Center's medical director, Fred Fisher maintains an active practice that occupies about half of his busy schedule. He sees outpatients through the Oppidania Medical Clinic, located in the doctors' office building adjacent to the hospital. Although the shifts in reimbursement, the rise of capitated care systems, and the efficiencies offered by the clinic administration have changed the circumstances of his practice, the gentle attention he gives to his patients and rapport he maintains with them has never altered.

He is on his way to a meeting in a private function room at a nearby Chinese restaurant frequented by the medical staff. The clinic's internal medicine physicians are gathering once again to discuss a reorganization of their practice; it seems to be a never-ending topic. Fisher's agenda for the meeting is the same one he has brought to every meeting in this series: he doesn't want anything imposed that will interfere with the care he gives his patients. He does not want to change his relationship with those patients, his colleagues, or his support staff.

The announced purpose of the meeting is to discuss the next step in the transition of the clinic away from a fee-for-service arrangement to the new array of payment methods, including blended capitation rates, episode-of-care payments, medical home models, global budgets, and pay-for-performance programs. As Fisher understands the distinctions from his reading of medical newsletters, this means that the group will be going from charging for services rendered to receiving a set fee for a covered *life*. "That's an odd term," he thinks. The less expensively and more effectively they are able to serve that life, the better off the organization will be financially. It all seems perverse to him.

Fisher takes a seat at the long table next to his old friend Dr. Ralph Rollins. This friendship began during their undergraduate days. They were together through medical school and their residencies and now at Oppidania. Rollins is one of the few friends with whom Fisher is able to show his boyhood sense of mischief. He turns to Rollins and whispers, "You know, Ralph, they are trying to turn us into an insurance company." He hesitates for dramatic effect and then adds, "Resist at any cost." Rollins considers the premise for a moment, then a smile breaks over his face as he goes into his trademark low-decibel laugh.

Rollins and Fisher practice the same kind of medicine, though Rollins tends to be much more low-key in his leadership and public activities. It is in keeping with their different styles that Fisher is in a high-profile position while Rollins is primarily in the clinic seeing patients. It is also typical that Rollins is more willing to accept change than Fisher is. In spite of their differences, Fisher depends on Rollins to give him an eye on what is happening within the medical staff.

"So our livelihoods are being turned upside down. What do you think of this wild new world?" In Fisher's usual style, he asks a question and, not waiting for the answer, gives his own opinion right away. "I think this whole idea of doctors assuming risk is a lousy idea. It changes the fiduciary relationship with the hospital and makes us out to be competitors in our clinical relationship with them and other physicians. I think it's a mistake."

Rollins is neither surprised by Fisher's attitude nor his compulsion to preach more than he listens. "It does change the fiduciary relationship, Fred, though it doesn't necessarily turn us into competitors. You can look at it another way, too." Rollins knows Fisher is ready to argue, even though he is listening closely. "We do in fact have a clear business relationship with the hospital. This arrangement merely brings it aboveboard, makes it explicit, and creates a different set of incentives. I wouldn't order this recipe if I had more of a choice, though in the long run I don't think it's as bad as everyone fears. And anyway, it's not a one-way street. We negotiate with them, and they negotiate with us. It's more balanced than you probably imagine."

"Oh, come on, Ralph," Fisher retorts, "that's a pile of you know what. What are we going to do, take our business elsewhere? Or what is the hospital going to do, stop admitting our patients? This is just giving work to a bunch of accountants and lawyers at our expense. Nothing is going to change, except our overhead costs."

Overhearing their conversation, Laura Lane, one of the younger members of the practice, decides to jump in. "Fred," she opens, "I am not going to defend the shift to these fancy reimbursement models. It's a product of too much of Washington meddling in our work. However, I am also not going to resist it, because to do so would be lunacy. It's simply the way things are happening now, and we either go along or—you're right, Fred—the hospital could take its business elsewhere. Not explicitly, because we wouldn't let them get away with that. But they could do it more subtly. Patients would just stop coming through our offices because insurance companies wouldn't send them our way. And the hospital would open up sources of care elsewhere, and we would wind up out of the loop. Look, Fred, the hospital hasn't coddled doctors for all these years because the administrators like us. It's because we send the hospital our patients, and that means dollars for the institution. The reason for looking at this new system is that it will ensure that we have patients. And it will ensure that we treat them well. That is our leverage with the hospital, and that is our lifeblood. It's the same thing as it used to be; it's just different."

Fisher looks at Lane as if she has said something that doesn't make sense. "Laura," he says, "I've been at this a few more years than you and here's what the difference is: It used to be that we were paid for providing a service. That is what we do, what we were trained to do. Now we make money for not providing a service. We're like those farmers who get money for not growing corn. Except this is not corn, it's medical care, and when we don't provide that service, it's not only wrong, it's dangerous. One of our patients gets sick and he can haul us into court. And you know where the insurance companies are going to be then?

Running for cover. Don't you see, Laura? Ralph? We hold both the financial risk *and* the legal liability. The insurance companies have manipulated medicine into a corner, and here we sit, eating Chinese food and going along."

"Fred, what's our job?" Rollins asks. "Keeping people well, right? You have confidence we can do that, right?" Fisher nods, though reluctantly, because he suspects he might be nodding about something with which he will ultimately disagree. "So that's what we are being paid to do—keep people well. And if we do a good job, we deserve the rewards. And if not, it's not doomsday, it's just not the cash cow we have become used to. You know it yourself, Fred; all our financial incentives were for ordering tests, doing surgery, making referrals. The more we did, the better off we all were. Yes, much of what we did was justifiable. Though you know yourself that many of the tests were ordered routinely without considering the cost or benefit. Now we must consider that cost-benefit balance. And to the extent that insurers are willing to pay more for better performance, well, that puts the incentives in the right place."

"Ralph, you are sounding like an ad for an insurance company," Fisher says disdainfully.

This annoys Rollins. It is tantamount to being called a traitor. "Fred, you are sounding like you were born yesterday. What's the alternative? This is the marketplace, Dr. Fisher"—Rollins is hoping to invoke his colleague's reservoir of professional common sense—"and you either play or call it quits. The medical groups that are going to survive are the ones who learn how to play the game. And those who are ahead of the game are going to thrive."

Fisher makes a grunt of acknowledgment and asks Rollins to pass the dim sum.

The waiters are clearing the plates and placing plastic-wrapped fortune cookies on the soiled tablecloth when Tim Thatcher rises to address the group. Thatcher has been the clinic's administrator for three years. A relatively young MBA, he has won the confidence of the medical staff by increasing efficiency while keeping the clinical practice intact. The management of the group had been pretty sloppy before Thatcher arrived, and he is well liked by the physicians.

Just as he is about to begin, Dr. Gloria Green, president of the clinic's internal medicine group, puts her hand on his arm in a delaying gesture. "Just a minute, everybody," she says, breaking into the many discussions around the table. "Before Tim starts up, I just want everyone to know that Tim and I have spoken about this issue of a new business model, and I am pleased with the work he has done to put together this proposal. He has a good deal of material for us to think about, so I hope you will listen carefully."

Thatcher listens with a sense of relief to Dr. Green's unplanned speech. He understands that she has realized that if this meeting turns into a doctor versus administrator contest, it will be counterproductive. By endorsing the proposal up front, she has discouraged divisive scoffing and pointed her colleagues toward serious consideration of some very complex issues.

Thatcher very briefly reviews what everyone already knows about changing reimbursement patterns and what it means for medical practices like theirs. He explains that in the current market, whether you are an insurer, hospital, or physician, you do what you need to do to ensure a steady supply of patients. The competition for patients is fierce, and they no longer come as individuals, they come in herds. The change is cost driven, and Thatcher emphasizes that this same factor affects everyone, though the implications are different for each. Patients and their employers want reasonably priced health care, and they recognize that they may have to sacrifice some, though not all, choice in order to get it. Given the high numbers involved, patients are likely to be more loyal to their pocketbooks than to their physicians. Insurers, Thatcher explains, are also under a great deal of financial pressure from their shareholders. They have to control the price of a service over which they have little direct control. They are essentially intermediaries, with expensive providers on one side and frugal buyers on the other. He explains that the rift between the Oppidania Medical Center and Community Health Plan is typical of what's going on around the country. And it is yet too early to tell how that jolt will be resolved.

Thatcher stops to catch his breath, and then continues, "And here we sit in the middle of all this." A faint smile forms on his face, revealing the anxiety he feels about this meeting. He goes on to explain that nothing is sacred in this new system. Tradition is neither reason nor excuse. After much investigation, he is recommending that the group reorganize to better fit into this changing market, negotiating competitive fees with a number of insurers to cover as many lives as possible. The future viability and size of the practice will depend on the number of patients it will be able to enroll and the overall good health of that group.

Thatcher has prepared as best he can for the question-and-answer period, but he is still dreading it.

The first question is one he had hoped would come later, after people started getting used to the idea. "What about our relationship with the specialists to whom we refer in the hospital? Who pays for that? And we are attached to OMC. What happens if we are forced to refer to Urbania by the insurance companies? That wouldn't be good."

Thatcher opens the explanation slowly. "That's perhaps the biggest change for you in your practice. Now when you make a referral, the patient's insurance company pays your bill as well as that of, let's say, the cardiologist. In this reconfigured system you get one lump sum to care for all the needs of your patient. Essentially, if you must make a referral to a cardiologist, then you pay for it. So, the more you are able to handle on your own, and the less you use referrals—or the smarter you are in shopping for them, the better off all of us will be financially. And we may have to put Urbania and its specialists more into our strategic mix."

Someone pipes up from the back of the room, "This is like a game of Russian roulette with all the chambers loaded. If we refer, we lose our money. And if we don't, and the patient has a heart attack, we lose our practice. If I were an insurance agent, it would make perfect sense to me." Subdued caustic laughter murmurs through the room.

Rollins comes to Thatcher's aid. He relishes the role of sage and plays it well. "Look, it makes no sense to put Tim on the hot seat for this. He didn't invent the system. You're right; it puts us at some disadvantage. And I think after we are done venting some steam, we have to understand this new reality. I don't think the question is whether or not we do it; the question is how to make the most of it." Rollins's remarks silence the room.

Thatcher picks up where he had left off. "There are two sides to this negotiation. We agree to a price with the insurers, and we budget accordingly. Then we go to the hospital and the specialty groups. We want to get as good a price as we can from them. If one of the cardiologist groups gives the same level of quality of care and a better price than the others, it's in our best interest to send business their way. Even more important, we'll want to send patients to specialists that get us the *most* for our money: good efficient care that is responsive to our continued involvement with the patient. The specialists need to be working with us, not wandering off in their own isolated world. If they are not with us, we don't send them patients, and soon enough the word gets out. We get a good level of service for our patients or we walk. We have some leverage in this system as well."

Gloria Green quickly asks the question that she knows is on everyone's mind. "What about the financials, Tim? How might the books look after this?" Green knows the answer but wants to give Thatcher the chance to tell it to the group before too much dissent surfaces.

"Financially we could do as well if not even better than where we are now," Thatcher announces. "Our advantage is that we will have control. We decide where the patient goes, who they see, and ultimately what it costs. Though we do carry some risk, it's like any financial deal. The rewards go to whoever takes the risk and manages it well. We could even be talking *lucrative*. It's just a matter of playing the game right."

Will Wainwright raises his hand. Dr. Wainwright typifies the aggressive, forty-year-old primary care physician who is working hard to establish a practice in spite of all the challenges imposed by the system. His practice is not nearly as solid as he had expected it would be at this point in his career. "I recommend we go forward with Tim's proposal as fast as we can," he declares. "A week doesn't go by without our hearing of some new merger, alliance, or consolidation. I say that every day we wait, we fall further and further behind. The fact is, if someone comes along and provides more cost-effective care, we could lose everything we have worked so hard to build. It wouldn't crack in one day. It would just fade away, and before we realized what had hit us, it would all be gone. And all the lamenting in the world wouldn't bring it back. Personally, I'm not interested in being around to turn off the lights on this group. I say we move fast.'' Wainwright's comments turn the mood in the room.

The discussion period continues for another forty-five minutes. As the meeting draws to a close, Thatcher hands out some stapled sheets showing current and projected financials for the practice, arranged in three columns: best case, worst case, and reasonable case. Thatcher explains that the group's strategy will determine the column in which they'll all end up.

''We have a lot of work to do, and we can't control the vagaries of the market,'' Thatcher concludes. ''But I think we can position ourselves for the best possible chance of success.''

After the meeting, Fisher and Rollins stand together in a corner of the coatroom, getting ready to venture out into the evening chill. Fisher laments, ''You know, Ralph, the biggest buildings in this town belong to the insurance companies. In this litigious, risk-averse society, our greatest architectural temples are built in their honor. That is their business—collecting lots of money, assuming risk, and paying out when there is a claim. I just think it's wrong for doctors to start taking over their function. It changes the texture of medical practice, and don't tell me it's for the better.''

''Fred, when you started off in your practice, weren't you concerned about cost?''

''Sure. It was different then. A good number of my patients were paying out of pocket, and I had to be sure that I kept their costs in line. It was just a part of what I did.''

''Well, Fred, think of it in those terms. You will still be providing the best medical care you can. You are just doing it with half an eye on the pocketbook. And just to make sure you don't forget, this time it's every patient's pocketbook, as well as your own.''

With that, each sent regards to the other's family, and they set off on their separate ways.

many, have you justly allocated your capacity for producing well-being? Have you used your know-how and resources to best achieve healthy people and a healthy society?

Circumstances, choices, decisions and actions, and consequences hang in a fluctuating balance. They each shift and then shift one another. When circumstances change, so too does the range of choices available to those charged with reaching decisions: when patterns of service reimbursement are adjusted, for example, so too must the inventory of service options be altered to ensure a workable flow of patients. If certain outcomes are no longer deemed acceptable, then choices must be reassessed to chart a course that reaches the desired objectives: thus mortality rates outside the range of acceptable for a treatment protocol, for a particular provider, or for an entire institution are a sentinel for corrective action. As these factors resonate with one another, you contemplate whether to be proactive or just reactive in formulating choices and decisions or in shaping outside circumstances and consequences.

What are the unique dynamics that influence these four factors in health care? How do you ensure that you are calculating correctly? What are the checks and balances that guarantee you do not swing too far in one direction or another? How do you appraise whether "what you do" is judicious?

The Essential and the Expendable

Health care occupies the domain of the *essential*. The essential frames how you align your priorities, assess your progress, and plot your game plan. For example, from the purview of orthopedists, it is essential that the orthopedic surgical suite have the optimum air filtration system, *or else* patients' prostheses are likely to become infected. From the standpoint of public health advocates, it is essential that lead be removed from the homes of young children, *or else* they risk neurological dysfunction and severe developmental impediments. In the opinion of leaders of nurses, it is essential that nurse-to-patient ratios be maintained, *or else* patient care will be compromised.

We live in a society that places considerable value on life and the quality of that life: virtue demands that people do what is necessary to enhance survival. We also live in a society with the technical capability to significantly extend and enrich life. Even death in this technological world has been transformed from a natural event to a conscious and calculated choice. And we live in a society that expects perfection. When that perfection is not achieved, those responsible live in apprehension of the retribution and legal actions likely to follow.

Because of these values, capabilities, and expectations, much of your work in health care is categorized as essential. The risks of overlooking a serious medical condition can be so ominous that you are careful not to be indifferent about anything for which you are responsible. Ensuring your professional or organizational survival dictates that diagnostic tests, medical procedures, safety precautions, and legal protections be transformed into the essential. Given the circumstances, choices, and consequences, prostate cancer screening, tobacco cessation initiatives, and infection control protocols all arguably are—or certainly could be—placed in the category of essential. Your decisions are framed foremost by the compulsion to promote and preserve life.

The converse side of essentialness is expendability. If you are not essential to the system, as a provider, administrator, or patient, then you can be expended in the rush to efficiency. The community outreach program can be closed if it is expendable. The nurse can be fired if she is extraneous. The evening clinic can be curtailed because it is unnecessary. Programs, services, and people's positions can be discarded when they are no longer deemed essential. This distinction will become increasingly important as health reform matures and pressures to control costs mean that affordability will be a factor in determining what is essential, what is expendable, and what is not.

The questions of who and what are essential or expendable will be the subtext of significant conflict and abundant negotiation. For example, people interested in cost will start with one set of imperatives and those delivering clinical care will start with another. Either consensus will be built or a struggle for dominance will erupt as all the involved parties advocate for their own definitions of essential and expendable.

There is nothing more professionally disenfranchising than being told you are expendable. The message can come in a number of shapes: the pink slip informing you of your dismissal, the subpoena announcing an impending lawsuit; the memorandum advising you and your department that the department is being closed, the letter from the insurance company informing you that reimbursement rates for your services have been cut to a near impossible amount, or the fact that your job is now being carried out electronically by a computer that is faster and more accurate, though less personable. To be informed of your expendability is to be told that you no longer belong and that your services are no longer necessary. Your past training and preparation seem meaningless, and your professional future is in doubt.

Just the peril of expendability strikes a chord of vulnerability. When you are the patient, for instance, you fear that those caring for you will ignore your needs because of your insignificance, omit necessary procedures because of their expense, and disregard telling symptoms because of other distractions. For patients, the apprehension in entering the depersonalized expanse of a large institution is the possible loss of individuality and the very identity that makes them valued and their well-being essential.

Although expendability is, taken at face value, ominous and offensive there are times when it can be judicious and humane. Accepting or even asserting expendability at an appropriate time and under legitimate circumstances is a vital principle of endurance, progress, and purpose.

Certainly for patients there is a time to let go—to let nature take its course. For the terminally ill patient whose condition is hopeless, when is it appropriate and ethical to shift from the essentialness of life-extending care to the comfort of hospice care? How do you balance appropriate intervention with a fair use of resources? When is it "too soon" to discontinue care, and when has it gone on far "too long"? In spite of our splendid technology and sincere intentions, life itself is a terminal condition. Yet in our present system, death is not an accepted option. Among the most contentious issues in the health care reform debate of 2009 was whether Medicare should pay for doctors to discuss end-of-life options with their patients. Rather than being seen as an opportunity for choices and preferences to be made clear among the parties, these visits were portrayed as "death panels": an attempt by the government to ration care and influence the elderly to forgo expensive life-extending treatments. The delusion that clinical intervention can overcome death itself skews the necessary balance of task, purpose, and humaneness. These questions were raised by the hospice movement, and hospice care has provided compassionate answers for those who have benefited from its services.

For those who guide and administer the health system, on the one hand there is the balance between life and the quality of life, and on the other hand is the balance between the essentialness of services and the limited resources society is willing to supply. You know that to ignore the health needs of a segment of the population—the poor, children, minorities, and immigrants—is to render its members expendable. The landscape of human history reveals the many groups who have been rendered expendable, either by acts of commission or by way of omission. If now, when you and your organization have the life-giving technology and capacity, you are unwilling or unable to share it, are you not doing the same? How do you select among the choices? As a responsible decision maker, you are compelled to reconcile priorities when you cannot do it all.

Having a Fluid Purpose

The health care opportunities and constraints you and your organization devise translate into services for people and employment for professionals. Priorities are manifest in the buildings you construct, the people you employ, the programs you offer, the machines you buy, and the medications you administer, as well as in how much you are willing to expend on each. These priorities define the context and circumstances of your work. As they change, so too do your responsibilities and, with them, your choices and decisions.

For those who work in the health care system, import and opportunity ascend and descend with the shifting tides that define what is considered essential and what is deemed expendable. Specialty care descends as primary care rises, and trailblazing nursing and medical schools change their curricula to stay ahead of the currents. Hospitalization recedes as outpatient care thrives, and responsive institutions close beds and open ambulatory care clinics with attached home care services. Integrated networks expand as solo practice fades, and providers band together to negotiate a place for themselves in the system. As primary care, deinstitutionalization, and integrated networks become essential, aspects of specialty services, hospital care, and solo practice become expendable. Fewer people are needed, which means that some people are not needed at all.

You are an extension of the essentialness of what you do and what you offer. Your importance derives from the significance of your tasks, skills, and knowledge. Your worth derives from the value of your contribution, both professionally and personally. At a time when services, priorities, and expenditures are at the center of the health care debate, the question of essentialness then becomes a matter of great personal as well as professional import. Will you have a job in this new system? Are your work and skills recognized and valued? Will your own professional values and personal goals fit the emerging contours of health care? How do you measure up among the others who champion their own essentialness? Will the verdict be made simply on the basis of power? Or will purpose and product also be legitimate items on the table?

Expendability and essentialness speak to your most fundamental interests as caregivers. They motivate your career aspirations and form the substance of what you hope to accomplish with your work. They speak to your membership in a community of caregivers and patients whom you hope will benefit from your endeavors. They are at the heart of much of what you negotiate in your day-to-day endeavors. And they are ever changing.

How do you craft a workable system to adjust this balance between the essential and the expendable so that the very process does not distort the fundamental question of what you do and why? How can you inspire circumstances, choices, decisions, and consequences that are just, principled, and fair so that the product is worthy of the effort? And how can you be confident that the end results, your accomplishments, reflect well upon you, your community, and your society?

Recrafting the Puzzle

Settling on what is essential and what is expendable is the pivotal conflict of health care. At times, it is a source for the creative tension that triggers the exploration of new and innovative ideas, the quest for more effective methodologies and treatments, and the construction of more efficient relationships and systems.

Conversely, it can be the crux of spiteful infighting that pits one group against another, that exploits the legitimate interests of patients, and that compromises the basic purposes of health care in the struggle. It speaks to how much the public and private sectors are willing to invest in basic research versus direct service. It was an unspoken torment in the early debates about responses to the AIDS epidemic. It is at the center of deliberation on infant mortality policy, violence prevention efforts, and what to do about the rising cost of health care.

The tone of a negotiation often reflects whether this conflict is producing creative tension or bitter infighting. Are the parties flexible, ready to express and recognize the range of legitimate concerns represented at the table? Or are they rigid, distancing themselves from one another in pursuit of narrow, self-centered objectives? Is it a matter of whole image negotiation or positional confrontation?

Whole image negotiation is most likely to occur when the parties honor each other's essentialness, when the operative premise is that my essentialness is not a function of your expendability. The intent of interest-based negotiation is not to dominate the pie or merely divide it up. Rather, the purpose is to find a way to understand, reshape, and expand it. Implied in this search for constructive options is respect for the essentialness of both sides. That understanding accepts that the parties will have their differences. There is only scant concern that those differences will be exploited by one side to destroy the other.

However, when the negotiation becomes a struggle that equates one party's essentialness with the other's expendability, then the interchange is likely to become positional. Each of the participants believes that whoever dominates the process will determine the outcome. The struggle for control assumes the urgency of survival itself. Participants seek to verify their position by contriving clear measures of their own ascendance and the other's downfall. They each believe their sustainability depends upon the eventual failure or vulnerability of the other.

At a time of significant change in the health system, when the very premises, people, and purpose of the work are open to question, the sensation of vulnerability rises. With the underlying topic of discussion revolving around who and what are essential and who and what are expendable, it is conceivable that everyone will become defensive of his or her own security. Leaping to the assumption that they are vulnerable, parties assume a positional stance, turning the process into one primed for destruction and defeat.

The system becomes mired in confrontation. How can this be turned around?

The key is having a negotiation purpose. If the parties intend to constructively build and rebuild the puzzle of which they are a part, then this ongoing, productive process facilitates the necessary and constant analysis, adjustment, and reconfiguration. They negotiate the size and shape of the pieces for a better fit and formulate the image they seek. Rather than a contest, their context is one of collaboration. The focus is not how can I defeat you. Rather, it is how can I balance what I am doing and what I consider essential with what you are doing and what you consider essential. Flexibility reigns as the parties focus more on fixing the problem than on fortifying their positions.

At times, successfully renegotiating the puzzle means not only reconfiguring the existing pieces but also opening the picture to new players, forums, and ideas. This is a fundamental aspect of rebuilding in order to have a system that is more responsive and more effective than before. And it is vital that these new players at the table are afforded valid participation in the process. This may mean including nurses in medical forums from which they were formerly excluded, patients in planning processes where they were once considered unnecessary, and physicians in administrative sessions in which they were previously objects of deliberation, not participants. These new players, forums, and ideas embody a new recognition, with beneficial returns for all who take part. This is not simply a matter of one side relinquishing and the other intercepting the power; it is not winners and losers. Rather, it is a process of enhancing the system's overall potency for resolving the daily predicaments of health care.

At other times, building new options means closing old ones. The expendability of programs, personnel, or participation must be considerately conceded and honorably conducted. It is not that I won and you lost. Insofar as we are in the same boat, your loss is mine as well as yours. Nonetheless, the consequences I feel, staying here while you leave, cannot be compared to your loss of a job, program, or professional dignity. When this occurs in an organization, it is a painful process. When this pain is fearfully avoided rather than tactfully managed, it can erupt into a tempest of new problems. How does this come about?

The very public nature of the process of identifying expendability is often disregarded. When the reconfigured puzzle requires the retention of some staff and the ouster of others, everybody watches. When one person or program becomes expendable, every person or program becomes vulnerable. People watch how the situation was handled. What led to the action? Were the criteria just? Was the process fair? In order to justify the action, were some people transformed into "the enemy"? A clear message is dispatched. Is it one that eases the process of putting the pieces back together? Or is it one that only heightens uncertainty and turmoil? Is the message "fight dirty or lose"? Or is it one of fairness and beneficence? Transparency and certainty around decision-making criteria and processes can alleviate much ill will, even when people disagree with the decision that is made.

We all hang in this precarious balance between essential and expendable. It is the nature of our work in health care. It defines our own job security. From

The Oppidania Medical Center hallways teem with their usual midday bustle. When Larry Lumberg and Fred Fisher converge in the crowded first-floor corridor that is the architectural backbone of the hospital, each instinctively knows where the other is going: lunch.

Fisher's greeting is uncharacteristically enthusiastic. Lumberg responds, "You're in a chipper mood today, Fred."

"You could say that." Fisher smiles and opens the door to the stairway that leads down to the cafeteria and the physicians' dining room.

Lumberg decides to have some fun with his longtime colleague and mentor. "Don't tell me, you won the lottery?" Fisher shakes his head and smiles. "I know, your daughter had another baby." Fisher's smile grows, and he again shakes his head. They reach the beginning of the cafeteria line, and Fisher hands Lumberg a tray before taking one for himself.

Finally, Fisher breaks his silence. "Two good guesses, Larry, though the second would have required Karen to give birth twice in a five-month period."

Fisher continues: "You know how you can wake up one day and see things slightly differently? Well, this was one of those days. I'm not sure exactly what provoked it. Maybe it was that meeting a few days ago, or this wholesale change in reimbursement, or that community health initiative meeting I went to. A few articles I've been reading maybe. I'm not sure exactly." Fisher places a plate of limp green beans, dreary mashed potatoes, and overcooked chicken on his tray. It's remarkable what gastronomical insults he puts up with just for the pleasure of having lunch surrounded by his colleagues.

Lumberg wonders where this is going.

"You know, Larry, sometimes we get caught up with our own baloney. We create illusions and hide behind them. And then one day, we wake up and realize that they are just illusions. We're not what we make ourselves out to be. We don't accomplish all the miracles we claim. But we have been taken with ourselves and who we are and what we do."

A small bowl of bright-red Jell-O cubes shakes as Lumberg places it on his tray. He looks quizzically at Fisher. "Fred, what are you talking about?" Lumberg has a hunch. He just can't believe these words are coming from a man devoted for so long to just the opposite sentiments.

Fisher expands on his thoughts as they wait at the end of the line to pay for their meals. "You know, Larry, we have fashioned such a complicated set of myths to insulate us. We appear to be one thing when we are something very different. We are far more secure in the myths we have created than in the reality of what we do."

They carry their trays into the doctors' dining room and sit across from one another at the far end of one of the long tables. Deep in conversation, they emit an unspoken message that they are not to be disturbed.

Fisher continues, almost excited to get his newfound thoughts out. "I became intrigued with figuring out exactly what we do, stripped of all that myth. Even look at this," he motions around the room. "Why do we eat in a separate room from the rest of the staff?"

Lumberg prods Fisher along. "So, what did you come up with?"

Fisher smiles. "You know I was a philosophy minor in college? I'm much better with questions than I am with answers."

Lumberg is quick on the return. "So what are the questions?"

"I think they're about patient care. Not necessarily the care we give patients but rather the care patients need. They are not always one and the same. And then I think of this complex roller-coaster on which we have placed a simple chariot. There is a certain simplicity to keeping people well and healing them in sickness. That is what we are supposed to be about. And yet we have created such a complex maze in which to make that happen, it's as if we forgot what we are doing and where we are going." Fisher pauses for a moment to consider the thought. "You know, Larry, trains get someplace. Roller-coasters, for all their jiggling around, never get you anywhere. There's a lot of push and pull and up and down. Ultimately, though, you just go around in circles. You think a lot has happened because you are so sick to your stomach. And yet you haven't made any genuine progress."

Lumberg laughs. "I've never been much for roller-coasters. But I take your point."

"We're in the midst of a revolution that could be as significant for medicine as the discovery of anesthesia. Technology is going to take over a lot of what we do. Yesterday, that scared me. Today, for whatever reason, I'm fine with it. Yes, we can learn the technicalities of interfacing with all this hardware. In the long run, though, that's a defined set of skills that will fluctuate with the introduction of each new invention. And there will be an army of technicians trained to do just that. But no computer can duplicate the human dimension of medicine, and on a human level, what could be more gratifying than keeping a fellow human healthy? The art of medicine derives from the synthesis of the human dimensions of our work. That synthesis, based on human understanding, relationships, and wisdom, is something we have turned away from. It's time we get back to those basics, understand them for what they are, and come out from the wizard's room, where we have concocted miracles that were in large part illusion. Do you remember the Wizard of Oz?"

"Sure," Lumberg says, "we watch it at home every Halloween. My kids love it too. So we're exposing the man behind the curtain?"

Fisher nods. "There is something very genuine about the practice of medicine. I've been burning out, like so many of our colleagues, because I lost that core value. It's time we honestly assess what we do, and do it well. If we don't, that curtain will get pulled back on us and we will be discovered and judged for what we are. Society won't put up with it."

"So, Fred, what are we, then?" Lumberg asks.

"It's not what we are, Larry. It's what we are becoming. It is a process of change. And if we manage that process correctly, then we will have a productive and satisfying place in whatever health care is becoming. And if we cannot adapt, then we will be like the dinosaurs. We will become extinct, replaced by technocrats who do not have the understanding or compassion that is at the heart of good medicine. Medicine can thrive alongside all the machines and efficiencies that are emerging. It just has to be a different kind of medicine. Most of the people who talk about it today see it only as a bad thing. It will be bad only if we let it become bad."

"This doesn't sound like the same Fred Fisher who was complaining the other night about becoming an insurance company."

"Oh, it is the same Fred Fisher. The only difference is one of perspective. I was responding to the business aspects of the arrangement. Now I'm thinking of the medical aspects. I am being paid to keep people healthy. If I succeed, my patients benefit, I benefit, and the insurance company benefits. Now, I might not like all the business aspects of the arrangement. Yet the core of my job is keeping people healthy. If the business office can handle the administrative aspects, and if I have the wherewithal to do my job well, then I am willing to give it a try. And if it doesn't work, let's constructively go back to the drawing board. Not to whine. We'll go back to refine. Big difference of attitude."

Their conversation continues through the end of lunch. They talk about the specifics, the politics, and the costs of change. They ponder their own careers, and how the difference in their ages so colors their experiences and expectations. When they finally finish their meal, they pick up their trays and head for the conveyor belt that will return their dishes to the inner dens of the kitchen.

The stale taste of the hospital carrot cake still lingers in Fisher's mouth. "You know, Larry, it's like this hospital food. It hasn't improved much in the many years I've been here. One day, we have to be wise enough to stand up and say we don't like it. And hospital administration needs to be wise enough to hear us."

Lumberg quips back. "Or else we all might realize the gastronomic deception. This has been feed posing as food."

As they part, Lumberg realizes for the first time that in terms of their work the two of them are somehow headed in a synchronous direction. He just feels more uncertain than ever before about their destination.

He also feels a renewed sense of self-confidence.

it we derive the satisfaction and hope that we anticipated when we chose our careers. Whether it is a constructive and creative process depends on how we play the game.

As we recraft the puzzle, some pieces change shape. New pieces are added. Some are discarded. It is a process that is at once fragile, precarious, and rewarding. How can you and your organization structure this evolution so that what you get on the other side is worthy of the effort?

Adapting Purpose and Process to Product

You, your colleagues, and your organization can strive for fit in many ways:

That your purpose fits what your surroundings expect; the expectations are those directly expressed to you by patients, staff, or colleagues. Resonance of purpose occurs when your personal direction corresponds with that of your surroundings.

That the choices available to you match those expectations so you have the capacity and means to select among feasible options. Legitimate choice occurs when you have the time, resources, and competence to do the job well.

That your decisions reflect your purpose, and your values and capabilities match the task. When the job is well done, the satisfaction is mutual among all involved.

That you have made a meaningful contribution for which you are appropriately rewarded; your work is part of an exchange for which you are fairly compensated.

That the process of creating fit abets your purpose so that your and others' shared understandings and interpretations of circumstances, choices, decisions, and consequences are symbiotic. You all negotiate and resolve differences in a constructive manner.

That this process helps you better assess your choices and collaboratively reach your decisions; you invest in the collaboration because your essentialness is recognized and honored.

That good process yields more good process based on meaningful participation; success begets more success.

That what you spend returns a positive sum back to society, and your efforts are recognized and duly rewarded.

That your priorities are sound and decisions judicious, and there is synchrony of expectation and product.

And that the consequences you reap in turn benefit society and offer you a sense of personal achievement so that your own purpose and product coincide.

Fit reflects what you do personally and what you do as part of a system. You reflect that picture personally when you speak and react to others. When you inform a patient that a procedure is not covered by insurance, when you commend the work of a colleague, or when you authorize the purchase of new equipment, what you say and do formulates others' experience with the system. Each individual is part of a larger whole, affecting that whole and being affected by it.

Just as a picture emerges when the pieces of the puzzle are placed together, your and others' combined work in health care creates a picture. It is the process you use to configure those pieces that will determine what picture will emerge.

Renegotiating the Balance

Compare two premises on which negotiation can be based: dichotomous thinking and balanced and integrated thinking.

Using dichotomous thinking, what you negotiate is either yours *or* mine: the notion of sharing is incompatible with this line of reasoning. Situations are clearly right *or* wrong: the possibility that truth may lie someplace in the middle is logically incongruous. People and services are either essential *or* expendable, and unambiguous lines define the distinction.

By contrast, balanced and integrated thinking affirms that ideas, skills, and expertise are naturally combined and adjusted in order to function: the care of a patient involves both clinical approaches and contextual and reimbursement matters. In most cases when attitudes toward a question have become polarized, the answer can be found someplace in between the extremes. And as situations change, what might have been true yesterday is no longer so today.

Because dichotomous thinkers have only two choices, they always advocate that which is in their best interest. Because ownership is yours *or* mine, they advocate to control as much as possible. Because a position can be only right *or* wrong, they always argue the rightness of their position. Because everything they do is essential, their concerns are important whereas those of others are trivial. It is two-dimensional, adversarial thinking (as described in Chapter Eight).

Balanced and integrated thinkers pursue shared interests, their own as well as those of others. Because they see themselves as part of a larger picture, they are amenable to sharing control with others. And because they grasp that no one person can be the repository of complete knowledge and expertise, they are simultaneously student and teacher, actively learning just as they are informing. They respect the disparities between their view of what is essential and expendable and that of others. It is the essence of multidimensional thinking.

And lest, in the course of making this distinction we make the very same error: yes! There is a time for dichotomous thinking, just as there is a time for balanced thinking.

So why is this distinction important?

It is important because as you renegotiate health care, you change not only what is on the table but also how you go about negotiating that substance. The product can only be as good as the process by which it was obtained.

For years, health care has been dominated by dichotomous thinking. Although this line of reasoning has benefited some, overall it has led the system into many of its current conundrums. The system is out of balance not because the people in it lack the knowledge, the expertise, or even the goodwill to make it work. And it is not for lack of money that so many people are without care: enough is spent to take care of everyone in the country. Rather, the system is out of balance because of the premises and processes that have been used to construct it.

Fostering a climate of change offers us an opportunity to generate a new congruence among the many services, staff, and resources that constitute health care. If we are to reliably frame a new arrangement, our method must be compatible with the task.

You are one of a collection of people working in the health care arena, and your and the others' aspiration is to weave a constructive balance that cultivates health in a socially responsible manner. To do so, you together formulate the picture—the image—that you all hope to achieve. It is not your picture; it is not my picture; it is our picture, with mutual investments, pursuits, and rewards. This template for thinking pertains to the particular relationship between a doctor and a patient and also to the broader interplay between policymakers and professional groups, administrators and providers, insurers and service systems, and nurses and other nurses. Our inevitable interdependence requires our movement in a congruent direction if the system is to get anywhere.

Because you are one piece of a larger vista, the whole, then it is a matter of fitting the exchange, the give-and-get of your negotiations, into some larger blueprint. The most trying task in getting a picture out of a puzzle is not getting all the right pieces on the table. Rather, the primary burden is tailoring those many pieces so that they fit together. And the task is all the more elusive in an emerging health system in which there is no box cover, no existing, exhaustively studied model, to guide your efforts. You are crafting this design as you go. You know that some precedents are valuable and should be retained. Likewise, you know that many need alteration. And it is those that need adjustment that are most resistant to finding their new place in this germinating design. That is why this process is so difficult, and why it is so wrought with conflict. It is why the dimensions of meta-leadership practice (discussed in Chapter Ten) can be so instructive to your work.

Balanced and integrated thinking is a puzzle-making process. It is not a matter of finding the winner or loser; it is a matter of uncovering the right combination of pieces to make the system work. Changes are deliberated. Ideas and people are reconciled and arranged to mold the best fit between purpose and outcome. And because changes in circumstances offer new sets of choices that must be accommodated by new decisions, adjusted expectations, and new sets of consequences, the process of balanced thinking becomes simply a means to an ever-fluctuating end.

Balanced and integrated work requires constant negotiation and a good deal of conflict resolution. It is not the path of least resistance. However, it is the means for achieving the most profound payoffs. Clinical understanding combined with administrative know-how enhances effectiveness without compromising efficiency. Nurses are not appendages to doctors; they offer a different set of eyes, understanding, and skills. When doctors' and nurses' eyes, understanding, and skills come together, they produce a more comprehensive view and more effective treatment for the patient. Similarly, doctors are not obstacles to good nursing; though not ever-present, the insight, knowledge, and authority of physicians are important pieces of holistic health care. With this kind of perspective, nurses and doctors, and others, can move beyond dichotomous images of one another as the enemy to realize complementary purposes and outcomes. It is an example of the cone in the cube phenomenon (Chapter One).

Balanced and integrated thinking not only successfully mixes different professions, organizations, and people; it also combines the old with the new. This is especially important during a time of change. It does not discard the past in its pursuit of fresh ideas and innovations. Tested ways and experiences blended with novel circumstances offer opportunities for trailblazing ingenuity based on solid reasoning and wise interpretation. Large-scale managed care operations that fuse administrative efficiency with the intimacy of a personal doctor's office will enhance the practice and experience of both patient and physician. Health programs that emphasize prevention and primary care while offering appropriate access to specialty treatment assure the provider, patient, and payer that a fair mix of services is available and accessible. Public health initiatives that address newly recognized "hot" issues, such as obesity prevention and chronic care, while not abandoning past hot topics, such as reducing teenage pregnancy, preventing smoking, and preventing and treating substance abuse, comprehend that many of these problems are intertwined, affecting the same populations and lending themselves to integrated solutions. In the rush to embrace the new, it is imprudent to abandon what is vital and practical from the past.

To achieve balance between pragmatism and pioneering, people and professions, the essential and the expendable, you negotiate on the basis of your interests. The process requires you to grasp well the frame you bring to the table. Likewise, you are challenged to discern the frames of others. And as you engage in this exercise of informing and discerning, you reach a deeper understanding of both your place in the picture and the places of others.

To the extent that you can remain flexible, your ability to spawn new and dynamic endeavors is propelled in positive directions. What is the importance of flexibility?

It is the interactive process of reframing that shapes differences and commonalities into resourceful perspectives that lead to new opportunities. These composite frames emerge from the participants' collaborative efforts: the essence of balanced and integrated thinking. The view you and the other participants take from the table is changed by the process. The reframe is the product, the outcome, the combined road map for what it is you all want to achieve. And as such, this outcome is in constant flux, adapting with time to the new opportunities and constraints of a changing health care system.

Whole image negotiation (Chapter Four) fits the challenges of assembling and reassembling the pieces of the health enterprise. It is a vehicle for moving not only organizations but this whole country away from dichotomous thinking and toward balanced, integrated, and collaborative achievement. It is a solution-based method for constructively guiding one another in distinguishing what is essential from what is expendable.

Similarly, mediation (Chapter Nine) fits the challenges of resolving the disputes encountered along the way. Mediation offers a fulcrum, a vehicle for articulating differences and finding what lies in between them. It is settlement oriented and assists those in conflict to advance beyond their differences to a balanced closure of their conflicts.

So what is it that you will achieve if you bring the system into better balance?

Two days after the meeting that brought the CEOs of the Oppidania and Urbania Medical Centers together, Iris Inkwater and Pete Patterson almost simultaneously call Manuel Mendez's office. They indeed have an interest in talking further about some sort of relationship. Each has spoken with his or her board and senior staff, and then they spoke again to each other. In that conversation they agreed to ask Mendez to stay on as their intermediary. Mendez arranges a conference call for the three of them, and during that call he suggests a meeting at a retreat center an hour outside of town. The two CEOs agree that such a meeting is a reasonable next step. Mendez offers to make the arrangements and to hire professional facilitators to lead them through a Walk in the Woods. Each hospital will send a delegation of about ten members. All three underline the importance of maintaining the confidentiality of these discussions. If the meetings were to be publicized, media sensationalism and staff anxiety would spoil the potential for any progress.

As this preliminary discussion continues, they decide to schedule a two-day session and to ask each participant to spend the night at the center. They all feel that the informality and intensity that can be achieved in such a setting will break the ice and enhance productive discourse. They further agree that each organization's delegation is to include individuals with decision-making authority: the board chair, CEO, chief financial officer, chief operating officer, hospital medical director, nursing vice president, two other administrators, and two other board members. The dean of the medical school is also invited. Mendez will be there with two members of his staff. Two facilitators will lead the meetings.

The time of the retreat quickly arrives, and in large part because the participants have come carefully prepared, the meeting is extremely productive, far beyond everyone's expectations. What becomes clear early on is that each hospital is, in fact, in trouble. There simply are fewer patients and there is less money.

By the end of the second day, the participants have reached an agreement, in principle, to ally the two hospitals, forming a new corporate entity to oversee the separate though coordinated operations of each. The new entity will bear neither of their names; it will be called the Oppidania Community Care Corporation (OCCC). They conclude by compiling a list of questions and issues that will have to be settled as the proposal moves forward, everything from finances to leadership, culture, administration, and clinical issues.

Each side sees a number of benefits to the arrangement. Certainly they will realize the economies of scale in purchasing and marketing. Together they will have far more leverage with insurers. More important, though, they will be able to reduce unnecessary duplications of services and purchases. In particular, the most expensive high-tech services will be limited to one facility and accessible to both. It is agreed that Oppidania will have the more acute services: this turned out to be a relief to Urbania, which had found over the past few years that it was investing large sums in underutilized and therefore ultimately unprofitable machinery.

With this understanding in principle in hand, each side agrees to open broader discussions with organizational leadership. The proposal will be reviewed by both boards as well as the key department heads of each institution. If no major stumbling blocks appear, the negotiations will be announced simultaneously, first inside each institution and then publicly at a joint press conference. The announcements will be intentionally vague, stating that the two institutions are "discussing the possibility" of some form of alliance. The press conference announcing these negotiations will involve the board chairs and CEOs of each institution, along with city health commissioner Manuel Mendez. It is decided to keep the mayor out of the picture until an actual alliance is formalized.

It takes nearly a year of concentrated work. The freshly sprouted alliance is heartily welcomed at a celebratory news conference attended by the newly aligned leadership, the mayor, and Manuel Mendez. After careful deliberation, it is decided to name Iris Inkwater CEO of OCCC, investing in that position general oversight of the overall operation as well as leadership for new ventures by this parent corporation. She outlines her aspiration to create new community outreach programs. Among her first initiatives is to announce a series of open meetings at which the public will be invited to offer their opinions and recommendations for the design of the health care organization of the future. Pete Patterson continues in his role as CEO of the UMC. Dr. Larry Lumberg is promoted to CEO of OMC. Janice Johnson is asked to work with her counterpart at Urbania to coordinate the collaboration of the nursing departments, and Dr. Fred Fisher is asked to do the same for the two medical staffs.

The new alliance is framed as an emerging and flexible integration that will grow over time, step by step. It is in large measure a learning process, by which the two institutions and their surrounding community can gradually come to better understand and link with one another. What is learned will be fed back into the system, serving as the basis for future decisions and directions.

The new organization views its mission as promoting a responsive agenda for the health and health care of Oppidania. With the mayor and health commissioner present, this vision is described as an active public-private partnership. The speakers observe that this effort had not been without its bumps and that genuine efforts are being made to hear and respond to the concerns of the many people and constituencies who are being affected by the changes. And they also acknowledge the widespread support expressed by staff, community, and business concerns.

A feeling of professional, personal, and organizational achievement pervades the room as the plan and vision are outlined. Having persevered to this point, all those involved can proceed together with the most important asset of all: a sense of confidence and coherence in what they are doing and where they are heading.

Conclusion

The purpose of this book is not to prescribe the correct model for health care. There are plenty of treatises available that attempt to do that. Rather, our intention is to offer a constructive means for moving toward that model and to remind you that once there it will be time to move on: health care by its nature is always changing. This is a travel guide for a journey that never ends.

Nonetheless, a few cautionary notes are in order to clarify exactly what *balance* does and does not mean.

Balance is not everyone and everything being equal. There are different levels of weight, import, experience, and know-how among the many people, skills, and problems on your organization's ledgers. To equate all of them would be naive. Calibrating their relative weights as part of negotiating a more balanced health system is what this book is all about.

To do so you and your organization will establish and apply a fair, transparent, and responsive checks and balances system: relevant parties should have a voice, and their messages should be heard, even if the relative influence of some is greater than that of others. You may work, think, and decide in hierarchical terms, or you may be in a more consensus-driven, team-based environment. Any structure in and of itself is not bad; it can be an efficient way to sort innumerable people and tasks. It is unjust only when it is used as a tool to silence some and insulate others.

Giving voice in order to craft a better balance is not just responding to a market survey or a staff-satisfaction questionnaire. It is deeper than that. It goes to a genuine understanding of what you are doing and what you are trying to accomplish. If the negotiation table provides you with an opportunity to gain better clarity on these means and ends, your chances of developing a worthy health system are greatly improved.

Balance means that in the change process, you negotiate ends and means; you define and redefine what you are doing; you are open to finding better ways to do it. The outcome is a system that represents the diversity of your organization's workforce, the population it cares for, and that population's health care needs. You promote health; you prevent illness—you deal. You assemble the pieces necessary to accomplish that noble endeavor.

This premise of balance is essential to transforming your organizational model and achieving priorities, and opportunities without sacrificing what is already excellent in the health care system.

Is this incremental thinking? Yes. Does it mean that change will be a bit slower, a bit more careful, a bit more reasoned than it would be if you totally abandoned the old order in order to bring in the new? Yes. What is the benefit?

It is better to change at a pace that offers the greatest likelihood of making the right choices than to refurbish the system with no idea whether you will succeed. Insofar as you take seriously what you do, how much do you want to experiment with systems that are untested and that may not work? Achieving balance means that you fix the big problems first and continue with the same commitment to the remaining problems. It means that you are bold enough to experiment with what might work and that your decisions will evolve from what is learned in the process. It means that society must be clear and reasonable in what it expects from the health system. It means that people must be reasonable in accepting what they get in the trade-offs bound to occur on the road to a more balanced health system.

Human life itself is a delicate balance of the chemicals, electricity, liquids, and frames that make up and hold together our anatomy. For our anatomy to work, all its components and systems must be in synchrony. If they are not, we become ill, and life itself is at risk. Similarly, our health care system, which intends to nurture our physical well-being, must itself be in healthy alignment.

CHAPTER 16

CONSTRUCTING A RESILIENT BALANCE

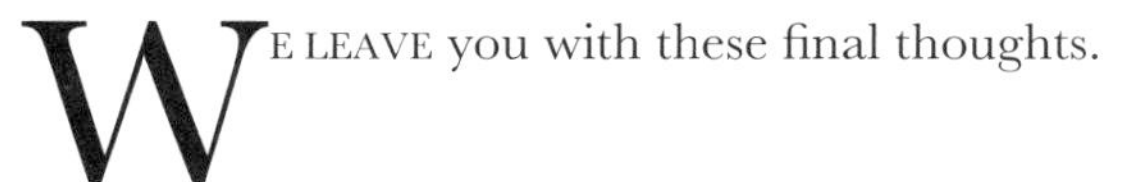

WE LEAVE you with these final thoughts.

On Conflict

Fundamental issues must be distinguished from cursory issues. The rhetoric, accusations, and demands shooting across the tables of conflict depict one representation of the issues. To understand what is really happening and how it might realistically be resolved, hear and understand what lies beneath the spoken assertions—the latent along with the manifest messages. What is the actual agenda of each side? Are there discrepancies between what is said and what is done? How might these underlying issues be configured or reconfigured to encourage settlement? Heed the message as well as the words.

At the heart of much conflict is vulnerability. Beneath the combat, rhetoric, and bravado of conflict, basic emotions and fears—the suspicions and insecurities of professional peril, physical risk, and personal uncertainty—motivate and impassion what ostensibly is on the table. At the core of the conflict, then, there is doubt, dread of betrayal, and fear of defenseless exposure. For some, vulnerability compels retreat. For others, inner vulnerability is masked by outward aggression; they attack others to secure themselves. Parties become locked in escalating defensive and offensive moves motivated and justified by their deep-seated fears. To uncover settlement options, discern these vulnerabilities and search for ways to understand, mitigate, relieve, and remove doubts that obscure resolution. This process is the gist of unearthing interests at a time when the conflict has intensified into hardened positions.

Conflict is inevitable. Strive for perfection—and know that in the long run it is unattainable, humans and natural events being what they are. Like life itself, the health system cannot be infallible; it cannot reliably address all the needs of all the people all the time, though we should never stop trying. Beware the conflicts that arise from the disappointments of imperfection; given the nature of your work, you will encounter expectations of infallibility even though all know that it is ultimately unattainable. What is reasonable is to expect that you will always diligently work toward optimal outcomes. Anticipate and prepare for the conflicts, knowing that from each conflict there is the potential for resilience: on the far side of your shared experience, you may well construct reconfigured expectations, relations, and outcomes that would not otherwise have been imaginable.

On Framing and Reframing

If it doesn't make sense, you probably don't have all the facts. People are assumed to operate on the premise of self-interest: usually some combination of money, advancement, satisfaction, security, and recognition. It is generally easy to understand motive when the incentives are relatively straightforward. Motive can become confusing, however, when the usual standards of self-interest are of secondary importance. It is particularly confounding when someone's self-interest is mingled with destructive purpose, either for themselves or others. In that case one person's safety depends on another's demise. Ironically, in the manner of a self-fulfilling prophecy, when a destructive impulse becomes an obsession, the outcome itself can become self-destructive. Likewise, when obsession for a mission overtakes common sense, the pursuit of the purpose may itself undermine that purpose. Notwithstanding these many intricacies, if only you could assemble all the revelatory pieces, you would ultimately be able to find a logical explanation for what happened and why. Negotiation is like good detective work. Being careful of decoys that might distract you from an investigatory pursuit, you look for motive and means, seeking clues to unravel the mystery.

There are always options: stretch to find them. Modify what you do. If you cannot change what you do, adjust when you do it. And if you cannot adjust when you do it, reframe how you do it. You are the mouse in the maze. Sometimes you retrace your steps to inform your journey. You are not deterred by dead ends. And you are flexible about how you respond to the destination you reach, even if it is not the piece of cheese you expected. Step back. Take another look. Turn the puzzle on its side. Try another angle. Seek realistic opportunity. You need not do it alone, and you need not give up the cause. There is aspiration and there is anticipation in the perseverance. They are yours to grasp.

Find ways to express differences without provoking contention. There will always be differences among people—in styles, attitudes, beliefs, methods, backgrounds, and skills. As a species we tend to the tribal: we coalesce in order to sustain ourselves. Like small republics congregating to fend off a common enemy, we sit in the congenial comfort of nurses' lounges, doctors' hideaways, and the inner dens of our administrative offices. The sense of familiarity we have when we're with our own—whether we define our own by profession, gender, age, ethnic group, race, religion, or alma mater—is not inherently troublesome if its prime purpose is simply to invoke that relaxing sensation of the customary. It becomes a problem when this coalescing is the rallying point for portraying outsiders as the enemy, a call for self-affirming aggrandizement and the disparagement of others, for building walls and not bridges between people who ultimately are or could be constructively intertwined. We can express our differences without denigrating the roots of those dissimilarities: different cultures, professional identities, or departmental affiliations. Those differences can be either a source of strength or an anchor of weakness; ultimately, you will be more vital and far more resilient if you shape them into a strength.

Turn jealousy into admiration. We spend boundless time and energy comparing ourselves to one another, measuring whether we are ahead or behind. If our work is merely a race to get somewhere, then this ceaseless comparison is understandable. However, if our intention is to accomplish something of value with others, we will find the constant equating and the jealousy it spawns to be more a hindrance than a boon to our work. When you perceive others' accomplishments as your loss, then you are caught in your own spiral of defeat, because you can never outdo all and will rank others only with your measuring stick. You become jealous of others. They become jealous of you. Conversely, if you can see each others' accomplishments as reflecting well on your common, collaborative efforts, you can turn this negative into a positive.

On Conflict Resolution

Conflicts always settle, over time. Time is that robust dimension of conflict and conflict resolution that often goes undetected for both its problems and its potential. Time offers perspective and a chance to bury that dagger of rage that overwhelms any appetite to settle. When the parties are not simultaneously ripe to resolve, one makes a move for the table of resolution while the other runs, only to return eventually and find that the bitterness over his or her retreat has killed any hope for rapprochement. Eventually, however, the conflict fades, settles, or is forgotten: people leave or die; the original issues are seen for their fruitlessness;

new opportunities cloud the sources of discord; the parties tire of the fight and relent. And so perhaps someone reflects on the time and energy devoted to the battle and wonders what could have been accomplished if those same resources had been devoted to the good that motivated each of the sides. In those hopeless moments of battle, it is wise to remember that life itself is short and fleeting and that in the long run we each possess little more on this planet than time itself. Our concern should be how best to use it.

Truth is usually found in the middle, not at the extremes. Truth is that rendition of reality that we have easily manipulated and crafted to reflect what we want to believe. Different parties to a dispute perceive it differently. No one owns it: there are fewer absolutes than we might desire. Keep your mind open, and cultivate the possibility that your version of the truth may deviate from that of others. Do not abandon your convictions; at the same time, do not allow them to blind you. Permit ideas and possibilities to commingle: multiple perspectives are more likely to reveal a perspective that meets the measure of many people's truths. Wisdom lies in tolerating that your version of the truth may be different than mine, and that for all practical purposes, they could both be true. And it also lies in recognizing that everything is relative: what may have been extreme yesterday is conventional today.

Mediation is like baking bread: you have to trust the process even though you can't see it happen. Take simple ingredients: facts, circumstances, people, choices, emotions, consequences. Blend them in a perceptive manner, and allow them to transform into something better than their individual parts. Know as you peer around the table that many of the deeply personal insights, changes, and discoveries that occur—and that transform the course of events—will be invisible to all except the person who has thought a new thought, gained a new understanding, and conceded on a point once dear. Resilience emerges from that collective yet often invisible series of realizations that, when brought together around the mediation table, offer a new range of possibilities.

On Trust

Trust is an essential element in the successful delivery of health care. Trust shapes the cooperation necessary to advance the purposes of health and health care. It must be present among clinicians, between clinicians and administrators, amid providers and patients, and across the system and those who pay for it. The opposite of trust is suspicion. When clinicians are suspicious of the motives and actions of their colleagues, it is impossible to fashion integrated and patient-focused care. When clinicians and administrators within an institution are suspicious of one another, strategic and operational congruity is undermined. Noncompliance, legal threats and actions, and distracted care result from suspicion between providers and patients. And when there is widespread suspicion across the health system, rules and institutions are gamed, distractions get in the way of good work, and countless dollars are spent to do little more than compensate for the lack of trust. And how can one comfortably put one's life, or the life of a loved one, in the care of someone or something that cannot be trusted?

It is time to reset expectations about trust. Trust comes naturally to us. Much as the brain is hardwired to take us to the emotional basement in a crisis, it is also hardwired for us to trust and form social bonds. At birth, we are unable to live on our own. We are dependent on parents and other caregivers for nourishment, warmth, and protection. Survival itself depends on forming and fostering close bonds, first as children and eventually as parents. As you grow personally and advance professionally, you develop your own trust continuum, determining whom you can trust and who not. Using our innate facility to emit and receive signals of trustworthiness, you transmit indicators to others that tell them whether you are a person whom they can trust; be intentional about what you transmit and understand the implications. You likewise receive clues about whether to trust others; be empathic about what is coming your way and what the person is really communicating. See beyond the suspicions, vulnerabilities, and fears that mask the hope for trust—we go through life seeking to find and recapture it. There is nothing more valuable than a trusting relationship and nothing that can inspire the resilience and the work of health care more than trust in the people, institutions, and systems that embody the health enterprise

Take steps to ensure you can trust in your technology. Trusting a human is one thing. Trusting a machine is another. It is natural to confer anthropomorphic qualities on the silicon, plastic, and wiring of the computers, robots, and sensors that increasingly are your companions in health care. Their consistency and dependability are the bedrocks for much of your work as diagnostics, record keeping, and procedures become increasingly mechanized. Although these machines sell themselves on their cost, speed, and ease of use, the question of trust is an additional critical component in the design and the acquisition of technology. If, for example, the ongoing security and privacy of the electronic medical record is questioned, a vital resource in your tool chest is compromised. If manufacturers are found to have covered up medical equipment defects, patients will lose confidence in the machines that are keeping them independent and alive. And as robotics bring remote surgery, minimally invasive surgery, and unmanned surgery to a growing patient population, the reliability of these machines will test just how far the balance between humans and machines can go. Trust is like a working component of these machines and must be incorporated intentionally

It is 11:00 P.M. The lingering smell of a day of hard work is still in the air as Ken Kavanaugh, chief of the ICU, and Dave Donley enter the deserted locker room to change out of their hospital greens. They make their way to a small alcove at the far end of the cramped room. Donley takes a seat in front of his open locker at one end of the bench. Kavanaugh prefers to stand, hanging onto his locker door, which dangles back and forth, squeaking, as he takes off his shoes. They both are exhausted, drudging through the routine of transforming back into their civilian lives.

"I know I'll get used to this leaner staff model eventually," Kavanaugh says. "I just hope I have the stamina."

"We'll get there, my friend." Donley slaps him on the back. "Change. It always gets me thinking." Donley suddenly lights up. "You know, Ken, I've been working on a whole new theory of the universe."

Kavanaugh barely has the energy to listen. "Here we go," he thinks, "from staff cuts to the universe being turned upside down." Before he has finished the thought, Donley is blurting ahead.

"You know how in those science fiction movies the alien creatures all look about our size and shape?" Donley pauses a moment to get Kavanaugh's assent. "I think they have it all wrong. I think even aiming telescopes into the sky may be inane."

"Tell me, why is it inane?" Kavanaugh says flatly, tries to convey his growing disinterest through the tone of his voice.

Donley plunges on, oblivious to Kavanaugh's indifference. "Have you ever looked at a picture of the universe? We look like an atom, with the sun as a nucleus and the planets like little protons spinning around the middle." Donley is gesturing in the air as he pulled his shirt over his head. His animated voice continues, absorbed in his own speculation. "And then, when you look at the whole Milky Way, it looks like a set of atoms assembled together to make up a molecule."

"Yeah, so what?" Kavanaugh grumbles. He is only half listening, trying to remember the stops he has to make on the way home.

"Well, have you ever considered that the universe as we know it may be a small piece of matter in a much larger particle? Say, all these atoms and molecules together are just a piece in some colossal being's thumbnail?"

Donley's diatribe finally catches Kavanaugh's attention. His face betrays his annoyance at his colleague's rambling. "Dave, you think we are an atom in somebody's thumbnail?"

"Well, perhaps." Donley hesitates. "And it gets more intriguing." His enthusiasm grows again. He is convinced that Kavanaugh is hanging on his every word.

"If *we* are a particle in someone's thumbnail, just as likely there could be whole universes in our own thumbnails." He points at his extended thumb. "There could be suns and planets, malls, gyms—the whole bit—right inside here."

Though Kavanaugh is beginning to find the prospect amusing, he doesn't want to encourage Donley. "Where do you come up with these crazy ideas?" he sighs.

Not attuned to Kavanaugh's signals, Donley continues unabated. "And then dimensions of time differ." Donley's arms wave theatrically around his head. "For the larger being, the billions of years of our planet's existence are only a millisecond. And for the beings in our thumbnail, why, whole civilizations could have come and gone in the course of this conversation, and we wouldn't know it." Donley stares at his thumb as if expecting one of the tiny beings to flash him a signal.

The two pick up their rumpled hospital attire and toss the clothes into the laundry hamper as they head out the door. "Am I going to see you wearing a colander on your head so you can communicate with little green men?" Kavanaugh asks with a laugh as they head down the brightly lit hallway toward the parking lot and home.

Stepping into the cool evening air, Kavanaugh decides to challenge Donley's fantastical line of thinking. "OK, Dave, let's say I have vast civilizations in my fingernails. What does that have to do with anything?"

Donley squints as if he is trying to squeeze a thought out of his brain. "A little five-year-old girl came in through emergency today—hit by a car, pretty bad trauma. I was in and out with her since this morning."

The introduction of an actual case captures Kavanaugh's attention. "Those are always tough. How long will she be in?"

"Three days if we're lucky," Donley replies. "With the new remote e-monitoring system, I can send her home to her teddy bears pretty quickly. I'll video chat with her and her parents every day for a few days after that."

"That's great. The sooner you get her home, the lower the chances of her picking up a secondary infection from a fellow patient. And never underestimate the medicinal value of someone's favorite teddy bear," Kavanaugh says with a smile.

Donley chuckles. "You'll never find evidence in a journal article to back that up, but I think you're right. But let me finish my story. When I was a kid, I got hit by a car too. That's how I got into medicine—I really admired everything they did for people. They ended up saving my life ... as you can see." Donley leans against his car. "I was in the hospital for ten days, and by the time they released me, I had convinced myself that one day I would be a doc too."

"So what does that have to do with planets in your thumbnail?"

"I was ten years old when it happened, and for some reason, it came back to me today. I dreamed up that wild idea right after the accident. Someone had brought me a book about the planets and the universe. All I could do was look at the pictures and think. I saw the sun and nine planets looking like an atom that's part of a larger molecule and all that."

Kavanaugh realizes that something has struck a deep chord for Donley.

Donley continues. "Anyway, as I was taking care of this little girl today, that image came back to me. And then a little later, while I was filling out some stupid insurance form on the computer, all my feelings about this vast health care cosmos we are a part of came bubbling up. You know, sometimes when I'm in the hospital, it feels like the whole world is right there in my hands. Every fiber of my being is invested in a particular procedure for a patient. Then at other times it feels like we are just some tiny little particle in a larger picture that I can barely fathom."

Kavanaugh pulls his jacket closer against the chill. He is anxious to go but remembers how Donley had listened to his long ruminations when he had separated from his wife a couple of years back. Payback time.

"And then I look at this little girl," Donley says. "She was scared and afraid. There were a dozen people swirling around her in emergency. Machines blinking and beeping. For her, this is an incomprehensible world. Today was a lifetime for her. She'll never forget what happened. She'll relive it over and over again—it will be with her forever. For us, it was just a few hours. When it's all over, we pack up and call it another day at work."

"So she's that world in your thumbnail?" Kavanaugh thinks he might be starting to see the point.

"That's right, Ken. She is that world in my thumbnail. It just brought it home how we always see things from our own perspective. We expect the universe to somehow be in our own scale, on our timeline and along our own dimension. It's very hard to step back and take another slant on what we are seeing. We are locked into our own biases, and we all see things through our own looking glass. We think we're seeing the same picture, but we're not."

Kavanaugh looks at his friend in the glare spilling down from the light tower between their cars. Donley has hit on some of Kavanaugh's own frustrations and fantasies about medicine. Sometimes you feel almost godlike, and other times it feels like you are being crushed under the pressure of an enormous bureaucratic superstructure. "I'm not sure I buy the thumbnail theory, though I'll grant you that we do get stuck on our own way of thinking. I had exactly that problem in the ICU today. Everybody was mired in their own mud, and we weren't working in sync."

"See," Donley says, "I'm not crazy."

"I'm not so sure about that," Kavanaugh continues with a warm smile. "But I am going to think about this idea of yours. It's lunacy, though I find it intriguing." He pulls out his car keys as he prepares to leave. "And by the way, tell me, in that mall in your fingernail, is there a multiplex?"

Donley looks down at his thumb to check. "Several," he says. "And they have the most amazing popcorn."

Kavanaugh grins. "Do me a favor? If they're showing any good sci-fi movies this weekend, text me. I'm bored with what's out here."

Donley unlocks his car door, excited that Kavanaugh understands what he is saying. "Ken, my friend, you've got a deal. And the popcorn's on me!"

into the design process. This is not only a message for those who devise and build these machines. This is also a dynamic question for those who use, encourage, and monitor the spread of technology into the health system. Trust lost is much harder to regain than trust earned and defended—and therefore protected.

On Change

There is little that is permanent: change is a given. The curve of the pace of change is climbing. Consider change over the past two hundred years and the quickening pace of that change in the most recent fifty years. And then consider the pace in the past fifty years in health care and the quickening pace of just the past five years. With sensational new technologies and expectations already in sight, we can be confident that the rate of transformation is likely to continue its ascent. And of course health reform sweeps the system with episodic regularity, bringing ambitious agendas with it. When you are caught up in this increasing pace of change, flexibility is the key to enduring achievement. On the interpersonal level of work relationships, nimbleness manifests as negotiation. Differences on the direction and pace of change manifest as conflict, then conflict resolution seeks to convey agility back into the process. What works today may not work tomorrow. For those who hate change and crave stability, this prospect offers little comfort. Let go. Your security rests more with your ability to be responsive than with your instinct to remain stationary. Further, your long-term achievement will soar higher when you can be ahead of the flow and highest when you can chart that flow's destination.

Individuals are defined by their context, and individuals define their context. People often discount their influence on others and the influence of others on them. On the personal level, in every conversation you reflect to someone something about themselves, from the appropriateness of their dress to the depth of their professional acumen or the place they hold in the pertinent social order. Likewise, your self-perceptions are often molded by what others resonate to you, whether that is overt, through direct comments, or oblique, through innuendo and body language. On the societal level, people are influenced and characterized by their culture of origin or the period in which they grew up. This web of subtle yet ever-present influence molds our negotiations. The negotiation expectations of others are shaped by the cues we give them, just as ours are shaped by those we get from them, the give-and-get of the process. This interplay excels when it is active and balanced, not dominated or controlled. Although the equation need not be exactly even, when one person eclipses or disenfranchises the other, constructive feedback does not work: the overbearing boss is not told bad news or learns it too late. An animated meta-leadership dynamic of exchange works best, moving up and down, down and up, and across. Fine-tuned organizations and individuals are so because they encourage conduits of influence that keep them responsive and resilient, because they have the wisdom to know the bounds, and because, when it is legitimate to do so, they have the courage to draw the line and hold it.

Distinguish the leader with a vision from visionary meta-leadership. The *leader with a vision*, on the one hand, has a specific objective, in pursuit of which he or she takes followers. That objective is molded and sanctioned by the leader. Followers, neatly lined up behind the leader, are uniformly directed. Anyone questioning purpose or method is a dissenter, to be silenced or cut down; there is no negotiation. The aspiration of the followers is to reach the vision of the leader: they passively have only marginal influence over either means or ends. *Visionary meta-leadership*, on the other hand, is an interactive process by which leaders bring together the contributions of many people and in the process enrich both the objective and the realization of that purpose. The objective is furthered because more people have contributed to it and are invested in it, and so it is broader in scope and relevance. It has been said that true leadership requires that the leader incorporate not only her interests but those of her followers (Burns, 1978). The means are enhanced because the scope of creative talent is broadened. The role of meta-leadership is to facilitate this process, diplomatically orchestrating efforts toward synthesized purpose. It is a modus operandi that requires constant negotiation and conflict resolution. Unanimity itself takes time to nurture, and at times it is elusive; visionary meta-leadership too has its challenges and pitfalls. Nonetheless, given the combined expanse of professions, knowledge, expertise, and interests in health care, visionary meta-leadership is an approach congruent with our field's purposes and processes.

On Meta-Leadership

We need conversations on health and health care. Amid all this change, it would be marvelous to engage in a national conversation about health care. Unfortunately, that isn't likely to happen. Often the polarized political debates that occur during periods of health reform are characterized as national conversations. However, these deliberations really only focus on limited aspects of the bigger questions: aspects such as financing, access, and compensation for services. These are critically important topics though only a slice of the questions that should be addressed. A more valuable conversation would examine the priorities and values that guide health and health care and consider how they translate into the operations and work of health care organizations, professionals, and the health of the population. Although this is difficult to do on a national level, there is no reason why you can't initiate and lead such a conversation within your own sphere of influence. Meta-leaders strive to frame the critical strategic and human questions, and then they open the opportunities and gather the people to seek new and generative solutions. You needn't wait to be asked to do it. You can take the initiative, see where it leads you and others, and as a meta-leader, explore where you might further drive the conversation. Placed together, these smaller conversations could meld into something much larger and certainly have enormous impact in clarifying priorities, developing robust strategies, and generating opportunities for constructive new ideas and programs. As a country, we must pay attention to what we are doing so that we do it well, do it intentionally, and at the end of the day, ensure that what we have fashioned is worthy of the people served and those who do the work.

Build innovative thinking, demonstrations, evidence, and a movement. Meta-leadership is a social phenomenon just as are managing, administering, and organizing health and health care. Whereas the rigors of laboratory science allow for controlled experimentation and measurement of complex hypotheses about ailments with physical bases, the social and societal aspects of health care cannot be confined in a test tube. Then how does one innovate and experiment in order to advance bold solutions to complex problems? Discuss an issue. Try an idea. Craft a business plan. Make it work. Measure the result. Advance it. This is how the most creative and important ideas have made their way into conventional health care. Hospice practice started as a marginal movement to care compassionately for terminally ill patients. Now it is a mainstream practice. The error prevention and patient safety movement was launched by mavericks willing to challenge long-held beliefs about quality of care and outcomes. Its leaders are now recognized for significantly raising the bar on patient safety and institutionalizing new and different ways of engaging in patient care. Evidence-based medicine itself was a movement that at its start failed to gain currency within a medical community convinced that it was not necessary. Now it is the standard for establishing protocols and policies for practice. It takes enormous meta-leadership to accomplish these feats of innovation and to forge resilient solutions to complex problems. When you find such a challenge, don't be afraid to fight for the cause. It could be the most fulfilling thing you do in your career. Be a meta-leader.

Build system connectivity to craft a values-driven health enterprise. Whatever we do as a whole in health care is a reflection of our national and community values. This is not simply about your personal values. The actions of the overall health enterprise reflect collective values, for the meaning of life, for the right of individuals to make decisions about their bodies and lives, and for the amount of the gross national product that we devote to health care. It is to be expected that people will differ on these values, and sometimes differ vociferously. Yet even on the most divisive of these issues, it is possible to find common ground and make progress on matters of shared interest. Moderates from both the right-to-life and pro-choice camps, for example, can agree on how to and how not to wage their differences and on the importance of women's health. There are times when these chasms and others far less divisive can be bridged. These are the times and the opportunities for your meta-leadership to engage parties across the divides to find common ground and temper the battles that can so distract those engaged in the work of health and health care.

On Health Care Systems

Build process to refine balance. The complex, high-consequence enterprise of health care requires fine-tuned checks and balances to ensure the proficiency of its work: What are *you* doing? What are *they* doing? How might *you all* do it better? The quality improvement movement has contributed substantive mechanisms to enhance this process: peer review procedures, data-gathering and communication techniques, and analytical models and management methods to transform both attitudes and practice. To be effective, these procedures must work both on the systems level and on the interpersonal level. This is where your negotiation skills come into play: systems are no better than what we are able to do with them. And because checks and balances naturally bring conflict to the fore, quality improvement in reality requires a good deal of conflict resolution. For a system of checks and balances to realize its objectives, one person must be sanctioned to check what another does, and the process must be affirmed so that the message is in fact accepted. There is neither beginning nor end to this cycle: you negotiate, raise differences, resolve differences, negotiate, and start all over again. It keeps everyone and everything proficient and in tune.

Strive for congruency of purpose and method. Good health care arises from healthy organizations and healthy negotiations. If the manner of conducting the business of health care is not consonant with its intention—healthy people—then you are eventually trapped in the very contradictions you have created. Negotiation that is genuine, honest, just, legitimate, moral, respectful, and mutually beneficial is congruent with your purpose. Your work is information intensive, and the authenticity of that information must be indisputable. You balance a multitude of criteria in your decision making, so your standards must be fair. The very essence of your work—life, death, and the quality of life—requires you to uphold moral principles and then guide your practice by them. Your endeavors concern healthy people and ailing patients, so fostering the interests and concerns of well-being is part of your obligation. And finally, your agreements must meet the measure of integrity if they are to endure, because in the long run, endurance amid the brevity of life is the nature of your work.

The bottom line of your work is healthy people—and time. There are many bottom lines in the negotiation of health care: professional reputation, political influence, personal vulnerability, and a balanced budget, to name a few. There is one bottom line everyone shares, and that bottom line justifies the recognition, power, prestige, and expense you and your colleagues claim at the negotiation table. That bottom line is the *best interest of the patient.* What is it after all that we produce in our work in health care? It is *time.* As living beings, time is really the only thing we have. How long will you live? What will be the quality of your limited time? The twenty-five-year-old, terminally ill patient who seeks health care and receives the treatment that cures her, so that she lives to fifty, seventy-five, or beyond, has been given time. That is what we produce. There can be no more sacred work or shared purpose that we can offer other human beings. It is the greatest justification for negotiating toward better solutions, resolving conflicts, and finding the best ways to provide people with more and better time.

So . . . negotiation and renegotiation are constants. Like breathing, negotiation is something you do all the time. As a negotiator, you are constantly learning and adjusting your strategy, methods, and moves. You know that what worked wonderfully yesterday could flop today. You understand that you have your own filters on reality, and that even though you might not always be able to control them, you can at least compensate for the ways in which they might skew your assessment of facts and options. You have a good sense of your own priorities and are willing to accept that others order their lists differently. You know that health care systems engage in moral conduct because people with a moral and ethical agenda place their perspectives persuasively on the table. You appreciate that the perfect system will not be created in one day and that you and others are on board for the long haul, a perspective that requires constant personal, professional, and systemic flexibility. And finally, you grasp that you are part of a bigger picture and that the quality of that picture depends on many individuals' joint capacity to assemble the pieces, one person, one problem, and one solution at a time.

Strength to you for all your journeys.

APPENDIX

LIST OF CHARACTERS

Names are listed in alphabetical order. OMC is the Oppidania Medical Center.

Arlan Abbington Chairman of the OMC board of trustees

Anna Ashwood Artie Ashwood's mother

Artie Ashwood Patient admitted to OMC with an enlarged heart

Bob Bennett Mediator with an agency that has a contract with the state board of medical registration to conduct mediation of medical practice disputes

Benjamin Bennington Retired physician and OMC board member

Beatrice Benson Attending physician in the emergency department

Benny Bourne Surgeon at a university hospital

Betty Brown Dr. Ted Tuckerman's patient who died of lung cancer

Cindy Carrington Artie Ashwood's girlfriend

Catherine Cartwright OMC board member

Charlotte Chung Triage nurse in the emergency department

Cliff Clemens A second-year resident

Charlie Collins A resident

Cathy Crow Nurse on Six West

Chuck Cummings Resident on Six West

Debby D'Alfonso Nurse on Six West

Diane Darling Operating room nurse responsible for room scheduling

David Dickenson Vice president of human resources at OMC

Dave Donley Resident in the emergency department

Evelyn Edelman Director of the dietary department

Eli Ewing Chief resident in the cardiac intensive care unit

Frank Farwell Chief of the surgical department

Fred Fisher Medical director of OMC

Gail Gonzalez Nurse in the cardiac intensive care unit

George Grant Chief information officer (CIO) for OMC

Gloria Green President of the internal medicine group at the Oppidania Medical Clinic

Heather Harriford Nurse in the cardiac intensive care unit, later transferred to the general medical floor

Helen Hayward A seventy-eight-year-old woman on Six West, suffering from colon cancer

Iris Inkwater Chief executive officer (CEO) of OMC

Judy Jameson Nurse on Six West

Janice Johnson Vice president for nursing at OMC

Ken Kavanaugh Chief of the intensive care unit

Katherine Knight Nurse manager in the cardiac intensive care unit

Larry Levine Ted Tuckerman's medical malpractice attorney

Lauren Lieber Chief resident for orthopedics at OMC

Leslie Long Betty Brown's daughter

Larry Larkin PhD social scientist

Larry Lumberg Medical director of the emergency department

Melinda Martin Director of the Harborside Youth Action League

Melanie McKenzie Chief of the surgical intensive care unit

Manuel Mendez City health commissioner for the City of Oppidania

Nathaniel Norquist Chief financial officer (CFO) of the Community Health Plan health maintenance organization

Nick Norton Chief of the orthopedics department

Oscar Ortiz Primary nurse on Six West

Pauline Patrick Nurse on Six West

Pete Patterson Chief executive officer (CEO) of the Urbania Medical Center

Patty Pinkerton An old friend of Janice Johnson and a leader in the regional nurse executive association

Perry Pudolski Chief operating officer (COO) for OMC

Rajeev Rao Chief financial officer (CFO) for OMC

Rusty Rice Chief of the hospitalist department

Ralph Rollins A senior physician at OMC and a close friend of Dr. Fred Fisher

Steve Schilling A second-year resident

Stuart Schilling Bioethicist at OMC

Sylvia Sheffield Nurse on Six West

Sarah Smith Lieutenant governor for the state, with responsibility for health reform

Tanya Tarrington Head nurse on Nine West

Tim Thatcher Administrator of the internal medicine group at the Oppidania Medical Clinic

Ted Tuckerman An internist

Mr. Ulrich A terminally ill patient at OMC about whom a do not resuscitate order was in question

Victor Vining A cardiologist

Will Wainwright A primary care physician

Will Walter An anesthesiologist

Wendell White An internist

Wendy Winchell A member of the nursing staff involved in the mediation between Chuck Cummings and Heather Harriford

Walt Wynn Mayor of the City of Oppidania

Ziva Zartman A social worker at OMC

REFERENCES

Alternative medicine goes mainstream. (n.d.). *Discovery Health.* Retrieved June 9, 2010, from http://health.discovery.com/centers/althealth/medtrends/medtrends.html.

American College of Healthcare Executives. (2006). *A comparison of the career attainments of men and women healthcare executives.* Retrieved on June 11, 2010, from http://www.ache.org/PUBS/research/gender_study_full_report.pdf.

Argyris, C., & Schön, D. (1996). *Organizational learning II: Theory, method and practice.* Reading, MA: Addison-Wesley.

Ashkenas, R., Ulrich, D., Jick, T., & Kerr, S. (2002). *The boundaryless organization: Breaking the chains of organizational structure.* San Francisco: Jossey-Bass/Wiley.

Ashkenazi, I. (2010, April). Top leadership mistakes to avoid. *Tale of Our Cities.* Symposium organized by the Centers for Disease Control and Prevention and the Harvard School of Public Health, Washington, DC.

Australian Public Service Commission. (2007). *Tackling wicked problems: A public policy perspective.* Retrieved November 5, 2008, from http://www.apsc.gov.au/publications07/wickedproblems8.htm.

Bacharach, S., & Lawler, E. (1981). *Bargaining: Power, tactics, and outcomes.* San Francisco: Jossey-Bass/Wiley.

Barker, C., Johnson, A., & Lavalette, M. (2001). *Leadership and social movements.* Manchester, U.K.: Manchester University Press.

Barnes, P. M., Powell-Griner, E., McFann, K., & Nahin, R. L. (2004). Complementary and alternative medicine use among adults: U.S. 2002. *Seminars in Integrative Medicine, 2*(2), 54–71.

Bass, B. M. (1985). *Leadership and performance beyond expectation.* New York: Free Press.

Bazerman, M. (1998). Can negotiation outperform game theory? In J. J. Helpern & R. N. Stern (Eds.), *Debating rationality: Non-rational aspects of organizational decision making.* Ithaca, NY: ILR Press.

Bazerman, M., & Lewicki, R. (eds.). (1983). *Negotiating in organizations.* Thousand Oaks, CA: Sage.

Bazerman, M., & Neale, M. (1992). *Negotiating rationally.* New York: Free Press.

Bazerman, M., & M. Neal. (1995). The role of fairness considerations and relationships in a judgmental perspective of negotiation. In K. Arrow (Ed.), *Barriers to conflict resolution* (pp. 86–106). New York: Norton.

Benderesky, C. (2003). Organizational dispute resolution systems: A complementarities model. *Academy of Management Review, 28*(4), 643–656.

Benko, C. (2007). *Mass career cultivation: Aligning the workplace with today's nontraditional workforce.* Boston: Harvard Business Press.

Bertalanffy, L. V. (1968). *General system theory: Foundations, development, applications.* New York: Braziller.

Berwick, D. (1991, December). Controlling variation in health care: A consultation from Walter Shewhart. *Medical Care, 29*(12): 1212–1225.

Big pharma spends more on advertising than research and development, study finds. (2008, January 7). *ScienceDaily*. Retrieved November 13, 2009, from http://www.sciencedaily.com/releases/2008/01/080105140107.htm.

Blagg, D. (2009, April 8). Clay Christensen on disrupting health care. *HBS Working Knowledge.* Retrieved December 31, 2010, from http://hbswk.hbs.edu/item/6149.html.

Blake, R., & Mouton, J. (1984). *Solving costly organizational conflicts: Achieving intergroup trust, cooperation, and teamwork.* San Francisco: Jossey-Bass/Wiley.

Blessing, L. (1988). *A walk in the woods.* New York: Plume.

Bodenheimer, R., Grumbach, K., & Berenson, R. (2009). A lifeline for primary care. *New England Journal of Medicine, 360*(26), 2693–2696.

Brams, S. J. (2003). *Negotiation games: Applying game theory to bargaining and arbitration* (rev. ed.). New York: Routledge.

Bransford, J., & Stein, B. (1993). *The ideal problem solver: A guide for improving thinking, learning, and creativity.* New York: Freeman.

Bryson, J. M. (2004). What to do when stakeholders matter. *Public Management Review, 6*, 21–53.

Buerhaus, P., Auerbach, D., & Staiger, D. (2009). The recent surge in nurse employment: Causes and implications. *Health Affairs, 28*(4), w657–w668.

Burkowski, N. (2009). *Organizational behavior, theory, and design in health care.* Sudbury, MA: Jones and Bartlett.

Burns, J. M. (1978). *Leadership.* New York: Harper Perennial.

Burt, C. W., & Hing, E. (2005, March 2). Use of computerized clinical support systems in medical settings, United States 2001–2003. *Advance Data from Vital and Health Statistics*, No. 353, 1–5.

Carpenter, S., & Kennedy, W.J.D. (1988). *Managing public disputes: A practical guide to handling conflict and reaching agreements.* San Francisco: Jossey-Bass/Wiley.

Childs, A., & Hunter, E. (1972). Non-medical factors influencing use of diagnostic X-ray by physicians. *Medical Care, 10*(4), 323–335.

Cloke, K., & Goldsmith, J. (2000). *Resolving personal and organizational conflict: Stories of transformation and forgiveness.* San Francisco: Jossey-Bass/Wiley.

Clyman, D. (2003). *Decision traps.* Presentation retrieved December 2, 2008, from http://www.darden.edu/varoom/documents/DecisionTrapsTalk-NOVA-v1–200304-Handout-3.pdf.

Cohen, J., Gabriel, B., & Terrell, C. (2002, September). The case for diversity in the health care workforce. *Health Affairs, 21*(5): 90–102.

Contandriopoulos, A., Denis, J., Touati, N., & Rodriguez, C. (2003). *The integration of health care: Dimensions and implementation.* Working paper, Groupe de recherche interdisciplinaire en santé, N04–01. Retrieved June 1, 2010, from http://www.gris.umontreal.ca/rapportpdf/N04–01.pdf.

Cooks, L., & Hale, C. (2007). The construction of ethics in mediation. *Conflict Resolution Quarterly, 12*(5), 55–76.

Coombs, J. G. (2005). *The rise and fall of HMOs: An American health care revolution.* Madison: University of Wisconsin Press.

Cooper, R. (2007). It's time to address the problem of physician shortages. *Annals of Surgery, 246*(4), 527–534.

Cooper, R. (2004). Weighing the evidence for expanding physician supply. *Annals of Internal Medicine, 141*(9), 705–714.

Crossley, M. (2005). Discrimination against the unhealthy in health insurance. University of Pittsburgh Law School working paper series, Paper 32. Retrieved June 3, 2010, from http://law.bepress.com/cgi/viewcontent.cgi?article=1031&context=pittlwps.

Crowley, T. (1994). *Settle it out of court: How to resolve business and personal disputes using mediation, arbitration, and negotiation.* New York: Wiley.

Cyert, R., & March, J. (1963). *A behavioral theory of the firm.* Englewood Cliffs, NJ: Prentice-Hall.

Daly, P., & Watkins, M. (2006). *The first 90 days in government: Critical success strategies for new public managers at all levels.* Boston: Harvard Business Press.

Dauer, E. (1993). *Health industry dispute resolution: Strategies and tools for cost-effective dispute management.* New York: Center for Public Resources, Health Disputes Project.

Deming, W. E. (1986). *Out of the crisis.* Cambridge, MA: MIT Press.

Deming, W. E. (2000). *The new economics: For industry, government, education* (2nd ed.). Cambridge, MA: MIT Press.

DeVol, R., & Bedroussian, A. (2007). *An unhealthy America: The economic burden of chronic disease—Charting a new course to save lives and increase productivity and economic growth.* Santa Monica, CA: Milliken Institute.

Deutsch, M., & Coleman, P. (2000). *The handbook of conflict resolution: Theory and practice.* San Francisco: Jossey-Bass/Wiley.

Donahue, J. M. (2006). A history of drug advertising: The evolving roles of consumers and consumer protection. *Milbank Quarterly, 84*(4), 659–699.

Donahue, J. M., Cevasco, M., & Rosenthal, M. B. (2007). A decade of direct-to-consumer advertising of prescription drugs. *New England Journal of Medicine, 357*(7), 673–681.

Dorn, B., Savoia, E., Testa, M., Stoto, M., & Marcus, L. (2007). Development of a survey instrument to measure connectivity to evaluate national public health preparedness and response performance. *Public Health Reports, 122*(3), 329–338.

Druckman, D., & Olekalns, M. (2008). Emotions in negotiation. *Group Decisions and Negotiation, 17*(1), 1–11.

Dubler, N. N., & Marcus, L. J. (1994). *Mediating bioethical disputes: A practical guide.* New York: United Hospital Fund.

Dubler, N. N., & Nimmons, D. (1992). *Ethics on call: A medical ethicist shows how to take charge of life-and-death choices.* New York: Harmony Books.

Dychtwald, K., Erickson, T. J., & Morison, R. (2006). *Workforce crisis: How to beat the coming shortage of skills and talent.* Boston: Harvard Business Press.

Eisenberg, D. M., Davis, R. B., Ettner, S. L., Appel, S., Wilkey, S., Van Rompay, M., et al. (1998). Trends in alternative medicine use in the United States, 1990–1997: Results of a follow-up national survey. *JAMA, 280*(18): 1569–1575.

Epstein, A. (2001). The role of clinics in preventable hospitalizations among vulnerable populations. *Heath Services Research, 36*(2): 405–420.

Expat Explorer Survey 2009 (2009). HSBC Bank International. Retrieved July 15, 2010 from http://www.offshore.hsbc.com/1/2/international/expat/expat-survey/expat-experience-report-2009

Facts and Figures (2008). Newton-Wellesley Hospital. Retrieved January 24, 2011 from http://www.nwh.org/your-community-hospital/about-newton-wellesley/facts-and-figures.

Feldman, M., & Pentland, B. (2003). Reconceptualizing organizational routines as a source of flexibility and change. *Administrative Science Quarterly, 48*(1), 94–118.

Fernandez, R. (1991). Structural bases of leadership in intraorganizational networks. *Social Psychology Quarterly, 54*(1), 36–53.

Fisher, R., & Brown, S. (1988). *Getting together: Building relationships as we negotiate.* New York: Penguin Books.

Fisher, R., & Ertel, D. (1995). *Getting ready to negotiate: The getting to yes workbook.* New York: Penguin Books.

Fisher, R., Kopelman, E., & Schneider, A. (1994). *Beyond Machiavelli: Tools for coping with conflict.* Cambridge, MA: Harvard University Press.

Fisher, R., & Ury, W. (1981). *Getting to yes: Negotiating agreement without giving in.* New York: Penguin Books.

Fisher, R., Ury, W., & Patton, B. (1991). *Getting to yes: Negotiating agreement without giving in.* New York: Penguin Books.

Folberg, J., & Taylor, A. (1984). *Mediation: A comprehensive guide to resolving conflicts without litigation.* San Francisco: Jossey-Bass/Wiley.

Folger, J., & Bush, R. B. (1994). Ideology, orientations conflict and mediation discourse. In J. Folger & T. Jones (Eds.), *New Directions in Mediation: Communication, Research and Perspectives.* Thousand Oaks, CA: Sage.

Ford, E. W., Menachemi, N., & Phillips, M. T. (2006). Predicting the adoption of electronic health records by physicians: When will health care be paperless? *Journal of the American Medical Informatics Association, 13*(1), 106–112.

Gawande, A. (2010). *The checklist manifesto: How to get things right.* New York: Metropolitan Books.

Gelfand, M. J., & Brett, J. (2004). *The handbook of negotiation and culture.* Stanford, CA: Stanford University Press.

Gellad, Z. F., & Lyles, K. W. (2007). Direct-to-consumer advertising of pharmaceuticals. *American Journal of Medicine, 120*(6), 475–480.

Gero, A. (1985). Conflict avoidance in consensual decision processes. *Small Group Research, 16*(4), 487–499.

Gilbody, S., Wilson, P., & Watt, I. (2005). Benefits and harms of direct to consumer advertising: A systematic review. *Quality & Safety in Health Care, 14*, 246–250.

Giuliani, R. (2002). *Leadership.* New York: Hyperion.

Goffee, R., & Jones, G. (2006). *Why should anyone be led by you? What it takes to be an authentic leader.* Boston: Harvard Business Press.

Goldberg, S., Green, E., & Sander, F. (1985). *Dispute resolution.* Boston: Little Brown.

Goldberg, S., Green, E., & Sander, F. (1987). *Dispute resolution: 1987 supplement with exercises in negotiation, mediation, and mini-trials.* Boston: Little Brown.

Goleman, D. (1996). *Emotional intelligence: Why it may matter more than IQ.* New York: Bantam.

Goleman, D. (1998). *Working with emotional intelligence.* New York: Bantam Books.

Goleman, D. (2001). *The emotionally intelligent workplace: How to select for, measure, and improve emotional intelligence in individuals, groups, and organizations.* San Francisco: Jossey-Bass/Wiley.

Gray, B. (1989). *Collaborating: Finding common ground for multiparty problems.* San Francisco: Jossey-Bass/Wiley.

Gray, B. H. (2006). The rise and decline of the HMO: A chapter in U.S. health-policy history. In R. A. Stevens, C. E. Rosenberg, & L. R. Burns (Eds.), *History and health policy in the United States* (pp. 309–340). New Brunswick, NJ: Rutgers University Press.

Green, D. D. (2007). Leading a postmodern workforce. *Academy of Strategic Management Journal*, *6*, 15–26.

Hackman, M., & Johnson, C. (2004). *Leadership: A communication perspective* (4th ed.) Long Grove, IL: Waveland Press.

Hader, R., Saver, C., & Steltzer, T. (2006). No time to lose. *Nursing Management*, *37*(7), 23–48.

Halvorson, G. C. (2009). *Health care will not reform itself: A user's guide to refocusing and reforming American health care.* New York: CRC Press.

Hammonds, K. (2005, August 1). Why we hate HR. *Fast Company*, retrieved June 14, 2010, from http://www.fastcompany.com/magazine/97/open_hr.html.

Haynes, W. W. (1959, August). Toward a general approach to organization theory. *Journal of the Academy of Management, 2*(2), 75–88.

Hazleton, V., Cupach, W. R., & Canary, D. J. (1987). Situation perception: Interaction between competence and messages. *Journal of Language and Social Psychology*, *6*(1), 57–63.

Heifetz, R. (1994). *Leadership without easy answers.* Cambridge, MA: Harvard University Press/ Belknap Press.

Hemp, P. (2009, September). Death by information overload. *Harvard Business Review*, pp. 82–89.

Hermalin, B. E. (1998). Toward an economic theory of leadership: Leading by example. *American Economic Review*, *88*(5), 1188–1206.

Hewitt Associates. (2010). Hewitt survey shows growing interest among U.S. employers to penalize workers for unhealthy behaviors. Retrieved June 3, 2010, from http://eon .businesswire.com/news/eon/20100317005918/en.

Hewlett, S., & Luce, C. B. (2005, March). Off-ramps and on-ramps: Keeping talented women on the road to success. *Harvard Business Review*, pp. 43–54.

Honeyman, C. (1990). On evaluating mediators. *Negotiation Journal, 6*(1), 23–36.

Honoroff, B., Matz, D., & O'Connor, D. (1990). Putting mediation skills to the test. *Negotiation Journal*, *6*(1), 37–46.

Hsiao, C. J., Burt, C. W., Rechsteiner, E., Hing, E., Woodwell, D. A., & Sisk, J. E. (2008). Preliminary estimates of electronic medical records use by office-based physicians: United States, 2008. Health E-Stat. National Center for Health Statistics. Retrieved December 31, 2010, from http://www.cdc.gov/nchs/products/pubs/pubd/hestats/hestats.htm.

Hughes, R., Ginnett, R., & Curphy, G. (2006). *Leadership: Enhancing the lessons of experience.* New York: McGraw-Hill.

Hurley, R. F. (2006, September). The decision to trust. *Harvard Business Review*, pp. 55–62.

Institute of Medicine, Committee on Quality of Health Care in America. (2001). *Crossing the quality chasm: A new health system for the 21st century.* Washington, DC: National Academies Press.

Isenhart, M., & Spangle, M. (2000). *Collaborative approaches to resolving conflict.* Thousand Oaks, CA: Sage.

Jaques, E., Clement, S., Rigby, C., & Jacobs, T. (1985). *Senior leadership performance requirements at the executive level.* Alexandria, VA: Army Research Institute.

Jones, T. S. (2005). The emperor's knew clothes: What we don't know will hurt us. *Conflict Resolution Quarterly*, *23*, 129–139.

Kaiser Permanente. (2009). *The future of health care: Six important questions and one promising answer* (2008 Annual Report). Retrieved December 31, 2010, from http://xnet.kp.org/newscenter/annualreport/docs/kpreport_2008.pdf.

Karrass, C. (1970). *The negotiating game.* New York: World.

Kellerman, B. (2008). *Followership: How followers are creating change and changing leaders.* Boston: Harvard Business Press.

Kelman, H. (1995). Contributions of an unofficial conflict resolution effort to the Israeli-Palestinian breakthrough. *Negotiation Journal, 11*(1), 19–28.

Kirkpatrick, S. A., & Locke, E. A. (1991). Leadership: Do traits matter? *The Executive, 5,* 48–60.

Kohn, L.T., Corrigan, J. M., & Donaldson, M. S. (Eds.). (2000). *To err is human: Building a safer health system.* Washington, DC: National Academies Press.

Kolditz, T. (2007). *In extremis leadership: Leading as if your life depended on it.* San Francisco: Jossey-Bass/Wiley.

Kolb, D., & Bartunek, J. (Eds.). (1992). *Hidden conflict in organizations: Uncovering behind-the-scenes disputes.* Thousand Oaks, CA: Sage.

Kotter, J. (1996). *Leading change.* Boston: Harvard Business Press.

Kotter, J. (1999). *What leaders really do.* Boston: Harvard Business Press.

Kressel, K., Pruitt, D., & Associates. (1989). *Mediation research: The process and effectiveness of third-party intervention.* San Francisco: Jossey-Bass/Wiley.

Kremenyuk, V. A. (2002). *International negotiation: Analysis, approaches, issues.* San Francisco: Jossey-Bass/Wiley.

Kritek, P. B. (1994). *Negotiating at an uneven table: Developing moral courage in resolving our conflicts.* San Francisco: Jossey-Bass/Wiley.

Kurtzberg, T., & Medvec, V. H. (1999). Can we negotiate and still be friends? *Negotiation Journal, 15,* 355–361.

Laue, J. (1987). The emergence and institutionalization of third party roles in conflict. In D. Sandole & I. Sandole-Starost (Eds.), *Conflict management and problem solving: Interpersonal to international applications* (pp. 17–29). New York: New York University Press.

Laue, J., & Cormick, G. (1978). The ethics of intervention in community disputes. In G. Bermant, H. Kelman, & D. Warwick (Eds.), *The ethics of social intervention* (pp. 205–232). Washington, DC: Halsted Press.

LeBaron, M. (2002). *Bridging troubled waters.* San Francisco: Jossey-Bass/Wiley.

Lee, R., & Dale, B. (1998). Business process management: A review and evaluation. *Business Process Management Journal, 4*(3), 214–225.

Leffall, L., & Kripke, M. (2010, May 6). *Reducing environmental cancer risk: What we can do now.* President's Cancer Panel. Retrieved December 31, 2010, from http://www.ph.ucla.edu/ehs/ehs100/other%20web%20posts/Reducing%20Environmental%20Cancer%20Risk%20Presidents%20Cancer%20Panel%20Report%20May%202010.pdf.

Levinson, W., & Lurie, N. (2004). When most doctors are women: What lies ahead? *Annals of Internal Medicine, 141*(6), 471–474.

Lewin, K., Lippitt, R., & White, R. K. (1939). Patterns of aggressive behavior in experimentally created social climates. *Journal of Social Psychology, 10,* 271–301.

Likert, R. (1967). *The human organization: Its management and value,* New York: McGraw-Hill.

Likert, R., & Likert, J. (1976). *New ways of managing conflict.* New York: McGraw-Hill.

Losa, F. B., & Belton, V. (2006). Combining MCDA and conflict analysis: An exploratory application of an integrated approach. *Journal of the Operational Research Society*, *57*(5), 510–525.

Luce, R. D., & Raiffa, H. (1957). *Games and decisions*. New York: Wiley.

Ludeman, K., & Erlandson, E. (2006). *Alpha male syndrome*, Boston: Harvard Business Press.

March, J., & Simon, H. (1958). *Organizations*. New York: Wiley.

Marcus, L. J. (1983). *The new organization: An implementation study of the Massachusetts Department of Social Services*. Waltham, MA: Brandeis University.

Marcus, L. (2003). A culture of conflict: Lessons from renegotiating health care. *Journal of Health Care Law and Policy*, *5*(2), 447–478.

Marcus, L., Dorn, B., & Henderson, J. (2006). Meta-leadership and national emergency preparedness: A model to build government connectivity. *Biosecurity and Bioterrorism: Biodefense Strategy, Practice, and Science*, *4*(2), 128–134.

Maslow, A. (1970). *Motivation and personality*. New York: HarperCollins.

Mayer, B. (2000). *The dynamics of conflict resolution: A practitioner's guide*. San Francisco: Jossey-Bass/Wiley.

McLaughlin, V., & Leatherman, S. (2003). Quality or financing: What drives design in health care? *Quality & Safety in Health Care*, *12*(2), 136–142.

McMullan, M. (2006). Patients using the Internet to obtain health information: How this affects the patient–health professional relationship. *Patient Education & Counseling*, *63*(1), 24–28.

McNulty, E. (2003, December). They bought in. Now they want to bail out (Harvard Business Review Case Study). *Harvard Business Review*, pp. 28–38.

Meisel, S. I., & Fearon, D. S. (1999). The new leadership construct: What happens when a flat organization builds a tall tower? *Journal of Management Education*, *23*(2), 180–189.

Mighty, J. E. (1991). Valuing workforce diversity: A model for organizational change. *Canadian Journal of Administrative Sciences*, *8*(2), 64–71.

Miller, D. (2006). A tribute to Sidney Farber—The father of modern chemotherapy. *British Journal of Haematology*, *134*(1), 20–26.

Moore, C. (1986). *The mediation process: Practical strategies for resolving conflict*. San Francisco: Jossey-Bass/Wiley.

Moore, G. M. (1965). Cramming more components onto integrated circuits. *Electronics*, *38*(8), 114–117.

Mullin, S. (2002). Communicating risk: Closing the gap between perception and reality. *Journal of Urban Health*, *79*(3), 296–297.

Murray, S., Rudd, R., Kirsch, I., Yamamoto, K., & Grenier, S. (2007). Health literacy in Canada: Initial results from the international adult literacy and skills survey. Canadian Council on Learning. Retrieved June 9, 2010, from http://www.ccl-cca.ca/ccl/Reports/HealthLiteracy/HealthLiteracy2007.html.

Needleman, J., Buerhaus, P., Stewart, M., Zelevinsky, K., & Mattke, S. (2006). Nurse staffing in hospitals: Is there a business case for quality? *Health Affairs*, *25*(1), 205–211.

Newport, F., & Mendes, E. (2009). About one in six U.S. adults are without health insurance. *Gallup-Healthways Well-Being Index*. Retrieved June 3, 2010, from http://www.gallup.com/poll/121820/one-six-adults-without-health-insurance.aspx.

Newton-Wellesley Hospital details. (2010, July). *U.S. News & World Report*. Retrieved January 24, 2011, from http://health.usnews.com/best-hospitals/newton-wellesley-hospital-6141530/details.

NIH. (2011). ClinicalTrials.gov. Retrieved February 4, 2011, from http://clinicaltrials.gov/ct2/home.

Northouse, P. G. (2004). *Leadership: Theory and practice*. Thousand Oaks, CA: Sage.

O'Brien, K., & O'Hare, D. (2007). Situational awareness ability and cognitive skills training in a complex real-world task. *Ergonomics*, *50*(7), 1064–1091.

O'Reilly, C.A.I. (1980). Individuals and information overload in organizations: Is more necessarily better? *The Academy of Management Journal*, *23*(4), 684–696.

Pear, R. (2009, April 26). Shortage of doctors an obstacle to Obama goals. *New York Times*. Retrieved June 11, 2010, from http://www.nytimes.com/2009/04/27/health/policy/27care.html.

Pearson, S. D., & Lieber, S. R. (2009). Financial penalties for the unhealthy? Ethical guidelines for holding employees responsible for their health. *Health Affairs*, *28*(3), 845–852.

Phillips, D., & Loy, J. (2003). *Character in action: The U.S. Coast Guard on leadership*. Annapolis, MD: Naval Press.

Potapchuk, W., & Carlson, C. (1987). Using conflict analysis to determine intervention techniques. *Mediation Quarterly*, *16*, 31–43.

Prensky, M. (2001). Digital natives, digital immigrants. *On the Horizon*, *9*(5), retrieved June 1, 2010, from http://web.me.com/nancyoung/visual_literacy/site_map_and_resources_files/Digital_Natives_Digital_Immigrants.pdf.

Pretz, J. E., Naples, A. J., & Sternberg, R. J. (2003). Recognizing, defining, and representing problems. In J. E. Davidson & R. J. Sternberg (Eds.), *The psychology of problem solving* (pp. 3–30). New York: Cambridge University Press.

Rahim, M. (1992). *Managing conflict in organizations* (2nd ed.). Westport, CT: Praeger.

Raiffa, H. (1982). *The art and science of negotiation: How to resolve conflicts and get the best out of bargaining*. Cambridge, MA: Harvard University Press, 1982.

Reed, D. (2008). *California's workforce: Will there be enough college graduates?* Public Policy Institute of California. Retrieved June 11, 2010, from http://www.ppic.org/main/publication.asp?i=809.

Reuben, D. B. (2007). Saving primary care. *American Journal of Medicine*, *120*(1), 99–102.

Robert Wood Johnson Foundation. (2010, May 20). Health reform's changes in Medicare. *Health Briefs*. Retrieved June 11, 2010, from http://www.healthaffairs.org/healthpolicybriefs/brief.php?brief_id=17.

Roberto, M. (2005). W*hy great leaders don't take yes for an answer*. New York: Pearson.

Robson, R., & Morrison, G. (2003, November). The final ADR frontier: Conflict resolution in health care. Mediate.com. Retrieved June 22, 2010, from http://www.mediate.com/articles/robmorr1.cfm.

Romzek, B. S. (1990). Employee investment and commitment: The ties that bind. *Public Administration Review*, *50*(3), 374–382.

Rosenthal, T. C. (2008). The medical home: Growing evidence to support a new approach to primary care. *Journal of the American Board of Family Medicine*, *21*(5), 427–440.

Rudd, R. E. (2010). *Literacy and implications for navigating health care*. Retrieved June 9, 2010, from http://www.hsph.harvard.edu/healthliteracy/files/overview_slides.pdf.

Rudd, R. E., & Keller, D. B. (2009). Health literacy: New developments and research. *Journal of Communication in Health Care*, *2*(3), 240–257.

Rules of engagement: Harnessing the power of the contingent workforce. (2009, October). Retrieved June 15, 2010, from https://candidate.manpower.com/wps/wcm/connect/

e4856280420bb00ea99aeda17e379a88/Contingent_Global_Key_Findings_FINAL .pdf?MOD=AJPERES.

Salsberg, E., & Grover, A. (2006). Physician workforce shortages: Implications and issues for academic health centers and policy makers. *Academic Medicine, 81*(9), 782–787.

Schelling, T. (1960). *The strategy of conflict.* New York: Oxford University Press.

Schrock, J. W., & Cydulka, R. K. (2006). Lifelong learning. *Emergency Medical Clinics of North America, 24*(3), 785–795.

Schuman, S. (2006). *Creating a culture of collaboration: The International Association of Facilitators handbook.* San Francisco: Jossey-Bass/Wiley.

Senge, P. M. (1994). *The fifth discipline: The art and practice of the learning organization.* New York: Doubleday.

Shell, G. R. (1999). *Bargaining for advantage: Negotiation strategies for reasonable people.* San Francisco: Jossey-Bass/Wiley.

Shenk, D. (1997). *Data smog: Surviving the information glut.* San Francisco: HarperEdge.

Sillence, E., Briggs, P., Harris, P., & Fishwick, L. (2007, May). Going online for health advice: Changes in usage and trust practices over the last five years. *Interacting with Computers, 19*(3): 397–406.

Singer, L. (1994). *Settling disputes: Conflict resolution in business, families, and the legal system* (2nd ed.). Boulder, CO: Westview.

Slaikeu, K. (1989). Designing dispute resolution systems in the health care industry. *Negotiation Journal, 5*(4), 395–400.

Slaikeu, K. (1996). *When push comes to shove: A practical guide to mediating disputes.* San Francisco: Jossey-Bass.

Slaikeu, K., & Hasson, R. (1998). *Controlling the costs of conflict: How to design a system for your organization.* San Francisco: Jossey-Bass/Wiley.

Stange, K. C. (2007). In this issue: Doctor-patient and drug company–patient communication. *Annals of Family Medicine, 5*(1), 2–4.

Steinbrook, R. (2009). Easing the shortage in adult primary care: Is it all about money? *New England Journal of Medicine, 360*(26), 2696–2699.

Stene, E. (1940, December). An approach to a science of administration. *The American Political Science Review, 34*(6): 1124–1137.

Sternberg, R. J. (2006). The nature of creativity. *Creativity Research Journal, 18*(1), 87–98.

Sternberg, R. J. (2007). A systems model of leadership: WICS. *American Psychologist, 62*(1), 34–42.

Strauss, A. (1994). *Negotiations: Varieties, contexts, processes, and social order.* San Francisco: Jossey-Bass/Wiley.

Stulberg, J. (1987). *Taking charge/managing conflict.* Lanham, MD: Lexington Books.

Susskind, L., & Cruikshank, J. (1987). *Breaking the impasse: Consensual approaches to resolving public disputes.* New York: Basic Books.

Szmania, S., Johnson, A., & Mulligan, M. (2008). Alternative dispute resolution in medical malpractice: A survey of emerging trends and practices. *Conflict Resolution Quarterly, 26*(1): 71–96.

Tannen, D. (1990). *You just don't understand: Women and men in conversation.* New York: Ballantine.

Tannenbaum, A. S., & Schmidt, W. H. (1973, May–June). How to choose a leadership pattern. *Harvard Business Review, 51*(3): 162–180.

Tekleab, A. G., Sims, H. P., Jr., Yun, S., Tesluk, P. E., & Cox, J. (2008). Are we on the same page? Effects of self-awareness of empowering and transformational leadership. *Journal of Leadership & Organizational Studies*, *14*(3), 185–202.

Thomas, S., & D'Annunzio, L. S. (2005, March). Challenges and strategies of matrix organizations: Top-level and mid-level managers' perspectives. *Human Resource Planning*. Retrieved November 12, 2009, from http://www.allbusiness.com/public-administration/administration-human/394122-1.html.

Thompson, L. (2001). *The mind and heart of the negotiator*. Upper Saddle River, NJ: Prentice Hall.

Thompson, V. A. (1965). Bureaucracy and innovation. *Administrative Science Quarterly*, *10*(1), 1–20.

Thorne, S. (1993). *Negotiating health care: The social context of chronic illness*. Thousand Oaks, CA: Sage.

Trompenaars, F. (1994). *Riding the waves of culture*. New York: Irwin.

Ury, W. (1991). *Getting past no: Negotiating with difficult people*. New York: Bantam Books.

Ury, W. (1999). *Getting to peace: Transforming conflict at home, at work, and in the world*. New York: Viking.

Ury, W., Brett, J., & Goldberg, S. (1988). *Getting disputes resolved: Designing systems to cut the costs of conflict*. San Francisco: Jossey-Bass/Wiley.

U.S. Bureau of Labor Statistics. (2008). Overview of the 2008–2018 projections. In *Occupational outlook handbook: 2010–11 edition*. Retrieved June 11, 2010, from http://www.bls.gov/oco/oco2003.htm.

U.S. Department of Health and Human Services. (2000). *Healthy people 2010*. Washington, DC: U.S. Government Printing Office. (The second edition of this report may be accessed at http://www.healthypeople.gov/2010/Sitemap.)

U.S. Department of State, Foreign Service Institute, Center for the Study of Foreign Affairs. (1987). *Conflict resolution: Track two diplomacy* (J. McDonald Jr. & D. Bendahmane, Eds.). Washington, DC: U.S. Government Printing Office.

Wadhwa, V. (2007, August 22). The reverse brain drain. Bloomberg Businessweek. Retrieved July 15, 2009, from http://www.businessweek.com/smallbiz/content/aug2007/sb20070821_920025.htm.

Wadhwa, V. (2009, Spring). A reverse brain drain. *Issues in Science and Technology*, *25*(3): 45–52.

Wagner, T. (2008). *The global achievement gap*. New York, Basic Books.

Watkins, M. (2002). *Breakthrough business negotiation: A toolbox for managers*. San Francisco: Jossey-Bass/Wiley.

Webber, A. (2004, February 23). Reverse brain drain threatens U.S. economy. *USA Today*. Retrieved July 15, 2009, from http://www.usatoday.com/news/opinion/editorials/2004-02-23-economy-edit_x.htm.

Weber, M. (1905). *The Protestant ethic and the spirit of capitalism*. New York: Penguin Group.

White, R. W., & Horvitz, E. (2009). Cyberchondria: Studies of the escalation of medical concerns in Web search. *ACM Transactions on Information Systems*, *27*(4), art. 23.

Winkler, D. (2002). Personal and social responsibility for health. *Ethics and International Affairs*, *16*(2), 47–56.

Yukl, G. (2002). *Leadership in organizations*. Upper Saddle River, NJ: Prentice-Hall.

INDEX

Page references followed by *fig* indicate an illustrated figure.

N

O

P

Y

Z